DYNAMICAL SOCIAL PSYCHOLOGY

Dynamical Social Psychology

Andrzej Nowak
Robin R. Vallacher

THE GUILFORD PRESS
New York London

© 1998 The Guilford Press
A Division of Guilford Publications, Inc.
72 Spring Street, New York, NY 10012
http://www.guilford.com

Printed in the United States of America

This book is printed on acid-free paper.

Last digit is print number: 9   8   7   6   5   4   3   2   1

Library of Congress Cataloging-in-Publication Data

Nowak, Andrzej.
    Dynamical social psychology / Andrzej Nowak, Robin R. Vallacher.
        p.   cm.
    Includes bibliographical references (p.   ) and indexes.
    ISBN 1-57230-353-0
    1. Social psychology.   I. Vallacher, Robin R., 1946–   .
II. Title.
HM251.N815   1998
302—dc21   98-30200
                                                                    CIP

About the Authors

Andrzej Nowak, PhD, is Professor of Psychology at the University of Warsaw, Poland, where he is also Director of the Center for Complex Systems in the Institute for Social Studies. He is the author and editor of three previous books and has published articles in a range of professional journals. Dr. Nowak's research interests include dynamics of social transitions, attitude change, self-control in neural networks models, dynamics of social judgment, and computer simulations of social processes. He is currently developing dynamical models of social psychological phenomena, with special emphasis on social change, dynamics of self-understanding, social judgment, and close relationships.

Robin R. Vallacher, PhD, is Professor of Psychology at Florida Atlantic University and an affiliate of the Center for Complex Systems, University of Warsaw. Dr. Vallacher has written and edited four previous books concerned with theoretical and topical issues in social psychology. His published research, funded in part by grants from the National Science Foundation and the National Institute of Mental Health, has addressed a wide variety of topics, including group dynamics, distributive justice, person perception, self-awareness, moral behavior, the mental representation and control of action, individual differences in goal-directedness, self-representation, moral judgment, and self-concept stability and change. Dr. Vallacher is currently developing dynamical models of social psychological phenomena, with special emphasis on the dynamics of self-understanding, social judgment, and close relationships.

Preface

T HE SUBJECT MATTER of social psychology is inherently dynamic. It is hard to conceive of action without movement, judgment without a flow of thoughts, emotion without volatility, social interaction without an ebb and flow of gestures and words, or social relationships without ongoing evolution of roles and sentiment. The self-evident dynamism of personal and interpersonal experience has not been lost on social psychology. Indeed, the nature of human dynamism provided a focal point in the earliest attempts to characterize experience in interpersonal contexts, as reflected in the seminal work of such figures as James, Mead, Cooley, Lewin, and Asch. Recent advances in the study of nonlinear dynamical systems have provided a set of concepts and tools that enable contemporary researchers to impose precision and rigor on the early insights that defined the field. Our aim in this book is to describe and illustrate with original empirical research what the new dynamical perspective has to offer the field of social psychology.

In general terms, to describe a phenomenon as dynamical is to note that it evolves and otherwise changes in time. Reliable patterns of change may arise from outside influences, of course, but what is of special relevance for personal and interpersonal experience is the potential for internally generated dynamics. Thus, thoughts, feelings, actions, and group-level processes may unfold according to their own rhythm in the absence of any external forces. This is not to suggest that external factors are irrelevant to the dynamics of interpersonal experience. A person's attitude may change in response to persuasive communication, a group may reverse a decision based on new information, and a society can undergo a transformation due to changing international conditions. But external factors do not cause changes directly in an otherwise passive system. Rather, such factors exert their influence by modifying the course of whatever internally generated dynamics are operative for the person, group, or society. Lacking insight into the ongoing processes within a person or social group, it is difficult to know what effect a given external influence is likely to have. Sometimes an external factor produces only resistance, with little or no change in the ongoing processes of the person or group. At other times, the person or group may show an exaggerated response to a lesser value of the same external factor. At yet other times, an external influence may simply initiate a process that unfolds according to its own pattern of changes, the effects of which may not be apparent for days, minutes, or years, depending on the phenomenon in question.

Research strategies that reduce dynamics to a single pass and focus on a stable outcome are clearly inadequate to capture such properties. The approach of nonlinear dynamical systems, on the other hand, is ideally suited to investigate internally generated dynamics, and to identify invariant properties of dynamics that transcend topical boundaries. Research on nonlinear dynamical systems has established, in fact, that the dynamics of highly diverse systems in areas as distinct as physics, chemistry, biology, and economics conform to a handful of basic patterns. And rather than simply evolving toward a stable equilibrium, these patterns can be self-sustaining as a result of repeated iterations of the mutual influences among variables internal to the system. This suggests the potential for developing general laws of social psychological dynamics that apply to all levels of social reality, from the flow of individual thoughts to societal transitions. Beyond providing coherence to an admittedly fragmented discipline, the discovery of such laws in social psychology may foster new levels of integration with other areas of psychology that have already embraced the dynamical perspective (e.g., developmental and cognitive psychology) and with other areas of science as well.

The dynamical approach should not be viewed as an alternative to more traditional approaches in social psychology. For the better part of the 20th century, social psychological research has attempted to isolate causal mechanisms with respect to distinct aspects of interpersonal experience. The methods spawned within this approach have been quite successful in identifying the key features of human thought and behavior. With the recent advent of the dynamical approach, it is now possible for investigators to assemble sets of such mechanisms into coherent systems. In contrast to a single causal relation, a system may be characterized by dynamic properties, such as emergence and self-organization, resistance to external influence, exaggerated response to minor influences, complex self-sustaining patterns of change, and seeming unpredictability. Beyond its value in integrating and verifying causal mechanisms, then, a concern with dynamics has value in its own right. Fascinating regularities in a system's dynamics may be discovered and important laws may be formulated concerning these regularities.

The focus maintained throughout this book is squarely on social psychological phenomena. Whatever shape dynamical social psychology ultimately achieves, such concepts as intrinsic motivation, self-awareness, planning, emotion, mental control, goals, and attitudes are certain to play a prominent role. We develop the implications of non-linear dynamical systems for the subject matter of social psychology in the context of experimentation and computer simulation, and in all cases we attempt to ground the approach in terms of classic and contemporary theories. For the most part, we present original research intended to illustrate how models within various domains may be constructed. At this early stage in the evolution of this perspective, we are in no position to claim that these models are superior to alternative models of the phenomenon in question. We do feel quite strongly, however, that an explicit focus on dynamics, whatever its specific manifestation, holds potential for generating integrative, yet rigorously supported insights into the nature of personal and interpersonal experience.

Of necessity, the book imposes a topical structure on the field, parsing the diverse subject matter of social psychology into more or less self-contained chapters. Any attempt to establish boundary conditions can ultimately be viewed as arbitrary, of course, but we feel that the chapter organization of this book resonates well with the dynamical perspective, in that it provides an orderly progression across different levels of social reality, from individual minds to large-scale social systems. We begin by establishing the context for the dynamical perspective in social psychology (Chapter 1) and outlining the basic elements of the dynamical approach (Chapter 2). After setting the stage in this manner, we explore the dynamic underpinnings for systems representing progressively broader units of analysis. Individual dynamics provide the focus in our treatments of social judgment (Chapter 3), the relation between mental dynamics and action (Chapter 4), and self-concept (Chapter 5). The unit of analysis is then expanded to characterize dynamics in dyads (Chapter 6), social groups (Chapter 7), and society as a whole (Chapter 8). Chapter 8 provides an explicit consideration of levels of social reality from a dynamical perspective, as well as a perspective on the current and projected identity of dynamical social psychology. This chapter progression was developed to provide coherence for the ideas and material we wished to present, of course, but we feel that it may also serve as a useful topical landscape for the field more generally.

The book is targeted to two primary audiences. It is intended, first of all, to serve as a primer for researchers who see the benefit of a dynamical perspective but who currently lack the necessary background regarding the relevant concepts, principles, and methods. In this sense, the book should have heuristic value, enabling social psychologists to establish research agendas concerning the dynamic underpinnings of social psychological phenomena. Equally important, the book is intended to serve as a primary reference source in graduate-level seminars and as a supplemental source in upper-level undergraduate social psychology courses. In this regard, we emphasize that the book is firmly rooted in social psychology. It is not a book on physics or math, and no such expertise is necessary to understand the concepts, research strategies, or data we present. Our goal was not to write a technical manual, but rather to introduce a new perspective that holds integrative and heuristic value for the field of social psychology.

Acknowledgments

PREPARATION OF THIS BOOK would not have been possible without the support we received from many quarters. The original research described in the book was supported by the National Science Foundation (Grant No. SBR 95-11657 to Vallacher and Nowak) and the Polish Committee for Scientific Research (Grant No. 1H01F07310 to Nowak). A number of people provided invaluable assistance in the conduct of this research program. Wojciech Borkowski, a biologist, and Michal Zochowski, a physicist, both of whom are associated with the Center for Complex Systems at Warsaw University, deserve special recognition for their direct contributions to the material presented in this book. Independently and at times collaboratively, Borkowski and Zochowski took part in the development of several of the dynamical models, wrote simulation programs, and prepared graphs and figures of the results. Dr. Zochowski also advised us regarding the physical aspects of nonlinear dynamical systems; this advice proved particularly crucial in the development of models of coupled logistic equations. Dr. Borkowski, meanwhile, served as our main simulation expert. In this capacity, he not only wrote and implemented several simulation programs, but he also developed a graphical library for visualization of the simulation results. We are also grateful to the conscientious assistance provided by our respective students at Florida Atlantic University and Warsaw University. Michael Froehlich, Jessica Markus, Jennifer Strauss, Kim Sussman, and Xiaojing Yuan at Florida Atlantic played an important role in the design and implementation of several studies in the research program on which this book was based. Agnieszka Guzik, Malgorzata Kozlowska, and Jakub Urbaniak played a similar role at Warsaw University.

We want to thank Maciej Lewenstein and Marek Kus, both of whom are physicists associated with the Center for Complex Systems at Warsaw University, for their advice on the application of dynamical concepts and tools to the subject matter of social psychology. Nowak expresses special gratitude to Drs. Lewenstein and Kus for introducing him to the work on statistical physics and nonlinear dynamical systems. Both had a significant impact on the development of Chapter 2. Dr. Lewenstein was also instrumental in developing the cellular automata and neural network models of social influence. Dr. Kus, meanwhile, provided invaluable advice regarding the work on the dynamics of close relationships. We also acknowledge Jacek Szamrej, a computer engineer at the Warsaw Center, who played a critical role from the outset in developing computer methods for simulating social processes. His contributions in this regard are greatly appreciated. And we are deeply grateful to Kasia Winkowska-Nowak, a mathematician at the Warsaw Center, who provided important advice and technical assistance during the preparation of the book.

We were fortunate to receive feedback from colleagues and friends at various points in the preparation of the book. We owe special thanks to Shelly Chaiken for her feedback on Chapter 3, and to an anonymous reviewer and Dan Wegner for their respective comments on a preliminary draft of the entire book. Both the reviewer and Dr. Wegner provided detailed and insightful observations on each chapter and offered constructive suggestions regarding matters of exposition and substance. The final version of the book incorporated the feedback we received from these individuals, and we feel that the quality of the book has been enhanced as a result.

We also wish to express our appreciation to Seymour Weingarten, Editor in Chief of The Guilford Press, who saw the value in preparing a volume such as this and approached us regarding this possibility. His advice also proved critical regarding the general tack and style of presentation represented in this book. Finally, we owe special thanks to our respective spouses, Kasia Winkowska-Nowak and Phyllis Merrill-Vallacher, for their support and constructive criticism during the preparation of this book.

Contents

1

&

Social Psychological Dynamics

SOCIAL PSYCHOLOGY HAS always thought of itself as dynamic. Pre-occupation with the nature of change in personal and interpersonal processes can be traced to the origins of social psychology in the early and mid-20th century, as reflected in the writings of such pioneering figures as James, Mead, Cooley, Lewin, Heider, and Asch. This focus has continued unabated ever since and is apparent today in the coupling of the word "dynamic" with the various literatures that define the topical landscape of the field. Thus, we talk of group dynamics, dynamics of attitude change, interpersonal dynamics, and so on, as if these topics each represented a different manifestation of a fundamental proclivity for evolution and change. With dynamism occupying center stage in theoretical treatments of interpersonal phenomena, social psychology stands as one of the most intriguing fields of scientific inquiry, and it has proven to provide considerable fascination for the lay public as well.

Although dynamism is a self-evident and widely acknowledged feature of social psychological phenomena, it has proven difficult to capture using traditional tools developed in the physical sciences. The nature of this difficulty is easy to appreciate when one considers the unparalleled richness and complexity associated with human social experience. An individual's thoughts, feelings, and actions are influenced by a large number of highly diverse factors, only a handful of which can realistically be investigated at a given time. The interdependency of different individuals in a social context, meanwhile, serves to amplify such complexity and to provide a universe of possible trajectories for each person's experience. Achieving complete description and precise prediction in the face of such intricacies is clearly a daunting task. Social psychology, of course, is not without its successes. During the relatively short existence of this field, a great deal has been learned about a wide variety of phenomena, from mechanisms of individual thought to the functioning of social groups. But because these insights are based on methods and tools that reflect traditional natural science assumptions, they necessarily fall short of capturing the rich complexity and subtle dynamism defining interpersonal experience.

In the 1980s, however, the natural sciences underwent a profound transformation that has had the effect of making it better equipped to deal with the dynamism and complexity of social psychological phenomena. The basis for this transformation was the realization that many phenomena in nature do not conform to certain longstanding assumptions regarding causality and reduction, but rather are more appropriately conceptualized as nonlinear dynamical systems. Broadly defined, a "dynamical system" is simply a set of elements that undergoes change by virtue of the connections among the elements. In nonlinear systems, the connections among elements generate global system-level behavior that displays remarkable variability over time, even in the absence of outside influences. When external influences are present, the system's behavior may change in a manner that is nonproportional to the magnitude of the influences. To capture such nonlinear dynamics, mathematicians and scientists in various fields have developed a variety of methods and tools, many of which are readily adaptable to social psychological concerns.

Our aim in this chapter is to develop the rationale for the use of such tools to investigate the subject matter of social psychology. We begin by developing the dynamic underpinnings of human social experience and then describe how such dynamism has been characterized in both classic and contemporary social psychology. The subsequent section outlines how the issues and concerns that have always been central to the field are beginning to be reframed within an explicitly dynamical framework. Our primary point is that the natural sciences have finally matured to the point that their concepts and methods can be meaningfully adapted to investigate the elusive nature of interpersonal dynamics. The dynamical perspective has already permeated virtually every other branch of science, and in so doing has revealed a set of invariant principles that transcend traditional boundaries of inquiry. There is reason to believe that the careful adaptation of the dynamical perspective to the subject matter of social psychology will provide integration for otherwise distinct facets of interpersonal experience, and may eventually serve to integrate social psychology with other areas of science as well.

DYNAMICS AND HUMAN NATURE

Even when viewed in strictly biological terms, nothing in nature comes close to matching the enormous complexity of human experience. The human brain is the most intricate structure in the known universe, consisting of approximately 100 billion neurons, each of which influences and is influenced by approximately 1,000 other neurons. The number of possible configurations of states of neurons at each moment in time, then, rivals the number of positively charged particles in the known universe (see Edelman, 1992). Because each neuronal configuration may correspond to a unique state of mind, the range of potential mental states is unimaginably large. Moreover, these configurations and their corresponding mental states display continuous change over time, forming a rich and varied stream of consciousness, the exact form of which may never reoccur (cf. James, 1890).

Complexity and Internal Causation

Perhaps of greater importance is the richness and complexity of human experience afforded by the social context in which thoughts, feelings, and actions develop and unfold. Throughout life, each individual's thoughts, feelings, and actions are influenced by a myriad of social stimuli that run the gamut from those that are momentary and trivial (e.g., a stranger's glance) to those that are persistent and significant (e.g., criticism from a loved one). This influence is apparent in everyday social interaction, with each person responding to the real or imagined thoughts, feelings, and actions of the other person. But even in the absence of interpersonal contact, an individual's experience can take on a variety of different forms as he or she reflects on past experiences or imagines those yet to take place. Patterns of thought, feeling, and action are generated as well by features of the larger social context, including the person's relationship with various groups, his or her position in society as a whole, the nature of various social institutions, and the assortment of beliefs, values, and expectations that collectively define culture.

The sheer number and variety of factors relevant to human experience guarantee that virtually all aspects of personal and interpersonal experience are constantly subject to change. This potential for dynamism is enhanced by several orders of magnitude when one considers the possible ways in which these factors can interact to influence an individual. The norms and beliefs of one's peer group during adolescence, for instance, may run contrary to parental expectations, societal norms, or standards of achievement. Which factor or blend of factors predominates, meanwhile, may depend upon yet other social influences and their interaction with prior experiences reaching back to childhood. Complex interactions of this type hold potential for generating diverse patterns of thought and behavior across individuals and for establishing different patterns within a given individual over time. In view of these bases for complexity and dynamism, one could well argue that the structure of human social experience is simply too intricate and multifaceted to admit to complete description, let alone precise prediction.

Even if we somehow managed to identify all relevant factors and specified how they can interact to influence thought and behavior, we may still be at a loss to explain or predict a person's beliefs, decisions, desires, or courses of action. Indeed, often the only explanation available for someone's action centers on the person's internal state—his or her goals, feelings, personality traits, motives, self-defined principles and values, sudden impulses, and so on. As noted by Cooley (1902), humans are born to action and are quite capable of charting their own direction without guidance from other people or from elements of the larger social context. The human potential for internal causation, in fact, not only confers upon people the capacity to resist external influences, but also an inclination to act in opposition to them. Unlike lower organisms, humans can disregard promises of reward, threats of punishment, social pressure from peers and authority figures, and other external inducements to action. In effect, then, the complex edifice of interacting causal forces permeating social life can collapse—seemingly without warning—in the face of personal desires, values, and momentary whims.

Complexity and internal causation arise as complicating forces in the depiction of social psychological dynamics because of the uniquely human capacity for conscious self-reflection. The remarkable complexity of the human brain enables people to process an amazing assortment of diverse and often abstract information, and as noted earlier, this capacity sets the stage for highly complex and dynamic patterns of personal and interpersonal functioning. What really sets the human mind apart from other systems in nature, however, is its ability to reflect on its own operations and output. The reflexive nature of human consciousness and its role in generating complex dynamics played a prominent role in early treatments of social psychology (cf. Allport, 1935; Cooley, 1902; James, 1890; Mead, 1934; Sullivan, 1953), and it continues to provide an important focus of theory and research in contemporary work (e.g., Baumeister, 1993; Carver & Scheier, 1981; Duval & Wicklund, 1972; Higgins, 1987; Kernis, 1995; Markus, 1983; Markus & Nurius, 1986; Sedikides & Skowronski, 1997; Steele, 1988; Suls & Greenwald, 1983; Swann, 1990; Tesser, 1988; Wegner & Vallacher, 1980). The fact that mental processes are reflected in consciousness makes them subject to evaluation and personal control. This means that humans not only display internal causation, but they are also capable of reflecting on their personal bases for action and evaluating them with respect to various personal and societal criteria. The self-evaluation afforded by self-awareness, in turn, can provide the impetus for people to modify their own psychological structure and thereby change their internal bases for action.

Dynamism and Unpredictability

The same qualities that make human social experience so fascinating also render it difficult to investigate with methods developed in the physical sciences. Humans, after all, are not like rocks or plants, or even laboratory rats, for that matter. Many of the unique features of human action, including complexity, internal causation, resistance to influence, and self-regulation, do not conform to simple cause–effect relations. This is not to say that causation is irrelevant to human experience. Rather, it is the pattern of causal relations that shapes the phenomenon in question, so that any causal mechanism in isolation is inadequate to characterize the resultant phenomenon in all its complexity. In such causal structures, moreover, even the basic distinction between cause and effect may become blurred because of reciprocal, or bidirectional, causality. In bidirectional causality, changes in variable A cause changes in variable B, but in turn changes in variable B cause changes in variable A. It is clearly the case, for example, that similarity in attitudes causes interpersonal attraction, but it is equally true that interpersonal attraction facilitates modeling and empathy, which can promote greater similarity in attitudes.

These difficulties are pronounced enough when the focus of theory and research is human action. Additional problems arise when the focus turns to an analysis of human thoughts and feelings, phenomena that go to the heart of personal and interpersonal experience. Not only is there a complex causal structure involving bidirectional influences associated with mental phenomena, but the elements of mental experience are highly idiosyncratic and difficult to characterize in a quantitative fashion. As noted by James (1890), mental process is an endless cascade of thoughts, memories, images, and fantasies vying for conscious attention in the stream of thought. The affective tone associated with the elements of thought, meanwhile, often proves difficult to verbalize, making this aspect of experience especially difficult to investigate.

These considerations point to the seemingly impossible task of providing complete description and prediction for social psychological phenomena. And in fact, it is widely acknowledged that social psychological theories are not as successful in explanation and prediction as are theories of biological and physical processes. It is customary for investigators to claim support for a theory based on a study in which the independent variables collectively account for less than 15% of the variance in the dependent measure. This means that the vast majority of the variability among participants has nothing to do with the theory being tested. In effect, the field is left trying to engender enthusiasm and optimism regarding a glass that is decidedly less than half full. In view of the notion of determinism in traditional natural science, this would seem to be a sobering state of affairs. After all, in a deterministic world *all* the variance should be accounted for. Classical mechanics, as epitomized by Newton's principles of dynamics, holds that nothing is left to chance, and that if all the initial conditions associated with a phenomenon were known, one should be able, in principle, to generate complete and precise knowledge of the phenomenon. Complete and precise understanding, in turn, sets the stage for complete and precise prediction, regardless of how far one looks into the future. The clear implication here is that the better one's theory, the closer one should come to explaining 100% of the variance. By this standard, accounting for a mere 15% generates the suspicion that a scientific understanding of something as complex and dynamic as human interpersonal processes is more a dream than a reality—and maybe an unrealizable dream at that.

This perspective on scientific social psychology is based on two assumptions that can be called into question. The first is that the physical sciences have in fact achieved Laplace's dream of complete and precise understanding. Some phenomena, to be sure, are fairly well understood, and it is fair to say that most biological and physical processes admit to more precise depiction than does even the most basic social psychological process. But despite a solid head start of two centuries or more, the scientific investigation of nature still leaves much to be explained. The second assumption, which goes to the heart of the scientific method, is that determinism implies prediction.

In the traditional approach to science, prediction commonly provides the criterion by which one assesses whether the causal variables in a study have a deterministic influence on the phenomenon being investigated. Only if the dependent measure varies in the predicted manner as a function of the earlier manipulations can the investigator claim support for the theory being tested. As we shall see, this assumption has been seriously challenged, if not outright rejected, as a result of developments in the physical sciences in the 1980s.

These points provide some solace for social psychology, but it still cannot be denied that the field has failed thus far to achieve as complete and precise an understanding of interpersonal phenomena as one would like. The subject matter of social psychology simply represents a serious challenge for the methods and tools developed within the traditional natural science paradigm. Although this assessment has led some to question the goal of framing interpersonal phenomena in scientific terms (see, e.g., Gergen, 1985, 1994; Parker & Shotter, 1990), we feel that the nature of the field's subject matter actually puts social psychology in a strong position to lead developments in science as we enter the 21st century. This is because many areas of science have undergone profound changes since the 1980s, changes that make these fields more in tune with what social psychologists have been talking about all along. Before discussing these changes and their relevance to social psychology, however, we discuss how social psychology has attempted to come to grips with the dynamism of interpersonal phenomena thus far in its relatively short tenure as a field of explicit scientific inquiry.

DYNAMISM IN SOCIAL PSYCHOLOGY

The special qualities of human dynamism were recognized and assigned a prominent role in early treatments of social psychological processes. As the 19th century came to a close, James (1890) theorized about the dynamic nature of human thought and action, with special emphasis on the continuous and ever-changing stream of thought. Soon thereafter, Cooley (1902) emphasized people's constant press for action, even in the absence of external forces and incentives, while Mead (1934) discussed people's capacity for symbolic representation and the enormous range of interpretation to which this capacity gives rise. Lewin (1936a, 1951), in turn, suggested that stability and variability in overt behavior reflect the persistent struggle to resolve conflicting motivational forces, including those that operate from within the person—an idea, of course, that is at heart of psychodynamic theories as well (cf. Freud, 1937). Asch (1946) suggested that social judgment reflects the dynamic interplay of thoughts and feelings, with this interplay giving rise to a unique Gestalt that is not reducible to the additive components of the elements themselves. And in one of the earliest attempts to systematize social psychology in a textbook, Krech and Crutchfield (1948) framed interpersonal thought and behavior in terms of Gestalt psychology, with an explicit emphasis on the constant reconfiguration of experience in response to conflicting fields of psychological forces.

Although dynamism was considered the critical feature of personal and interpersonal process by the founding fathers of social psychology, this emphasis was not always apparent in subsequent phases of the field's development. With some notable exceptions, theory and research became more concerned with forces toward stability than with those underlying the penchant for constant change and evolution. This redirection of focus was inevitable in view of the prevailing methods for investigating personal and social processes. To an important extent, these methods reflected widely held assumptions in the natural sciences concerning the primacy of external causal factors in promoting change in physical, chemical, and biological phenomena.

Early Insights into Dynamics

Of all the insights generated during social psychology's formative years, the most important may be the recognition that psychological states within the person are subject to constant change and transformation. This does not simply mean that a person's thoughts, feelings, moods, desires, and plans are subject to temporal variation, but also that the causes of these changes are located within the person. Human dynamics, in other words, were said to be internally generated. This means that cognitive, affective, and behavioral tendencies unfold and undergo change even in the absence of any environmental influences. Thus, people think without being prodded to do so, act without the inducements of rewards and punishments, and experience a succession of different emotions without provocation. Even in a stable, unchanging environment, psychological processes never come to a rest. What might be termed *intrinsic dynamics*, then, represents a fundamental feature of human experience.

To say that a process displays intrinsic dynamics is tantamount to saying that the only causal agent for the process is the process itself. Causation of this kind is made possible by constant interactions among the elements or variables defining the process. The state of each element at each moment, in other words, influences the states of other elements at the succeeding moment, and the state of each element at that moment influences the states of other elements at the next moment, and so on. Through successive iterations of this process, the state of all the elements and of their configurations undergo a sustained process of change. This idea provides a perspective from which to understand persistent claims from different quarters in psychology that people are not simply passive respondents to external forces, but rather are active agents defined in terms of psychological forces that operate independently of instigation. Thus, human agency, personal causation, self-determination, and the like are consistent with the potential for sustained patterns of change and growth that occur as a result of interactions among internal forces, often without guidance from cues in the social and physical environment.

The potential for intrinsic dynamics exists at all level of social psychological analysis, from individual minds to social groups. If one's focus is the individual, various thoughts, memories, and impulses interact over time to produce a sequence of judgments and acts that may display considerable temporal variation. If a social group provides the focus, it is the interaction among individuals over time that produces change and evolution of group-level properties. To learn about individual- or group-level processes, then, one should let these processes unfold on their own, undisturbed by external influences. Only later may we see how these processes are affected by external factors. To be sure, individuals and groups are responsive to external influence. An individual's attitude may change in response to persuasive communication, a group may reach a new decision based on new information, and a society may undergo transformations due to changing international conditions. External factors do not cause direct changes in an otherwise passive system, however, but rather exert their influence by modifying the course of whatever intrinsic dynamics are operative for the person, group, or society.

At the level of the individual, this point refers to the uncontroversial notion that incoming stimuli are cognitively processed and that the results of such cognitive mediation determine the actual impact of the stimuli. Messages, after all, do not enter empty minds. The notion of intrinsic dynamics goes beyond this recognition, however, to suggest that the cognitive–affective system is always in motion (see Port & van Gelder, 1995), so that even in the absence of external stimuli, there is the potential for constant evolution and change. There are always plans, feelings, thoughts, and action tendencies in the person, and whatever happens does not put an otherwise passive system in motion, but rather impinges on the ongoing process. This can take many distinct forms, such as stopping, reshaping, or replacing the ongoing processes. Responses to environmental influences, in fact, sometimes only consist of resistance, with little change in the state of the person or group. At other times, meanwhile, the person or group may show an exaggerated response to external factors. At yet other times, an external influence only initiates a process that then unfolds according to its own intrinsic dynamics, the effects of which may not be apparent for days or even months. The well-documented "sleeper effect" in attitude change provides an example of delayed response to external factors (e.g., Hovland & Weiss, 1951; Kelman & Hovland, 1953; Pratkanis, Greenwald, Leippe, & Baumgardner, 1988).

The importance of considering intrinsic dynamics and their interaction with external factors can be illustrated by considering the classic demonstration of conformity to group pressure in the Asch (1956) paradigm. Compliance in this study was not mechanically produced by the observation of incorrect statements by the other group members. Participants were engaged in a task that had its own dynamics involving perceptual, judgmental, and response processes. Another set of processes reflected their participation in a group situation involving consideration of the experimental setting, the other group members, and their judgments. It is also likely that some processes not directly relevant to the experimental setting were engaged as well (e.g., planning for behavior upon of the completion of the experiment). The observation that others are providing incorrect judgments may alter the process of perception and judgment, or it may simply influence the process of generating a response in that situation. Moreover, even if conformity is not demonstrated by participants, this does not mean that the experimental manipulation failed to affect their internal processes. It is quite likely that the manipulation strongly affected their thinking about group members, the experimental setting, and perhaps even their perceptual process (e.g., repeated perception of the stimuli to reduce their uncertainty). All of these considerations are lost when one rejects consideration of intrinsic dynamics and concentrates solely on the outcome of the manipulation.

The intrinsic dynamics of social psychological processes may follow very rich and diverse courses. An obvious course of intrinsic dynamics is simply gradual change in the magnitude of some psychological state. A person's happiness, grief, or preoccupation with someone, for example, may grow progressively stronger for a period of time and then begin to dissipate. Intrinsic dynamics, however, can follow more intriguing temporal courses. For example, a person's psychological state (e.g., happiness, anger) may show little change for a notable period of time, followed by a sudden and catastrophic change. Such a course of dynamics is well documented, for example, in Gestalt psychology as reflected in such notions as perceptual reorganization and insight. At yet other times, the intrinsic dynamics of a process may be observed as the oscillation between two or more states. Ambivalence regarding a course of action, such as the approach–avoid conflict described by Miller (1944), represents a clear example of this course of intrinsic dynamics. Another example is the oscillation between affection and rejection that can come to characterize intimate relationships. Finally, intrinsic dynamics may follow very complex and irregular patterns. The stream of consciousness, as described by James (1890), represents an example of this type of intrinsic dynamics.

Despite the variety and richness of possible forms that intrinsic dynamics can take, there is reason to believe that there are strong rules underlying these forms. It might be possible, therefore, to discover general laws governing the dynamics of social psychological phenomena. Support for such optimism comes from work in other areas of science. Recent discoveries have shown that the intrinsic dynamics of various physical, chemical, biological, and economic systems, at some level of abstraction, conform to only a handful of possible temporal patterns that transcend topical boundaries (see Cohen & Stewart, 1994; Glass & Mackey, 1988; Pietgen & Richter, 1986; Prigogine & Stengers, 1984; Schuster, 1984). This suggests the potential for developing general laws of social psychological dynamics that apply to different levels of analysis, from the temporal pattern of individual thoughts to the coordinated interplay of nonverbal behavior in dyadic and group interactions. In each case, the dynamic patterns may be reliably associated with meaningful psychological properties, such as ambivalence in judgment or group solidarity. The discovery of such laws, in turn, might foster the integration of the subject matter of social psychology with the subject matter of seemingly distant disciplines.

The Ebb and Flow of Dynamics in Social Psychology

Despite the explicit focus on internally generated dynamics in the classic treatments of social psychology, this concern was diluted a great deal in subsequent years. It seems, in fact, that the primary legacy of the early dynamic perspectives has been an emphasis on tendencies toward achieving a stable equilibrium rather than on self-sustaining dynamics (e.g., Kruglanski, Clement, & Jost, 1997; Messick & Liebrand, 1997). This is apparent in theory and research on the cognitive underpinnings of social behavior. James (1890), for instance, underscored the dynamic nature of conscious experience in his stream of consciousness metaphor, but subsequent cognitive models in social psychology tended to emphasize the achievement of stable attributions, categories, beliefs, and other mental structures. By the early 1980s, in fact, the dynamic properties of cognition were difficult to discern in mainstream theory and research (cf. Markus & Zajonc, 1985). Lewin (1936b, 1951), meanwhile, offered a broad metatheory that framed human experience in terms of a field of ever-present and conflicting internal forces, but for the most part, this perspective inspired a host of cognitive theories centering on such notions as cognitive balance, the reduction of cognitive dissonance, and the elimination of incongruity.

The dynamics of action have also been reframed so as to emphasize the achievement of stability. So although Cooley (1902), for instance, argued that action is an ongoing process that can follow any number of paths, subsequent models and research programs reduced action dynamics to the attainment of goals, the maintenance of standards, the reduction of discrepancies between beliefs and behavior, or the elimination of tension. Especially in the 1980s, it became commonplace to suggest that the defining feature of action is its goal-directedness. Presumably, once a goal (or some other end state) is obtained, the press for action came to a halt until a new goal or action endpoint was engaged. Even conflict theory (Miller, 1944), with its emphasis on the simultaneous prepotence of incompatible goals, tended to generate research focusing on the tendency to establish an equilibrium point between the conflicting forces. It is somewhat ironic that the early attempts to express the intrinsic dynamics of psychological process ultimately generated research emphasizing instead the static features of these processes.

The focus on stability is understandable in view of the difficulties inherent in characterizing and analyzing the complex intrinsic dynamics of social psychological processes with the traditional tools of natural science. In adapting these tools to the field's concerns, social psychology developed an approach to change that was not well suited to capture dynamics that were internally generated and self-sustaining. In the typical research paradigm, first of all, change is usually conceptualized and operationalized as a discrete difference between two arbitrary points in time. Any variability that occurs within this time interval is totally lost. Before reaching a moderate decision, for example, a person or group may swing between the most extreme positions, but such variability will go unnoticed if the process at work is only sampled at one point in time. In focusing on a discrete difference, in other words, dynamics are effectively reduced to a single step of what usually is an ongoing iterative process. Although, in principle, the process could be recorded as many such discrete differences, in practice, the focus is usually on a single step of the process, thereby obscuring any patterns of change that may have occurred. In social judgment, for example, the most interesting and informative aspect of the process may lie in the pattern of oscillation between different considerations (see, e.g., Vallacher, Nowak, & Kaufman, 1994). In some cases, judgmental oscillation may be of a continuous nature, persisting well beyond the arbitrary time constraints imposed by the experimental design. The stability observed at the endpoint of a psychological observation thus may be imposed by the experiment's measurement strategy; were it not for this artificial constraint, this presumed endpoint might be experienced simply as a stage of an ongoing continuous change process.

Of course, the natural course of intrinsic dynamics may be constrained by real-world considerations, such as the need to make a decision or undertake an action, a point we develop in detail in Chapter 4. Even if one's goal is predicting how a judgment will stabilize under such conditions, however, insight into the pattern of changes in judgment may prove more informative than a single static measurement. If repeated measurements indicate that the judgment is more or less stable over time, then it is safe to extrapolate from the observed value to the final state. If, on the other hand, one observes sustained oscillation between conflicting judgments, the judgment is likely to stabilize on one of the observed values, and probabilities may be assigned to each value based on the relative frequency with which they occurred in the stream of judgment. In yet another case, the difference between two conflicting judgments may diminish over time due to ongoing integration processes, so that the average of the judgments may represent the final value. Even here, however, early measurement may force formation of a judgment based on only one of the conflicting values that has yet to be integrated with the other. In short, a single measurement not only cannot distinguish between the different dynamic scenarios, but may also lead to a misleading prediction. Identifying the pattern of judgment, in turn, indicates the conditions under which a static characterization of judgment is meaningful and offers means of providing a dynamic characterization when static characterization is inappropriate.

The very nature of psychological experimentation makes it unlikely that any intrinsic dynamics will be observed, regardless of the temporal density of measurement. In the typical paradigm, a presumed cause or set of causes is manipulated at one point in time, and the result of this intervention is assessed at some convenient (hence, arbitrary) later time. Although this approach is obviously well suited to capture the effects of environmental causes on a process in a person or group, it loses sight of the intrinsic dynamics at work. Intrinsic dynamics per se might be better revealed by observing the process as it unfolds on its own, in the absence of external influences. The research on thought-induced attitude polarization (Tesser, 1978), which reveals the extremification of initial attitudes with the passage of time, provides a clear example of how intrinsic dynamics may be captured by examining a process at only two points in time.

Paradigmatic assumptions are notorious for biasing one's selection and interpretation of facts, and the widely held view that external factors drive behavior is no exception. A particularly telling instance of this is the way Asch's (1956) classic research on judgment in a social context is reported (Levine, 1996). Asch's aim in this research was to demonstrate the internal workings of the mind when people were confronted with bizarre sets of informational elements. And, in fact, the results of this research revealed that conformity to bogus judgments by the majority occurred only a little more than one-third of the time. In the majority of cases, in other words, the external influence provided by the other group members was resisted rather than embraced, suggesting that the intrinsic dynamics serving to resist the pressure were the most salient aspect of participants' experience in this setting. Textbook presentations of this research convey a far different image of what this research demonstrated. In line with the prevailing metatheory concerning external causation, the results obtained in the Asch paradigm are invariably presented as evidence of the power of social forces to influence thought and behavior.

Dynamics, of course, never completely disappeared from mainstream social psychology. Even in the heyday of behaviorism, there were a variety of research programs focusing on the internal workings of psychological mechanisms. The legacy of Lewin and others was felt especially in research in the 1950s and 1960s that focused on people's attempt to deal with cognitive and affective inconsistencies engendered by the receipt of new information or by their own behavior (see Abelson et al., 1968). Dissonance theory (Festinger, 1957) garnered the most attention and arguably had the most enduring impact (see Aronson, 1992, and commentaries). For the most part, though, this research was conducted within the constraints of the natural science paradigm available at that time and thus could not adequately capture the dynamics per se that presumably generated the outcomes observed. The trajectory of thoughts and feelings that produced adoption of a counterattitudinal position in forced compliance research (e.g., Festinger & Carlsmith, 1959), for instance, was never directly assessed. Then, too, the assumption that internally generated dynamics always evolve toward a stable equilibrium ruled out consideration of a host of temporal trajectories that do not have this particular property.

The 1980s saw a particularly noteworthy resurgence of interest in the nature of various cognitive and affective processes within the individual. Among the key insights generated during this period was a distinction between judgments that occur more or less automatically in response to information or influence and those that reflect deliberate conscious processing and consideration of salient (and presumably relevant) information (cf. Bargh, 1989). The distinction between automatic and controlled processing played a prominent role, for example, in research on persuasion (cf. Chaiken, 1980; Petty & Cacioppo, 1986; Petty, Ostrom, & Brock, 1981), attribution (e.g., Gilbert, 1993), and stereotyping (e.g., Devine, 1989; Fiske & Neuberg, 1990). A host of other insights regarding the nature of internal mechanisms, meanwhile, were generated in research on unwanted thought, rumination, thought suppression, and mental control (cf. Baars, 1988; Martin & Tesser, 1989; Pennebaker, 1988; Uleman & Bargh, 1989; Wegner, 1994; Wegner & Pennebaker, 1993). This line of work is noteworthy in demonstrating that cognitive processes can be self-sustaining, continuing to unfold long after the external instigation to thought has ended. The potential for sustained intrinsic dynamics is also evident in theory and research on thought-induced attitude polarization (cf. Liberman & Chaiken, 1991; Tesser, 1978). The results of this research are notable in that they imply the operation of feedback mechanisms serving to amplify the initial state of the cognitive system over time.

Human action was also conceptualized in terms of internal dynamics during this period. Beckmann and Gollwitzer (1987), for instance, explored the cognitive processes at various stages of goal-directed action. The potential for mental dynamism was said to be especially strong during the predecisional phase of action, during which people consider the possible courses of action and weigh the likely effects and implications associated with each. Vallacher and Wegner (1985), meanwhile, discussed the processes by which people come to identify their past, present, and future actions. This work was a particularly strong precursor to the dynamical perspective, in that it pointed out the potential for reconfiguration of basic action elements in service of emergent action identification. Newtson, Hairfield, Bloomingdale, and Cutino (1987) were even more explicit regarding dynamics in their treatment of action, providing evidence that both individual and interpersonal action involve the coordination of basic components in a time-dependent manner. Indeed, Newtson's work qualifies as the first line of theory and research in social psychology to be couched in terms of nonlinear dynamical systems.

For the most part, these research programs were conducted within the constraints of the traditional natural science paradigm. So although a potential for intrinsic dynamics was implicit in the underlying theoretical models, the temporal trajectory of changes in the judgment state in question was not the primary focus of conceptualization or empirical investigation. By and large, dynamics were reduced to a single pass, and participants were assumed to generate a stable judgment by the time the experimenter decided to institute measurement procedures. Some programs did follow features of a process over time. The research concerned with issues of thought suppression, for example, sometimes focused on the appearance of unwanted thoughts in stream of consciousness protocols (e.g., Pennebaker, Hughes, & O'Heeron, 1987; Wegner, Schneider, Carter, & White, 1987; Wegner, Shortt, Blake, & Page, 1990). However, the interest here was the content of participants' thoughts, not the nature of the temporal pattern associated with the appearance of these thoughts in consciousness. As we shall see, there are means available for characterizing such patterns and using such characterizations for making inferences about the structure and function of the underlying cognitive–affective system.

THE REEMERGENCE OF DYNAMICAL SOCIAL PSYCHOLOGY

Since the early 1990s, there has been a renewed interest in identifying the dynamical aspects of social psychological processes (see Kunda & Thagard, 1996; Kruglanski et al., 1997; Messick & Liebrand, 1997; Read, Vanman, & Miller, 1997; Smith, 1996; Tesser, McMillen, & Collins, 1997). What was once represented in a few scattered papers and chapters has expanded to the point where it now qualifies as a new paradigm for the field. To a substantial degree, the reemergence of this paradigm has been made possible by discoveries concerning the behavior of nonlinear dynamical systems in other areas of science during the 1980s. In essence, these discoveries have enabled social psychologists to achieve precise understanding of the dynamical aspects of social experience that provided the key insights for the field during its formative years.

Cyclic Phenomena

There is a long-standing interest in the temporal patterns associated with various biological phenomena. Considerable research, for example, has focused on the biological clocks in animals and humans (Brown & Graeber, 1982). Perhaps the best known clocks are circadian rhythms, which dictate the timing of activity cycles and other processes. These rhythms are coordinated with external cues, such as patterns of light versus darkness, the gravitational tug of the moon, barometric pressure, and so on. Interest in circadian rhythms in humans was in part inspired by the phenomenon of jet lag and the need to cope with this desynchronization of one's internal biological clock. It was observed, for example, that pilots who fly on routes from south to north, which tend to be associated with climate changes but not with time-zone changes, experience much less stress and exhaustion than do pilots who fly on east–west routes, which do entail time-zone changes but often little change in climate (Graeber, 1982). The desynchronization of internal clocks is also an issue for shift workers in industry, who must reverse their daily cycle of sleep and work (Naitoh, 1982). Research has shown that synchronization is provided by the day–night cycle and is mediated by melatonin concentrations in the brain.

There is also evidence that internal clocks can dictate rhythms of biological function even in the absence of environmental cues. Evidence for this in humans comes from investigations in which volunteers spend several weeks in bunkers or underground facilities that are devoid of environmental cues to the day–night cycle—and, of course, devoid of external clocks (Wever, 1982). The volunteers in these studies maintained a fairly stable sleep–wake cycle, although they did begin to drift from the 24-hour cycle to a certain extent after a few days without external sources of synchronization. Research has also demonstrated that the various internal clocks tend to be synchronized with one another, often in the form of embedded cycles. Embedded within the 24-hour sleep–wake cycle, for example, are various biological and psychological characteristics (e.g., body temperature, hormone secretion, arousal level, concentration). The sleep–wake cycle, in turn, is embedded in larger monthly and seasonal rhythms.

More recently, there has been a growing appreciation of cyclicity in social psychological phenomena (Gottman, 1983). It now appears that periodic structure is a fairly ubiquitous feature of personal and interpersonal experience, reflecting cyclic variation in cognitive, emotional, and behavioral processes. Moods, for example, tend to show periodicity (cf. Mandell & Selz, 1994), often corresponding to a weekly cycle (e.g., Brown & Moskowitz, 1998; Larsen, 1987; Larsen & Kasimatis, 1990). Among college students, weekly mood variation can be approximated by a sinusoidal wave that explains 40% of the variance. Moods tend to peak on Fridays and Saturdays and to bottom out on (blue) Mondays and Tuesdays. It is not clear to what degree the weekly mood cycle reflects biological underpinnings or instead is socially generated. In support of the biological interpretation, a 7-day pattern of immune responses has been observed and this pattern is not necessarily coordinated with the Christian calendar. Research has also revealed individual differences in the strength of weekly mood patterns. Extroverts, for example, are more likely to show mood variation in response to external influences than are introverts, and so experience greater disruption in the regularity of this pattern (Brown & Moskowitz, 1998). Penner, Shiffman, Paty, and Fritzche (1994) have established that intraindividual variability in mood is a stable and distinct dimension of individual difference, with some people reliably demonstrating greater temporal variation than others.

Periodic structure also appears to be a defining feature of human action (Newtson et al., 1987), and it has proven useful in the investigation of social interaction as well (e.g., Beek & Hopkins, 1992; Buder, 1991; Gottman, 1979; Newtson, 1994). When one analyzes the temporal aspects of human activities, meanwhile, the strongest effect is daily periodic structure (e.g., Nezlek, 1993; Nezlek & Wheeler, 1984). This work has revealed both daily and weekly rhythms in social encounters. Interestingly, there are indications in Nezlek's data that greater periodicity in social contacts is characteristic of people who are poorly connected with others. A plausible interpretation is that those who show high regularity are synchronized by prescheduled activities and routines, whereas those who show more irregular patterns of contact are driven by impulses and desires to interact with others. High regularity may therefore reflect a lack of freedom of choice and little opportunity to engage in spontaneous interactions in accordance with one's preferences. In a related vein, the variation in positive versus negative feelings in close relationships may have a periodic structure (e.g., Vallacher, 1995; Wiggins, 1979), although this possibility appears not to have received a great deal of empirical attention to date.

There is clearly abundant evidence showing the existence of rhythms of both a biological and social nature. Until recently, however, this evidence was primarily descriptive and not well integrated into theory. In most cases, it was not clear what the existence of such temporal patterns might reveal about underlying mechanisms of human cognition, affect, and action. Tools developed in research on nonlinear dynamical systems, however, have allowed more detailed understanding of the "rhythms of life" (Glass & Mackey, 1988). We now know, for example, that the temporal evolution of a system may be governed by the superimposition of different periods (e.g., weekly and seasonal rhythms in addition to daily rhythms). This form of periodicity is referred to as "multiperiodic evolution." The most complex case of multiperiodic evolution is quasiperiodic evolution, in which each of the system's variables exhibits different periods, and these periods are incommensurable (i.e., they are not multiples of a single basic period). In such instances, the values of all the variables repeat with some period, but the system as a whole (the combination of all the variables) never returns to exactly the same value.

Fourier analysis is a mathematical technique designed to identify different periods and their relative importance in a system's behavior (see Schroeck, 1994). Newtson (1994), for instance, has used this approach to expose periods in seemingly aperiodic human movement. Beyond identifying complex temporal patterns in diverse human phenomena, theory and research on nonlinear dynamical systems are showing that internal rhythms can provide an important source of information concerning the internal workings of mechanisms generating the temporal patterns. Both the observation of internally generated rhythms and the relative resistance to disruption of such rhythms provide insight into the nature of biological and psychological systems. Dynamics and structure, from this perspective, represent complementary aspects of human experience and serve to enlighten the nature of one another.

Cellular Automata

Cellular automata models are used to investigate collective phenomena reflecting the interaction of individual elements in complex systems (cf. Gutowitz, 1991; Ulam, 1952; von Neumann, 1966; Wolfram, 1986). Cellular automata are discrete dynamical systems, in that they are composed of a specified number of elements, each of which can adopt a discrete number of states at discrete points in time. The basic unit is a cell representing an individual component of the system in question. Thus, each cell represents a single particle of fluid in models of hydrology, a single particle with magnetic orientation (spin) in models of magnetic phenomena, and a single tissue cell in models of biology. Regardless of the particular application, each cell can adopt one of a limited number of discrete states (often only two). The cellular automata is composed of a large number of such cells, which are arranged in a well-defined spatial configuration, such as a one-dimensional line or a two-dimensional lattice. The state of a cell depends on the states of neighboring cells and is dictated by so-called updating rules. One of the simplest updating rules is the majority rule, which specifies that a cell at time $t + 1$ will adopt the state characterizing the majority of its neighbors at time t. Different neighborhood structures are possible for cellular automata models. In a two-dimensional lattice, for example, there may be four neighbors (one on each side) or eight neighbors (the original four plus an additional four in the diagonals). Cellular automata with different updating rules can exhibit a wide variety of spatial and temporal patterns characteristic of dynamical systems (Wolfram, 1986).[1]

In social science applications, cellular automata are primarily used to study the emergence of group-level phenomena from individual-level interactions. In such applications, each cell corresponds to a single individual, and states of the cell may represent individual characteristics such as opinions and attitudes, decision, and so forth. It is usually assumed that each individual's interactions are limited to neighboring cells and that the outcomes of these interactions determine the state each individual adopts. Against this general backdrop, two distinct classes of cellular automata models have been applied to social psychology, each designed to provide insight into a different set of issues. The elements in both classes correspond to individuals who interact with their neighbors. In one class, each individual's characteristics change as a result of the updating rules. This class of models is useful, then, for understanding changes in attitudes, opinions, and so forth, as a result of social interaction. In the other class, the characteristics of individuals do not change over time, but the individuals may change their physical location. This class of cellular automata is used primarily to investigate the emergence of spatial patterns on the basis of stable values, preferences, strengths, and so forth. In an early example, Shelling (1969, 1971) formulated an updating rule simply stating that an individual who has more dissimilar than similar neighbors will move to a different random location. This simple rule has proven sufficient to produce patterns of social segregation.

For both classes of models, one commonly observes the emergence of regularities and patterns on a global level that were not directly programmed into individual elements. These emergent properties often take the form of spatial patterns, such as the social segregation observed by Shelling or the emergence of coherent minority clusters from an initial random distribution of opinions. Emergent properties can also take the form of temporal patterns (cf. Wolfram, 1986), including evolution toward a stable equilibrium (fixed-point attractor), alternation between different states (periodicity), and apparent randomness (chaos), each of which is discussed in detail in Chapter 2. Cellular automata are thus proving useful in understanding the effects of different rules of social interaction and the generation of societal-level phenomena as a result of such rules. Several distinct and theoretically meaningful aspects of this linkage between microrules and macroprocesses have been investigated in recent years. These include the nature of social influence (e.g., the spread of new attitudes in a population), discussed in Chapter 7, social interdependence (e.g., cooperation vs. competition), discussed in Chapter 8, and key features of social change (e.g., social and political transitions), also discussed in Chapter 8. We emphasize, though, that cellular automata are not restricted to group- or societal-level phenomena, but can be used to model individual-level phenomena as well. In Chapter 5, in fact, we introduce a cellular automata model of self-concept.

Connectionism

The basic feature of connectionist models is that the state (activation) of each element in a system is determined by the total influence (excitatory minus inhibitory) from other elements across connections. Connectionist models are also known as artificial neural network models because their architecture resembles that of the nervous system. Elements are analogous to neurons, and connections are analogous to synapses. Connectionist models are good illustrations of the basic principles of dynamical systems because the state of elements at one moment in time depends on the state of the elements to which they are connected at the preceding moment in time. Beginning in the mid-1980s with the publication of *Parallel Distributed Processing* by McClelland and Rumelhart (1986), this approach has emerged as one of the leading paradigms in the study of cognitive processes (cf. Smolensky, 1988).

Although this approach has only recently been introduced to social psychology, its assumptions resonate with many of the early insights regarding interpersonal thought and behavior we have noted in this chapter (e.g., Smith, 1996). Connectionist models enable one to capture directly the classic Gestalt notions of structural dynamics, for example, including the idea that the same elements can be reorganized into different wholes (see Read et al., 1997). This approach is also well suited to model the experience of competing forces within the individual. In principle, social reality at all levels of analysis can be described within a connectionist framework. Thus, the mind can be viewed in connectionist terms, with nodes representing cognitive elements and connections corresponding to associations or other types of functional relations among these elements. In a connectionist model of social groups, each node might represent a single individual, with connections representing social relations. Societal dynamics could also be modeled in a connectionist framework, with each node corresponding to a particular social group and the connections corresponding to intergroup relations. As testament to the utility of this perspective, such issues as person perception, stereotyping, social categorization, causal attribution, personality dynamics, attitudes and beliefs, and social influence have recently been recast in terms of connectionist models (cf. Kunda & Thagard, 1996; Read & Miller, 1998; Smith, 1996).

The connectionist approach clearly represents a highly general and flexible approach, one that is well suited to illuminate invariant principles across a wide variety of topics and levels of analysis. Indeed, one could extend the connectionist approach beyond the domain of social psychology to model phenomena in sociology and political science. In such an approach, an entire nation could be represented as a node, and various aspects of international relations (political alliances, trade arrangements, etc.) could represent instantiations of connections among the nations. In principle, one could build a connectionist model in a hierarchical form, with different levels of social reality represented simultaneously. In such a model, investigation would center not only on the mutual influences among nodes within each level, but also on the influences between different levels of description. Although analytical models exist that formally capture some types of connectionist models, progress in the understanding of these models and their application to social psychological phenomena is mainly due to computer simulations (see Nowak & Vallacher, 1998; Nowak, Vallacher, & Burnstein, 1998).

Nonlinear Dynamical Systems

A dynamical system can be defined in general terms as a set of interconnected elements that undergoes change. The ability to evolve in time, in fact, is the most important characteristic of a dynamical system. The primary task of dynamical systems theory is to describe the connections among a system's elements and the changes in the system's behavior to which these connections give rise. The state of a system at a given point in time is described by dynamical variables, which are numbers that change in time and that characterize the relevant properties of the state of the system at that moment. The state of the system at time t is fully described by specifying actual values of all the dynamical variables, $X_1(t)$, $X_2(t)$, . . . , $X_n(t)$.

To capture the dynamics of the system, one needs to describe how the dynamical variables change. In mathematics and physics, this description is usually given in the form of either difference or differential equations. Systems described by difference equations are referred to as discrete dynamical systems or discrete maps. In difference equations, time is treated as a discrete variable that can be divided into innumerable instants. The value of each variable X_i at time $t + 1$ is described as a function, f_i, of the values of all variables at time t,

$$X_i(t + 1) = f_i[X_1(t), X_2(t), \ldots, X_n(t)].$$

Differential equations are employed whenever it is more appropriate to use continuous time instead of discrete time. Differential equations express the rate of change of dynamical variables as a function of the state of the system (i.e., the values of the variables). For a system that can be described by n dynamical variables, $X_1(t)$, $X_2(t)$, $\ldots$, $X_n(t)$, the dynamics are governed by a set of n differential equations, each of which specifies the rate of change of one of the variables as a function, f_i, of the state of the system (i.e., all the other variables):

$$\frac{dX_i(t)}{dt} = f_i[X_1(t), \ldots, X_n(t)].$$

For both difference and differential equations, knowledge of the state of all the system variables enables prediction of the state of the system at succeeding points in time.

The rules underlying the evolution of a system may be described alternatively in geometric terms. The set of numbers, $X_1(t)$, $X_2(t)$, $\ldots$, $X_n(t)$ may be considered a set of coordinates in an n-dimensional space, referred to as a *phase space*. Each coordinate of this space corresponds, then, to one dynamical variable describing the system. Each point in the system's phase space corresponds to a unique combination of values of all the dynamical variables and thus describes a unique state of the system. The dynamics of the system correspond to motion in the phase space, with the succession of points representing the succession of states. This motion draws a curve in the phase space, referred to as a *trajectory*, that is simply a set of points visited by a system in its time evolution.[2] Plotting the phase space trajectory of a system's evolution is a common first step in understanding the mechanisms responsible for a system's behavior. In the physical sciences, it is commonly observed that diverse nonlinear systems composed of a small number of variables tend to evolve along only a few types of trajectories. Through visual inspection of a trajectory, then, one may identify resemblance to some established trajectory for which the underlying equations governing its evolution are known. In social psychology, however, one can rarely identify, much less measure, all the dynamical variables that would be required to construct a phase space for a phenomenon. In Chapter 2, we discuss the concept of *state space*, which enables one to generate a geometrical description in the form of trajectories, even without complete knowledge of all the dynamical variables in the system.

Prior to the advent of the mathematical theory of nonlinear dynamical systems, the natural sciences assumed that the relations among variables in nature could be approximated as linear. A linear relation between any two variables exists if changes in one variable can be expressed as a direct proportion of changes in the other variable. The greater the change in magnitude of one variable, in other words, the greater the resulting change in magnitude of the second variable. In causal terms, this simply means that the magnitude of the effect is always proportional to the magnitude of the cause. It is also the case that a linear system consists of additive relations. This means that the description of such a system can be decomposed into separate influences, each of which can be analyzed independently. Because linear equations in general can be solved analytically and the influences of linear variables can be analyzed independently, an analytical treatment of even fairly complex phenomena is possible.

For dynamical systems to display complex properties, it is critical that the elements or variables in the system influence one another in a nonlinear rather than in a linear fashion. When relations are nonlinear, even precise approximations based on linear assumptions can lead to very false and misleading conclusions. In a nonlinear system, the effects of changes in one variable are not reflected in a proportional manner in other variables. The behavior of a nonlinear system, moreover, often cannot be decomposed into separate additive components. Rather, the relations among variables usually depend on the values of other variables in the system, and thus are interactive in nature. Thus, one cannot ignore the effects of other variables when describing the relation between one's variables of interest. Changes in any one variable, however, tend to reveal the influence of changes in all the other variables in the system. Because of this effect, repeated observation of even a single variable may be informative about the structure of the system as a whole (Grassberger & Procaccia, 1983; Kaplan & Glass, 1992; Takens, 1981).

In the 1990s, the relevance of nonlinear dynamical systems to various topics in psychology became recognized by a growing number of researchers (e.g., Abraham, 1990; Abraham & Gilgen, 1995; Barton, 1994). It emerged as a dominant paradigm in the psychology of motor control (e.g., Kelso, Ding, & Schöner, 1991; Kelso, Scholz, &

Schöner, 1986; Saltzman, 1995; Turvey, 1990), for example, and it is providing insights into a wide variety of other topics, including perception (e.g., Gilden, 1991; Hock, Kelso, & Schöner, 1993; Hock, Schöner, & Voss, 1997; Jones, 1976; Petitot, 1995; Turvey & Carello, 1995), attention (e.g., Jones & Boltz, 1989), speech production (e.g., Tuller, Kelso, & Harris, 1983), linguistics (e.g., Elman, 1995), and human development (e.g., Fischer & Bidell, 1997; Smith & Thelen, 1993; Thelen, 1992, 1995; Thelen & Smith, 1994; van Geert, 1991, 1995). Cognitive science has especially embraced the dynamical perspective, not only in the form of numerous connectionist models, but also in the form of direct applications of the underlying theoretical perspective (see Port & Van Gelder, 1995). This perspective is particularly well suited to capture the dynamism and complexity inherent in social psychological phenomena (Vallacher & Nowak, 1994b). People and social groups, of course, are not the same as lasers, weather systems, and other phenomena investigated from this perspective in the physical sciences. But the discoveries concerning internally generated dynamics and the emergence of complexity in nonlinear dynamical systems suggest that this approach can provide important insights into the nuances of human experience.

This perspective is in fact gaining momentum in social psychology. A growing number of researchers are reframing their theories to incorporate dynamical assumptions and are utilizing dynamical concepts and tools to investigate diverse aspects of personal and interpersonal experience. Thus, research has begun to explore the dynamical underpinnings of attitudes (e.g., Eiser, 1994b; Latané & Nowak, 1994; Ostrom, Skowronsky, & Nowak, 1994), social relationships (e.g., Baron, Amazeen, & Beek, 1994; Tesser & Achee, 1994), cognitive consistency (e.g., Read et al., 1997; Shultz & Lepper, 1996), action (e.g., Newtson, 1994), social judgment (e.g., Kunda & Thagard, 1996; Smith, 1996; Vallacher et al., 1994), the mental control of behavior (e.g., Vallacher, Nowak, Markus, & Strauss, 1998), goal attainment (e.g., Carver & Scheier, 1990, 1999; Hsee & Abelson, 1991; Hsee, Abelson, & Salovey, 1991), social influence (e.g., Nowak, Szamrej, & Latané, 1990), altruism and cooperation (e.g., Messick & Liebrand, 1995), decision making (e.g., Busemeyer & Townsend, 1993; Kaplowitz & Fink, 1992; Richards, 1990; Townsend & Busemeyer, 1995), and group dynamics (e.g., Losada & Markovitch, 1990). The potential of this approach for providing conceptual and methodological integration for the field as a whole has also been articulated by a number of social psychologists (see Vallacher & Nowak, 1994a, 1997, and associated commentaries).

Dynamics and Causation

We wish to emphasize that the traditional approach to social psychology and the dynamical approach are not in opposition, but rather may be seen as complementary. For its part, the traditional approach concentrates on isolating one-directional causal links between variables. Research in social psychology has thus focused primarily on the development of single-step models that do not track processes over time. The dynamical approach, meanwhile, tries to characterize the ongoing dynamics of a system, where the dynamics are produced by sequences and reciprocal loops of causal mechanisms. In this perspective, an essential causal factor in a psychological process is the process itself (cf. van Geert, 1997). This means that the state of the system at any moment in time is determined by the state of the system at the preceding moment, so that an effect at one time may operate as a cause the next.

To illustrate the interplay between causal mechanisms and dynamic processes, consider the following causal relations: Similarity in attitudes causes attraction, physical proximity increases social influence, and lack of distinctiveness from others produces efforts toward self–other differentiation. At first glance, these seem to be three unrelated causal mechanisms, each of which bears no obvious relation to system dynamics. When these mechanisms are considered together, however, prediction concerning the system's dynamics becomes possible. Because attraction involves increased contacts between people, it tends to increase physical proximity. The increased influence due to proximity, in turn, facilitates the development of greater similarity in attitudes, which creates a base for even greater attraction. These two mechanisms thus form a positive feedback loop that moves the relationship to increased values of attraction, similarity, and proximity. As a result, the system evolves in a unidirectional fashion. The third causal mechanism, however, suggests that at very high values of similarity, a desire to distance oneself is initiated. Ironically, then, the positive feedback loop between similarity and attraction may produce conditions that ultimately undermine the relationship. In particular, after similarity reaches a critical threshold due to repeated cycling of this feedback loop, the relationship partners are likely to experience forces toward differentiation, even to the point of terminating the relationship. At this point, a similar temporal sequence is likely to be repeated with a different—or perhaps even the same—partner. When viewed in a longer time frame, a repetitive pattern may emerge in which an individual slowly increases his or her proximity to like-minded others, only to suddenly increase the distance and terminate the relationship.

Observation of system dynamics may therefore enable verification of specific causal mechanisms and the way in which they are related to one another. In this sense, an analysis of dynamics is informative about how parts, in the form of causal mechanisms, are assembled to form a functioning system. Beyond verifying specific causal theories, a dynamical analysis can also indicate the types of causal mechanisms that might be operating in the system, even when there are no *a priori* hypotheses in this regard. Thus, one may start with an analysis of the patterns of system dynamics and work backwards to identify the causal mechanisms responsible for producing these patterns. From this perspective, analysis of system dynamics provides a new way to formulate as well as test hypotheses regarding specific causal mechanisms in the system. The utility of the dynamical approach, however, goes beyond shedding light on causal mechanisms. Specific laws may be discovered that characterize dynamic properties per se. One can specify the conditions, for example, under which a system is likely to reach an equilibrium versus display a sustained pattern of changes. As demonstrated in the subsequent chapters of this book, the dynamical perspective allows for the formulation of laws concerning important properties of a system, types of temporal patterns, and the scenarios of change in system properties and temporal patterns.

The availability of powerful tools makes dynamical analyses not only insightful, but precise and informative. Our aim in the subsequent chapters is to illustrate how the dynamical perspective in social psychology may be implemented with such tools. For each topic under consideration, we characterize both the dynamical properties on a global level and the underlying causal mechanisms. The linkage between these two aspects goes to the heart of the dynamical approach. Although it is possible to discuss both structure (as reflected in causal relations) and process (as reflected in a system's dynamics) separately, dynamical tools are ideally suited to characterize the linkage between structure and process.

The specific dynamical models and lines of research we present are not intended to be comprehensive. They are intended instead as illustrations of how the dynamical approach can be applied to various issues and topics that define classic and contemporary social psychology. In large part, these illustrations represent original lines of research we have developed over the last several years. We stress that those phenomena for which we present illustrative research of our own can be, and in some cases have been, investigated with respect to very different types of dynamical models. In considering social judgment, for example, we build models in the form of low-dimensional nonlinear dynamical systems, although social cognition and judgment have been successfully analyzed within the framework of the connectionist approach (cf. Kunda & Thagard, 1996; Read et al., 1997; Shultz & Lepper, 1996; Smith, 1996). Although our intent is not to provide a comprehensive survey of all relevant research within a dynamical framework, we try to summarize the essence of the dynamical perspective in each domain of social psychology and refer the reader to original sources for more detailed discussions.

INSIGHT AND RIGOR IN SOCIAL PSYCHOLOGY

As a scientific discipline, social psychology has always been faced with a seemingly intractable dilemma: whether to pursue the deep insights provided by the founding fathers of social psychology concerning the nature of human experience, or whether to impose strict canons of science in order to bring the field in line with the physical sciences. Voices have been raised in recent years that essentially come down on the side of preserving insights, even if this means abandoning accepted scientific methodology (cf. Gergen, 1985, 1994; Harré & Gillett, 1994). This perspective has not taken hold in mainstream social psychology. This is not to say that contemporary social psychology has abandoned any hope of capturing the subtleties of phenomenology and process. In the context of the demands imposed by the prevailing metatheory of scientific explanation, however, the field has often restricted itself to methods that were not designed to reveal the dynamic and complex nature of interpersonal functioning.

When attempts to apply traditional scientific methods and tools to social psychology fail to capture the deep essence of human thought, emotion, and action, it is understandable that advocates should blame either the scientific approach or the subject matter of social psychology. Those who side with the traditional scientific approach point to the soft and tentative nature of social psychological data. Unlike "hard" sciences such as physics and chemistry, the argument goes, the subject matter of social psychology is inherently ambiguous with respect to causality, and the concepts of social psychological theory are typically vague and ill-defined, making the derivation of precise and objective measures next to impossible.

The perspective provided by the theory of nonlinear dynamical systems helps resolve this long-standing dilemma. The discoveries made within this approach have shown that linear models of dynamical systems, which were used predominantly until the 1980s, are inadequate to model much beyond the simplest physical phenomena. It is hardly reasonable, then, to expect such models to provide satisfactory characterization of the complex phenomena defining the subject matter of social psychology. The frustration associated with persistent attempts to apply models and tools developed in the physical sciences to social psychology, in other words, may be attributed to the inherent weakness of those models and tools rather than to the purported weaknesses of social psychology. The nonlinear dynamical systems perspective does not share these limitations; to the contrary, it was developed as a means to capture the complexity and dynamism that heretofore had stymied scientific analysis. This perspective thus offers hope that one can combine the most sophisticated and precise theories and tools in the physical sciences with the deepest insights concerning the nature of human thought, emotion, and action.

There is reason to believe, in fact, that the most advanced tools, methods, and concepts of contemporary science may ultimately have the greatest application to social psychology. Such notions as spatial–temporal chaos, self-organization, and unpredictability may prove to be even more useful in the social sciences than in the physical sciences. There is a clear precedent for this scenario in the neural sciences. Although network theories were developed in physics, it turned out that the brain—a well-entrenched topic of biological and psychological inquiry—provided the most appropriate exemplar. It is reasonable to expect that continued developments in the study of nonlinear dynamical systems will make this perspective increasingly applicable to the subject matter of social psychology.

NOTES

1. Perhaps the best-known example of cellular automata is the "game of life" (see Gardner, 1983; Sigmund, 1993). In this automata model of artificial life, each cell may be either alive or dead, depending on the number of neighboring cells that are alive. Different initial configurations of living and dead cells may give rise to very complex spatial–temporal patterns.

2. In discrete dynamical systems, the trajectory is a sequence of points rather than a curve.

2

⤛⤜

The Dynamical
Perspective

T HROUGHOUT THE HISTORY of social psychology, there have been repeated attempts to borrow insights and tools from the physical sciences. As noted in Chapter 1, however, the classical paradigm in the physical sciences was too simplistic to provide meaningful characterization of the complexity and intrinsic dynamism inherent in interpersonal processes. Social psychology was thus correct in avoiding many of the oversimplifications that would have been required to embrace the traditional scientific approach in its entirety. It is noteworthy, for example, that radical behaviorism, with its strong emphasis on logical positivism, never achieved mainstream status as an approach to interpersonal dynamics. Social psychology may have experienced difficulty capturing, in practice, the elusive nature of thoughts, feelings, and actions, but the field remained steadfast in its commitment, in principle, to the unique qualities of human experience that simply cannot be ignored.

This patience and persistence has been rewarded. As it happens, the physical sciences have now evolved to the point where they can begin to appreciate the insights that have defined social psychology since its inception. The approach of nonlinear dynamical systems that swept through the natural sciences beginning in the late 1970s radically transformed understanding of the nature of dynamism and complexity inherent in many natural phenomena. The enormous popularity of this approach reflects the fact that similar, often identical, models of dynamical systems apply to many diverse phenomena in science, from fluid turbulence and weather patterns to brain function, laser pulsation, and chemical reactions (see Haken, 1982; Kelso, 1995; Prigogine & Stengers, 1984). The invariant nature of dynamical systems, in fact, has fueled optimism that dynamical systems theory may represent an integrative perspective for science as a whole (see Gleick, 1987). For this reason, and because of certain exotic phenomena such as chaos, strange attractors, and butterfly effects that are associated with nonlinear dynamical systems, this approach has also captured the fascination of the lay public in recent years.

Broadly defined, a dynamical system is simply a system that evolves over time. This means that the state of a system at one point in time determines the state of the system at the next moment in time. Thus, dynamical systems have the capacity to display internally generated dynamics and to evolve even in the absence of external influences on the system. The source of change lies in the mutual influences among components of the system. This approach has been used for centuries to describe simple phenomena, such as the motion of a pendulum or the revolution of planetary bodies around the sun. Generally speaking, it was assumed that the complexity of a system's behavior was a direct reflection of the number of interacting elements and the complexity of their mutual influences. The more complex the phenomenon, the greater the number of elements and the more varied the rules of interaction among them. It was recognized that many natural phenomena involved nonlinear relations, but it was believed that such relations could be approximated with adequate precision by linear equations. The revolution in the 1980s reflected a realization that even simple systems consisting of few elements typically exhibit behavior of enormous complexity when the interactions among the elements are nonlinear as opposed to linear. Thus, a nonlinear system may display such features as irregularity and unpredictability, the emergence of patterns, and self-organization. These features of nonlinear dynamical systems clearly resonate with the insights concerning social processes developed nearly a century earlier. Perhaps even more important, the discoveries concerning the sources of complexity provide hope that we may be able to find relatively simple explanations for the extremely complex phenomena that define social psychology.

In this chapter we highlight the primary features of nonlinear dynamical systems that are especially relevant for social psychology. We discuss the principal insights from the dynamical perspective and suggest how they might be manifest in various aspects of interpersonal functioning. As it happens, many phenomena in social psychology already express properties one would expect within a dynamical perspective. We focus in particular on the nature of intrinsic dynamics, the relation between complexity and simplicity in phenomena characterized by nonlinearity, the meaning of stability and change within dynamical systems, and the distinction between determinism and prediction. We conclude by describing the research strategies and analytical tools associated with nonlinear dynamical systems, and we illustrate how these can be adapted to investigate the unique nature of social psychological dynamics.

INTRINSIC DYNAMICS

A defining feature of dynamical systems is their tendency to display internally generated changes that often conform to identifiable patterns. This means that systems evolve according to some rule rather in direct response to external influence, so that the state of a system at time 1 determines to some extent the state of the system at time 2. As noted in Chapter 1, this capacity for intrinsic dynamics captures the idea that people are often the source of their own thoughts, feelings, and actions.

Intrinsic Dynamics, Feedback, and Causality

In a dynamical system, the values of the variables at time n depend on the values of these variables at time $n - 1$, and in turn they determine the values of the variables at time $n + 1$.[1] The same variable can thus act as a "cause" one moment and as an "effect" the next. This feedback process is at odds with traditional notions of causality that assume asymmetrical one-directional relationships between cause and effect. For the same reason, it does not fit well with the standard division between independent and dependent variables in social psychological research. There is reason to think, though, that bidirectional causality is in fact a fundamental feature of social psychological phenomena (Bandura, 1986). It may be appropriate, then, to describe the relationships in social psychology as multiple feedback loops between variables.

Because feedback mechanisms internal to a dynamical system are sufficient to promote sustained dynamics, a change in the state of such a system does not necessarily indicate the presence of an external causal factor. External factors, in fact, rarely bring about changes directly in a system's behavior. If such factors do promote change, they do so by interacting with the system's internally generated dynamics. In some cases, a very slight change in the value of an external factor can change dramatically the system's intrinsic dynamics and thereby affect the behavior of the system. But in other cases, even a large change in the value of an external factor may have minimal or no influence on the system's intrinsic dynamics and thus fail to change the system's behavior. The lesson here is simple: The causal effects of external variables are difficult to describe without taking into account the system's internally generated sources of change. In attempting to model and predict change, then, it is necessary to consider the interaction of both external and internal forces.

This perspective on causality has clear parallels in social psychology. It is hard to imagine, in fact, how any "situational factor" or "stimulus" could influence a person's thoughts, feelings, or actions independently of the person's internal mechanisms—his or her motives, goals, concerns, and so forth. In this regard, it has become commonplace for psychologists to emphasize the importance of "person by situation" interactions in discussions of behavioral prediction. An appreciation of internal sources of change also helps one understand how and why people actively resist external influences under some circumstances (e.g., Brehm & Brehm, 1981) but demonstrate dramatic change in response to minimal instigation in other circumstances. Unfortunately, a conceptual framework based on traditional cause–effect assumptions does not lend itself to research strategies that can fully exploit the various ways in which external factors influence the intrinsic dynamics of personal and interpersonal processes.

Intrinsic dynamics may be observed at all levels of social reality—from the interaction among thoughts, plans, and impulses within a single individual, to the interaction among individuals, social groups, and organizations within a society. In each case, the successive interactions among the system's elements promote continual change in the system, and the nature of this change will mediate how external factors (e.g., persuasion for an individual, an international threat for a society) impact on the system. In effect, the concept of "person by situation" interaction can be generalized to different levels of analysis, so that one may speak of, say, a "group by societal context" or a "society by international context" interaction. In each case, the external factor affects the system's behavior by virtue of its interaction with the dynamics at work within the system itself.

Patterns of Intrinsic Dynamics

The internally generated behavior of a dynamical system often can be characterized in terms of a pattern of changes. If a reliable pattern can in fact be discerned, the unit of analysis is no longer the discrete changes constituting the pattern, but rather the pattern itself. In trying to understand the weather, for example, one is not concerned with each momentary change in temperature, humidity, and the like, but rather with the pattern of such changes over some time scale (e.g., day, season, decade, millennium). In the context of social psychology, this suggests that focusing on stability versus variability in the features of some phenomenon—a person's expressed attitude, for example, or a dyad's level of affection—may be a case of overlooking the forest for the trees. The value of any given feature (attitude expression, intimacy) may well vary a great deal over time, but if this temporal variation conforms to a reliable pattern, the phenomenon can be nonetheless characterized as stable and predictable.

The tendency for internally driven changes to conform to patterns helps clarify how interpersonal thought can be characterized with equal validity as a stream of consciousness (James, 1890), with specific thoughts coursing past one another in a whimsical fashion, and as an organized structure, with specific thoughts fitting together in a stable and coherent manner (e.g., Heider, 1958). Specific elements of cognition may indeed come and go, but social thinking can nonetheless be represented as a stable structure if the succession of elements reoccurs in a regular manner. Hence, it may be misleading to characterize a person's thoughts and feelings about someone in terms of an average value collapsed over time. Thus, a person's feelings toward an intimate other may reliably alternate between love and hate; averaged over time, one might conclude erroneously that the person feels neutral toward the target.

A focus on temporal patterns in intrinsic dynamics is also relevant to the perennial issue of behavioral consistency in theory and research on personality (cf. Bem & Allen, 1974; Epstein, 1979; Mischel & Peake, 1982). Assume that a person displays considerable variation over time in his or her degree of extroversion—he or she is very outgoing and sociable at some times, but quiet and reserved at others. It is tempting to conclude that the person lacks a disposition to behave in a consistent manner with respect to this dimension. His or her behavior might be viewed as under the control of situational forces or as simply unstable and unpredictable. One could average the person's behavior over time, but this would lead to the curious conclusion that the person is moderately outgoing—a tendency he or she may never display. An approach based on pattern recognition, in contrast, might well identify remarkable consistency in the person's behavior—not with respect to his or her degree of extroversion, but with respect to a recurring temporal pattern. Thus, the person might show a reliable pattern of alternation between periods of talkativeness and silence in social settings. If so, the person's behavior could be characterized as stable and predictable despite the inconsistency from one assessment to the next.

It is noteworthy that personality research in the 1990s began to characterize personality—as well as other features of personal experience, such as moods—in terms of patterns rather than central tendency. A perspective emphasizing patterns as the unit of analysis for personality has been forwarded, for example, by Mischel and Shoda (1995; Shoda, Mischel, & Wright, 1994). This model holds that stability resides in the internal mechanisms producing behavior, not in the behavior itself, and that these mechanisms produce reliable and personally distinctive patterns of behavior across psychological contexts. In yet other research programs, trait-relevant behavior and moods have been characterized in terms of periodicity and other aspects of temporal variation (e.g., Brown & Moskowitz, 1998; Larsen, 1987; Penner et al., 1994). With the benefit of dynamical methods and tools, it may be possible to uncover temporal patterns in internally generated aspects of experience that are difficult to discern by traditional means.

A recurring temporal pattern, even one involving large variability in behavior, does not necessarily reflect the operation of an external cause. A person who oscillates on some time scale between love and hate toward someone, for instance, may do so without learning anything new about the target. In like manner, a person who alternates between talkativeness and silence may do so without consideration of the situational appropriateness of either behavior. In both cases, the pattern may reflect the operation of mechanisms internal to the person. On the other hand, a change in a temporal pattern may indeed suggest the presence of an external causal agent. Thus, if a person switched from love–hate oscillations to a consistent sentiment, or if a person's alternation between talkativeness and silence gave way to sustained periods of one behavior or the other, one might suspect the operation of some salient external factor (e.g., new information, social pressure) prompting the change. External factors that hold potential for qualitatively changing the intrinsic dynamics of a system are called *control parameters*. The identification of a system's control parameters is an important part of dynamical analyses and is discussed in greater detail in the section on complexity later in this chapter.

Pattern recognition is clearly central to an understanding of dynamical systems. A variety of analytical tools have been developed for identifying patterns in what might otherwise be interpreted as random temporal variation. Such tools, which include Fourier analysis, wavelets, coherent state analysis, and grammatical complexity, may prove especially valuable and necessary in social psychology, where the data are inherently noisy and subject to multiple random influences (Schroeck, 1994). Beginning in the 1990s, several research programs have provided evidence that these methods can in fact be applied to social psychological phenomena. Thus, insight has been generated into the often complex patterns characterizing individual and interpersonal action (e.g., Beek & Hopkins, 1992; Newtson, 1994; Schmidt, Beek, Treffner, & Turvey, 1991), social judgment (Vallacher et al., 1994), attitude change (Kaplowitz & Fink, 1992), decision making (Busemeyer & Townsend, 1993; Kaplowitz & Fink, 1992; Richards, 1990), and choice behavior (Selz & Mandell, 1994).

NONLINEAR RELATIONS

A prerequisite for the emergence of complex properties in a dynamical system is nonlinearity in the relations among the system's elements or variables. Because a primary task of theory construction is providing simple explanations of the complexity of human experience, the concept of nonlinearity is highly relevant for understanding social psychological phenomena. In a nonlinear world, many phenomena may happen that are virtually impossible in a linear world. Models based on linear dynamics alone cannot adequately describe the turbulent flow of water, the pulsation of lasers, or the unpredictable nature of weather patterns. How could we have expected such an approach to capture the complexity and dynamism of human behavior?

Linear versus Nonlinear Relations

As noted in Chapter 1, nonlinear relations are simply relations in which changes in the value of one variable cannot be described as a linear function of changes in the values of the other variables. This general feature of intervariable relationships is well represented in social psychology (see, e.g., Vallacher & Nowak, 1997, and commentaries). Threshold phenomena provide a clear example of nonlinearity. A threshold relation is simply one in which changes in variable A do not have any effect on variable B until a critical value of A is achieved. This value in effect triggers variable B, and no further increments in the value of A affect the value of B. Decisions of a binary nature (yes vs. no, act vs. don't act, etc.) typify this type of nonlinearity. Thus, when there is a clear preponderance of evidence favoring a particular decision, the receipt of new arguments against the decision is likely to have little or no impact. When the arguments for and against the decision are relatively balanced, however, even seemingly minor influences can drastically influence the decision and resultant action. Such a scenario is exemplified in Latané and Nowak's (1994) consideration of attitude distributions. They suggest that whereas attitudes on personally unimportant issues tend to be normally distributed, attitudes on important issues tend instead to have a binary "either–or" nature. This reasoning suggests a threshold effect in attitude change for important issues. When the arguments clearly favor one position over another, the addition of contradictory arguments tends to have little impact until a point is reached that promotes a dramatic shift to the other position.

Nonlinearity also characterizes situations in which the effect of variable A on variable B depends on the current value of B. This is evident, for example, in power functions with exponents less than 1.0. When the value of B is low, B will react strongly to changes in A, but when the value of B is high, even large changes in A will have little effect on the value of B. In psychophysics, for instance, subjective experience is a power function of the objective intensity of a sensory stimulus (see Stevens, 1961). There is evidence for relationships of this form in social psychology as well. With respect to social influence, for example, it has been observed that when the level of influence is minimal, even the addition of one person arguing for a particular position tends to have a notable impact on the opinion of the influence target. When the level of influence is relatively high, however, the addition of someone arguing for a particular position has negligible impact on the influence target (see Latané, 1981). More generally, practically all relationships involving ceiling effects are nonlinear in nature. The form of such relationships is simple: Up to a certain value of B, increases in A promote changes in B; beyond that value, further increases in A have little or no effect.

Nonlinearity also includes relations that show reversals in sign (i.e., from positive to negative or vice versa) depending on the values of the variables. Perhaps the most familiar form of this relationship is the inverted-U function. The Yerkes–Dodson (1908) law, for example, holds that performance effectiveness increases with increases in arousal up to a point, beyond which further increases in arousal promote performance decrements. The simplest type of relationship that shows a reversal in sign is the quadratic function, $B = A^2$. When A is less than 0, increases in A produce decreases in B, but when A is greater than 0, increases in A produce increases in B. The form of the relation between A and B in this case is not monotonic but parabolic. Just such a relationship was forwarded by Atkinson (1957, 1964) in his formulation of achievement motivation. In this model, the value attached to a particular goal, V, increases with the difficulty of achieving the goal and thus can be expressed as inversely proportional to the probability of success, P. Since motivation to achieve a goal is expressed as the value of the goal (V) times the probability of success (P), the value of the motive to achieve scales as $P(1 - P)$, which is equivalent to $P - P^2$. This quadratic function takes the form of an inverted U and produces a maximal value of achievement motivation when $P = 0.5$. When the probability of success is either 0 or 1, the value of achievement motivation is at a minimum (i.e., equals 0).

As noted in Chapter 1, nonlinear relations often have a nonadditive nature, in that the relation between any two variables is dependent on the value of one or more other variables. This feature is captured by the notion of statistical interaction, which goes to the very heart of theory and research in social psychology. It is difficult, in fact, to find a relationship between two variables that is not dependent on the value of a third variable when one examines published research in social psychology. In principle, of course, interactions are not limited to two-way or even three-way interactions, but also can be extended to encompass all the variables relevant to the phenomenon under investigation. Although interactions imply that the system in question is nonlinear, the absence of interactions does not imply that the system is necessarily linear. Even when two variables are considered divorced from the other variables in the system, the relation between them may be nonlinear, as in the threshold and ceiling effects discussed above.

The Logistic Equation

Dynamical variables whose time evolution is governed by quadratic relations may produce very interesting dynamics. The *logistic equation* is a prime example, having been employed often to investigate the nature of deterministic chaos (see Feigenbaum, 1978; Schuster, 1984). The logistic equation involves repeated iteration of the quadratic function in which the values of B vary as a square of the values of A. Iteration, which is basic to all discrete dynamical systems, simply means that the output value at one step is used as the input value at the next step. The logistic equation is expressed as $X_{n+1} = CX_n(1 - X_n)$, where X_{n+1} is the value of a dynamical variable at one time, X_n is the value of the same variable at the preceding time, and C is a variable that influences changes in the system's state (i.e., a control parameter). As long as X is not 0 or 1, the value of X at one moment will result in a new value at the next moment. For starting values of X between 0 and 1, and values of C between 0 and 4, X will take different values in the interval between 0 and 1 as the equation is iterated. Depending on the value of the control parameter C, we may observe different patterns of temporal evolution (e.g., increases in X followed by decreases). The logistic equation captures diverse phenomena, including evolution to a stable attractor, periodic attractors, certain types of bifurcations, and chaos and unpredictability, all of which are described in subsequent sections. The key point is that a system described by this simple equation evolves through a sequence of values without any influence from outside. It is in this sense that the system displays intrinsic dynamics.

To illustrate the potential for intrinsic dynamics in the logistic equation, consider how attendance at a new restaurant might change on a week-to-week basis. For simplicity, assume that the restaurant provides good service and good food, so that with a certain probability each visitor is likely to advise his or her friends about the restaurant's desirability. This mechanism suggests a linear growth pattern, such that the number of visitors in a succeeding week, $X(t + 1)$, can be expressed as some constant, R, multiplied by the number of visitors in the current week, $X(t)$, so that $X(t +1) = RX(t)$. $X(t)$ is a dynamical variable, and the constant, R, can be interpreted as the rate of information transmission. To simplify calculations, we can express the number of visitors, $X(t)$, as a proportion of the maximal number of visitors the restaurant can accommodate in a given week. This means that $X(t)$ can vary between 0 and 1. It is reasonable to posit a second mechanism that works in the opposite direction to limit the growth in the number of visitors in succeeding weeks. In particular, with increased number of visitors at the restaurant each week, the wait for a table becomes longer and customers become less satisfied as a result. According to the second mechanism, the number of visitors at $t + 1$ is a linear function of the difference between the maximum and actual number of visitors, and thus is proportional to $1-X(t)$. When these two mechanisms are combined, the expression describing the attendance at $t + 1$ becomes $X(t + 1) = RX(t)[1 - X(t)]$. which has the form of the logistic equation.

Different patterns of growth and decay are possible for this general scenario. Which scenario is actually observed depends on the value of R, which plays the role of a control parameter (discussed in detail under "Complexity"). We can thus consider the patterns of growth and decay for different values of R in the restaurant example. The results of these calculations are presented in Figure 2.1 (a–d). Let's start with a small value of R, say, 0.5. Suppose that during the first week, attendance is relatively small, say, 20% of the restaurant's capacity, so that $X(1)$ equals 0.2. To determine the attendance during the second week, the first week's attendance, 0.2, is used as input in the equation. The resultant value, $X(2) = 0.08$, is then used as input into the equation to calculate attendance during the third week. The resultant value, $X(3) = 0.037$, is used as input to determine the fourth week's attendance, and so on, for predicting attendance in succeeding weeks. In this process of iteration, diminishing values of X quickly converge to values close to 0, so that the restaurant eventually goes bankrupt (Figure 2.1a). If the process is repeated with a relatively high starting value of X—say, $X(1) = 0.6$—the restaurant will experience the same fate, as values of X converge toward 0. In general, for low values of R (i.e., less than 1.0), X will converge toward 0 regardless of its starting value.

If, however, the value of R is greater than 1.0 but smaller than 2.95, the attendance will stabilize at some nonzero value for almost all starting values of X. If $R = 2.3$, for example, attendance will stabilize at approximately 0.57, which is slightly greater than half the restaurant's capacity (Figure 2.1b). There are some initial values of X, however, for which the fate of the restaurant will be different. If attendance during the first week is 0, for example, there is no one to spread the word about the restaurant's quality and attendance will remain 0 forever. For values of R between 2.95 and 3.56, meanwhile, the attendance will go through a repeating (i.e., periodic) sequence of values in successive weeks as the equation is iterated. When R equals 3.2, for example, attendance will alternate between two values, 0.51 and 0.80 (Figure 2.1c). Thus, after a week of low attendance in response to previously overcrowded conditions, the growth tendency dominates, which leads to high attendance and the return of overcrowded conditions and a subsequent drop in attendance. With increasing values of R within this range, attendance will go through a repeating sequence involving more than two values (i.e., 4, 8, 16, . . . , values).

Finally, consider the implications for the restaurant when the spread of information takes on yet higher values, within the range of $R = 3.56$ to 4.0. For most of these values, X will exhibit a very irregular and nonrepeating pattern of changes. It should be noted that for values of R within this range, very similar starting values of X will go through very different sequences of successive values, despite the fact that the overall pattern is of the same type for all starting values. This sensitivity to initial conditions is portrayed in Figure 2.1d, which presents the results of iteration for $R = 3.95$. In addition to the starting values of 0.6 and 0.2, we have included a starting value of 0.21. Note that the nearly identical starting values (0.2 and 0.21) initially display the same (roughly periodic) evolution but begin to diverge noticeably after the 6th week. From then on, the similarity in their respective patterns is no greater than the similarity between each of these patterns and the pattern associated with a very different starting value (0.6).

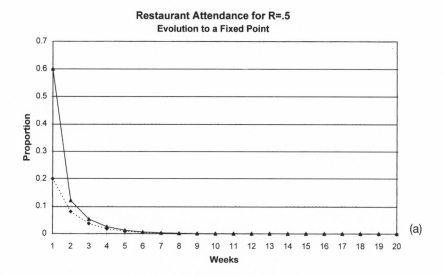

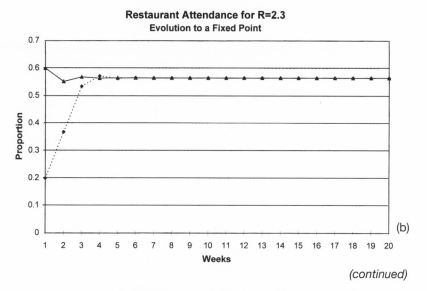

FIGURE 2.1. The logistic equation.

(continued)

In summary, the long-term pattern of behavior of the dynamical variable, $X(t)$, may exhibit qualitatively different fates depending on the value of the control parameter, R, and relatively independently of the initial value of $X(t)$. The asymptotic values of the dynamics are called *attractors*, because they attract the long-term dynamics of the

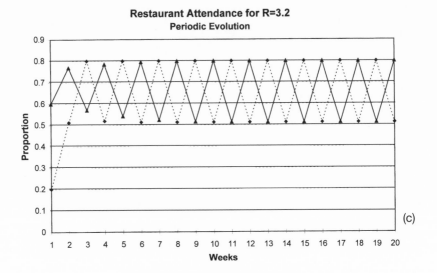

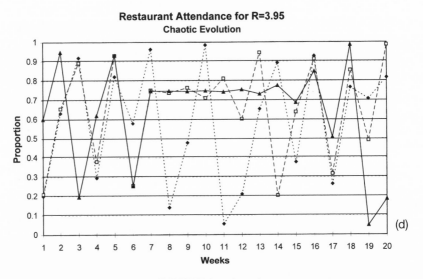

FIGURE 2.1. *(cont.)*

system. When $X(t)$ converges to 0 (or some other stable value), the dynamics are referred to as evolution toward a *fixed-point attractor*. When $X(t)$ repeatedly cycles through the same sequence of values (e.g., 2, 4, or 16 different values), the dynamics are referred to as evolution on a *periodic attractor*. Finally, when $X(t)$ displays irregularly and seemingly random evolution, the dynamics are referred to as evolution on a *chaotic attractor*. In each of these cases, although the dynamics ultimately converge on an attractor, there is an initial period called the *transient regime*, during which initial values of the dynamical variable dictate the system's trajectory. The concept of attractor is clearly central to dynamical systems and thus holds potential for the development of dynamical social psychology. In a subsequent section of this chapter ("Stability and Change"), we discuss this concept in greater detail and suggest some ways in which it can be used to understand the dynamics of personal and interpersonal experience.

The logistic equation can have diverse interpretations, both in different areas of science and within social psychology (see, e.g., van Geert, 1991). This is because the evolution of a system described by the logistic equation does not depend on the specificity of the system, or the identity of system elements, but rather on the form of the relations among variables describing the system. Any system that can be described in terms of the logistic equation, then, is capable of displaying sustained intrinsic dynamics for some range of values of the control parameter. A system in which the same factor has two opposite ways of influencing its future state may under certain circumstances display sustained and complex intrinsic dynamics.

Coupled Logistic Equations

An especially promising application of the logistic equation for social psychology is the modeling of coordination among people and groups. The fact that logistic equations are capable of displaying qualitatively different types of intrinsic dynamics makes them ideal for modeling an individual's thoughts, feelings, and behaviors. When such equations are coupled, then, they provide very simple, yet very rich formalisms for studying the emergence of coordination among people. The coupling between equations is introduced by making the value of the dynamical variable, X, in each equation partially dependent on the previous value of the dynamical variable in the other equation (in addition, of course, to being dependent on its own prior value).

Different types of collective phenomena may be observed within this framework (e.g., Kaneko, 1989). The exact nature of such phenomena depends on how strongly the two equations are coupled, the magnitude of the difference between their respective intrinsic dynamics, and in some circumstances, the starting values of the dynamical variables. By setting these variables in different combinations, one can produce qualitatively different forms of coordination of the dynamical variables in the respective equations. For some combinations of these variables, the two equations will evolve in synchrony, traversing complex trajectories together. For other combinations of these variables, however, the dynamical variables of the two equations will be negatively correlated in their respective behavior as they evolve over time. Under yet other conditions, the coupling will provide for stability of otherwise chaotic dynamics within the respective systems described by the equations. This latter possibility portrays a means by which highly complex individuals who might otherwise follow erratic and irregular trajectories in their thoughts and actions may achieve relative stability by forming social relationships—even with other potentially erratic individuals.

We should note that the coupling of logistic equations has only recently been introduced to physics (e.g., Kaneko, 1984, 1993) and to our knowledge has not yet been adapted to the subject matter of social psychology. In Chapter 6, we present an initial attempt in this regard. Specifically, we use the framework of coupled logistic equations to conceptualize coordination in close relationships. Multiple coupled equations (Zochowski & Liebovitch, 1997), meanwhile, may provide a generative framework for investigating coordination issues within the context of group dynamics. Indeed, in view of the formal simplicity and theoretical richness of this framework, it is likely that it will become one of the primary tools of choice for investigating social coordination at different levels of social reality.

Hysteresis

Hysteresis is a feature that is common to otherwise distinct manifestations of nonlinearity (e.g., Hock et al., 1993). This phenomenon refers to the fact that variable B may be in two different states for a single value of variable A. Which value of B is observed for a given value of A depends on the history of changes in B. If B has a history of low values, A must take on relatively high values to cause increased values of B, whereas if B has a history of high values, A must take on relatively low values to cause decreased values of B (see Figure 2.2). The range of values of A for which B can be in two different states is referred to as the hysteresis region.

As Figure 2.2 illustrates, changes in B are marked by both continuity and discontinuity. With increases in A, there is a linear change in B until some critical value of A is reached, at which point B jumps abruptly to a new value. After that, further increases in A are associated with further linear changes in B. This same mix of continuity and abrupt change occurs when the value of A is gradually reduced from a high value, except that a different value of A is involved. Before a de-

B

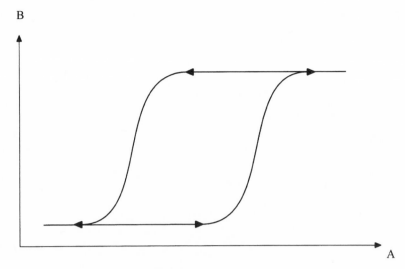

FIGURE 2.2. Hysteresis.

crease in A can promote an abrupt decrease in B, it must pass the value of A that promoted the qualitative increase in B when A started at low values. The hysteresis region corresponds to the difference in values of A associated with the abrupt changes in B observed in these two directions. As discussed later, the phenomenon of hysteresis is critical to research designed to probe the relative stability of a dynamical system. In general, the more stable a system, the greater the hysteresis it displays.

Hysteresis may prove to be a common feature of social psychological systems. Primacy effects illustrate the potential for momentum in social judgments, for instance, and have been observed in impression formation (e.g., Asch, 1946; Hamilton & Zanna, 1972; Hodges, 1974; Luchins, 1957), assessments of ability (e.g., Jones, Rock, Shaver, Goethals, & Ward, 1968), and persuasion (e.g., Miller & Campbell, 1959). Commitment theory (Kiesler, 1971) is also compatible with hysteresis. When people commit themselves to a decision or course of action, they tend to maintain this position in the face of increasing social pressure to change. To discern whether these (and other) instances meet the criteria of hysteresis, one would have to show that at some point the person's judgment or decision shows a qualitative change to a very different judgment or decision. In the case of commitment, for instance, increasing social pressure might eventually undermine commitment, with the person displaying a sudden jump to a position in line with the pressure. Changes in the opposite direction would have to follow the same pattern, but with change occurring at a different value of the information or pressure than that associated with qualitative change in the original direction. From the symmetry in psychological momentum, one could compute the region of hysteresis and gain insight into the dynamical properties of the system under consideration. Just such an approach has in fact been advocated in recent years. To date, manifestations of hysteresis have been observed in social psychology with respect to social perception (Hanges, Braverman, & Rentsch, 1991), attitude change (Latané & Nowak, 1994), and commitment in close relationships (Tesser & Achee, 1994).

COMPLEXITY

The goal of science is to find the simplest possible explanations for phenomena. As noted at the outset, however, the remarkable complexity of human thought, behavior, and relationships makes this a difficult goal to achieve in scientific social psychology. We also noted, though, that the success of dynamical systems theory in the natural sciences is due in large part to its ability to provide simple explanations for complex phenomena that had previously resisted theoretical understanding. Indeed, the major accomplishment of the nonlinear dynamical systems approach is the discovery of how complexity can arise from simplicity. In this section, we discuss important features of complexity, both within the system and with respect to the myriad external influences relevant to a system's behavior, and the various ways in which complexity mirrors simplicity. We first consider the concept of control parameter, which greatly simplifies the task of specifying the multiple and varied influences on a system. We then discuss the concept of order parameter, which has proven essential to understanding how complexity within a system can be simplified. Attention is then given to the means by which system-level properties emerge in complex systems through the self-organization of elements connected by nonlinear relations.

Control Parameters

As indicated earlier, the external variables influencing the behavior of a dynamical system are called control parameters. Some control parameters are more important than others. A wide range of variables produce quantitative effects on the system's behavior, but usually only a relatively small subset of them promote noteworthy qualitative changes. For example, a system might tend toward stability for some values of a control parameter, but begin to display a breakdown in stability above a certain value of the same variable. Describing the effect of such a variable is clearly more enlightening about the system than is describing the effect of variables that produce only quantitative effects. The identification of important control parameters thus provides a means by which complex social psychological phenomena may be described in relatively simple ways. Focusing only on the subset of factors representing critical control parameters, in other words, may prove sufficient for making qualitative predictions of behavior. Of course, it may be necessary to account for the influences of less crucial control parameters if more precise quantitative predictions are desired.

The identification of a system's most important control parameters is a crucial step in understanding a phenomenon. This task often requires two steps. The first is isolation of variables that influence the system. Social psychology has been quite successful in this regard, having identified a large number of independent variables in different domains. The second step is distinguishing those factors that influence the system in a quantitative way from those that cause qualitative changes. Social psychology has not been particularly successful at this task, and current research strategies are not very promising about future progress in this regard. Thus, although the tradition of reporting significance levels is well suited to identifying causal factors, it does not allow one to distinguish critical control parameters from the background of multiple external influences. Social psychology, moreover, lacks qualitative descriptions of the possible classes of behavior (e.g., the type of temporal patterns characterizing different types of phenomena). It is difficult, therefore, to tell which external factors merely affect behavior quantitatively and which factors instead change the class of behavior (e.g., change the system from one type of pattern to another).

Consider, for example, the distinct ways in which attitudes can be distributed in a social group. Research and analytical considerations have revealed four such distributions: complete unification, where everyone eventually adopts the same position; stable clusters, where localized islands of minority sentiment exist; fluctuating clusters, where the islands of minority sentiment change position in the larger group; and chaos, where the distribution remains highly irregular (Latané & Nowak, 1997; Lewenstein, Nowak, & Latané, 1993; Nowak & Lewenstein, 1996; Nowak, Lewenstein, & Szamrej, 1993). Some external influences have been shown to change the degree of each of these tendencies (e.g., the rate at which unification is achieved, the amount of fluctuation in minority islands). Other influences, however, have been shown to change the type of distribution itself. In particular, four such factors have been identified: nonlinearity of attitude change, the magnitude of individual differences, the geometry of the social space, and the degree of randomness in attitude change rules. Each of these factors thus represents an important control parameter for the system. In Chapter 7, we describe this line of research and discuss how these control parameters influence the distribution of attitudes in groups.

Order Parameters

Because social psychological phenomena are complex, it is unlikely that we will ever be able to incorporate all the variables operating on all levels of social reality into a single theoretical model. A complete description of even a simple social interaction can be understood with recourse to myriad situational, dispositional, and historical factors that may interact in nonlinear fashion, and the nature of such interactions may themselves change with successive iterations of the process (Vallacher & Nowak, 1994b). Social psychology, then, is faced with the challenge of how to choose among relevant variables when constructing dynamical models.

This problem is faced in the physical sciences as well. A full description of a system composed of many simple interacting elements may require enormous amounts of information. Even if we know that the system's evolution is governed by the interactions among its elements, the number of such elements and their interactions render the task of describing such evolution practically impossible. Consider, for example, a bottle filled with gas. The dynamics in this case reflect individual gas molecules bouncing off each other and off the walls of the bottle. A full description of the system would require one to specify values of six variables (position and velocity in three dimensions) for each molecule. The number of molecules in a 1-liter bottle of gas is on the order of Avogadro's number, 10^{23}. As unimaginably large as this number is, it does not begin to do justice to the number of possible interactions among these molecules. Not surprisingly, the dynamics associated with the basic properties of such a system are difficult to describe with general laws and may appear to be random for all practical purposes.

In dynamical systems, however, regularities and patterns are usually exhibited at a global level and may be described in terms of macroscopic as opposed to microscopic variables. Variables that serve this function are commonly referred to as *order parameters*. Order parameters do not describe individual elements, but rather properties of the system as a whole. In classic statistical physics and thermodynamics (Landau & Lifshitz, 1964), order parameters refer to global emergent properties of a system stemming from the interaction of system elements. The values of these emergent properties distinguish between qualitatively different states of the system (e.g., gas vs. liquid). In the approach of nonlinear dynamical systems (e.g., Haken, 1978), the notion of order parameter has been generalized to capture collective variables that provide characterization of the system's evolution on a macroscopic scale. In this sense, order parameters are dynamical variables, so that regularities in the system's temporal evolution can be expressed as changes in the value of order parameters over time. Such evolution can be described in the form of difference or differential equations or as trajectories in phase space. Characterizing a system in terms of order parameters eliminates or reduces most of the idiosyncracies associated with individual variables, putting one in a much better position to formulate general laws concerning a system's dynamics. In fact, identifying appropriate order parameters of a system is a major step in the construction of a successful theory.

In this regard, it is important to note that not all global properties of a system are order parameters. Only those properties that reflect the critical aspects of a system's macroscopic states and dynamic patterns constitute the system's order parameters. In the case of gas in a bottle, for example, a relevant order parameter is the density of the substance. By tracking variation in density, one can observe qualitative changes in the macroscopic state of the substance, such as the transition from gas to liquid. Although the color and odor of the gas, as well as the sheer number of particles, are also global properties, they do not uniquely characterize the system's macroscopic states and dynamic patterns. Finding appropriate order parameters can prove quite difficult to accomplish (Beek, Verschoor, & Kelso, 1997; Landau & Lifshitz, 1964). In systems defined in the form of differential or difference equations, it may be possible to derive appropriate order parameters through analytical methods. Although this is feasible in mathematics and physics, it is rarely useful when dealing with biological and social systems (see, however, Lewenstein et al., 1993). In these disciplines, the description of individual elements and their dynamics is often insufficiently precise for analytical solutions to be useful. Indeed, the identity of individual elements may not even be known. This represents a particularly salient issue in social psychology, where the focus is on elements that are often elusive and difficult to specify with a high degree of certainty (e.g., thoughts and feelings).

When analytical solutions are inappropriate, one may be able to discover order parameters by examining the system's behavior (e.g., Beek et al., 1997). The key property of order parameters in this regard is that they distinguish between qualitatively different system states and types of dynamics. A macroscopic variable can thus be considered an order parameter if it demonstrates a rapid change from one qualitative state or dynamic pattern to another in the presence of a smooth and gradual change in the value of a variable controlling the system's behavior (i.e., a control parameter). To find order parameters within this approach, one needs to identify the possible qualitatively different types of states or dynamics for the system and to concentrate on the transitions between these states or dynamic patterns. Those variables that exhibit rapid change whenever the system's changes its macroscopic state but remain relatively stable within each state are the likely order parameters for the system.[2]

Order parameters may be specific for a given system. Thus, each class of phenomena in social psychology can be understood in terms of its own particular order parameters. In the mental system, for example, evaluation represents a likely order parameter for individual thoughts and feelings (Chapter 3), whereas polarization is a likely order parameter for the dynamics of attitudes in social groups (Chapter 7). Some variables, however, are likely to play the role of order parameters across different levels of social reality. A plausible candidate in this regard is a system's coherence. Coherence is manifest in different ways, of course, depending on the phenomenon in question. In mental systems, coherence can be described as the evaluative congruence of relevant cognitive elements (see Chapter 3). In action systems, coherence can be viewed in terms of the match between mental representations and task demands (see Chapter 4). In the self-system, coherence refers to compatibility among different subsets of self-understanding (see Chapter 5). In close relationships, coherence takes the form of coordination of each person's thoughts, feelings, and actions (see Chapter 6). In groups, coherence takes the form of spatial clustering of like-minded individuals (see Chapters 7 and 8). In each case, the order parameter characterizes the degree of order and organization in the system. We hasten to add that although coherence seems to be an order parameter at different levels of social reality, complex systems are commonly characterized by more than one order parameter. In social psychology, then, it is likely that more than one order parameter will prove necessary to provide full description of a system's macroscopic properties.

Order parameters are somewhat analogous to dependent variables in social psychological research, in that both enable description at some level of globality. In studying social interaction, for example, the investigator is unlikely to track, let alone attempt to predict, every individual utterance or gesture. Instead, the focus is on some global variable (e.g., consensus in attitudes, the degree of cooperation or competition, mutual liking) that captures the overall state of the interaction. In like manner, the study of human action typically focuses on goals and other higher order structures rather than the multitude of specific movements (e.g., Carver & Scheier, in press; Gollwitzer, 1990; von Cranach & Harré, 1982), social cognition research is usually concerned with global variables such as evaluation, certainty, and integration, rather than with individual thoughts (cf. Eiser, 1990; Fiske & Taylor, 1991; Vallacher & Nowak, 1994c; Wegner & Vallacher, 1977; Zebrowitz, 1990), and research on close relationships focus on such things as trust, affection, and commitment rather than the content of every specific exchange (e.g., Baron et al., 1994; Brehm, 1992; Clark & Mills, 1979; Duck, 1988; Levinger, 1980).

Apart from their common globality, however, order parameters and dependent variables differ in important respects. Whereas dependent variables may be chosen at will for a variety of reasons (practical implications, personal preferences, etc.), order parameters are uniquely capable of providing quantitative characterization of qualitatively different states of the system under investigation. It is also the case that many global properties of a system are not essential for the system's dynamics, so that knowledge of their values does not allow one to predict future states of the system. Because order parameters are dynamical variables, however, they not only describe the response of a system, but they also determine the state of the system in succeeding moments in time, even in the absence of other sources of influence (i.e., independent variables).

Finding appropriate order parameters involves identifying the most important features of a system's state or dynamics. Like other aspects of theory construction, this process is based on theoretical considerations and often requires insight into the phenomenon under investigation. In introducing the concept of order parameter, for example, Haken (1978) describes thoughts as order parameters of the brain. Such a conclusion clearly follows from theoretical considerations and intuitions about the crucial properties of the human brain, not from an analysis of instabilities in brain function. It is also the case that whenever one can write a formal model of the phenomenon, order parameters can be determined by analyzing the dynamics of the equation without having to rely directly on empirical methods (Haken, 1978). With respect to the cognitive system, for example, this suggests that one may disregard the rapid turnover in individual thoughts when describing the global properties of the mind, and focus instead on global evaluation as a likely order parameter for the system (Vallacher & Nowak, 1994c).

Order parameters may have a recursive structure, in that the parameters at one level of description may become dynamical variables at a higher level of analysis. Extending Haken's example, thoughts may be order parameters for brain states, evaluation may be an order parameter for thoughts, and mode of integration may be an order parameter for evaluation (Vallacher & Nowak, 1997). Yet higher level order parameters can be defined if one broadens the scope to consider the coordination of evaluation among interacting individuals. Thus, the degree of clustering of attitudes in a group may be considered an order parameter for group-level evaluations (Nowak et al., 1990). The idea that order parameters can be arrayed in a functional hierarchy is reminiscent of models in social psychology that attempt to depict the structure of various phenomena, such as self-regulation (Carver & Scheier, 1998; Powers, 1973), action identification (Vallacher & Wegner, 1987), and social cognition (Fiske & Taylor, 1991).

This provides another instance in which social psychology has shown appreciation for the complexity of phenomena without the help of nonlinear dynamical systems. Hierarchical models in psychology, however, often have a somewhat arbitrary feel to them (e.g., the number of levels specified, the label attached to each level) and are correspondingly difficult to validate. With the insights and tools provided by such models as synergetics (Haken, 1978), it may be possible to develop functional hierarchies for individual- and group-level phenomena with greater certainty and precision. The ordering of levels, for example, may be derived from the time scales found to be associated with the various elements in the system under investigation as well as from the nature of the interdependencies among the elements (Vallacher et al., 1998).

Emergence and Self-Organization

From its beginning, social psychology has been concerned with the means by which the individual elements of a phenomenon (e.g., thoughts, behaviors, individual actors) are assembled into orderly and complex structures capable of performing complex functions (judgment, meaningful action, group processes). Although there are notable exceptions, social psychological theory has tended to address this question by assuming that some higher level agent is necessary to impose structure and order on lower level elements. With respect to group dynamics, for example, it is commonly assumed that leadership and social norms are necessary to impose order on the interactions among individuals comprising a given group. In a similar manner, intergroup relations are commonly assumed to achieve coherence by virtue of cultural values, customs, and laws backed by formal authority. The notion that higher level processes are necessary to coordinate the interaction of lower level elements can be problematic and has not gone unchallenged. With respect to the human mind, for example, this assumption leads to the philosophically untenable notion of the homunculus—the mind-within-the-mind that itself cannot be explained without invoking an infinite regress (cf. James, 1890; Ryle, 1949).

The principle of self-organization provides a very different picture of the relation between lower level elements and higher order structure. The basic idea is that the interaction among low level elements, where each element adjusts to other elements, may lead to the emergence of highly coherent structures and behavior that provide coordination for the lower level elements (Haken, 1978; Kelso, 1984, 1995). No higher order agent is necessary for the emergence of such coordinative structures (Haken, 1982). Rather than being imposed on the system from above or from outside the system altogether, the higher order structures emerge from the internal workings of the system itself. In this process, the system loses degrees of freedom, and the state of the system may be described by a small number of variables. Ironically, then, complex systems can sometimes be described by fewer variables than can relatively simple systems.

To illustrate how systems lose degrees of freedom due to the interaction among elements, consider the task of characterizing the preferences of n individuals for a weekend's activities. If they are strangers, each individual must make an independent decision, and the system can be characterized with respect to n variables, where each variable describes the preference of a single individual. If, however, the individuals constitute a circle of friends who not only influence one another's preferences, but also prefer to engage in joint activities, their decisions are not independent of one another. In the extreme case, they all may decide to engage in the same weekend activities, so that their behavior may be described in terms of a single variable. If the influences among the individuals are somewhat weaker, and different subsets of them decide on different activities, one variable for each subset would be necessary to achieve full description of the system. Thus, with increasing influence among individuals, there is a reduction in the degrees of freedom in the group as a whole, so that the group can be described by a small number of collective variables. The coordination of preferences among individuals may also lead to the emergence of group norms (e.g., Festinger, Schachter, & Back, 1950), providing for additional coordination in the group by influencing each member's future choices.

Many phenomena studied as dynamical systems have been shown to have emergent properties. Emergence has been demonstrated in fields as diverse as hydrodynamics (Ruelle & Takens, 1971), meteorology (Lorenz, 1963), laser physics (Haken, 1982), and biology (Amit, 1989; Basar, 1990; Glass & Mackey, 1988; Othmer, 1986). Emergence is especially evident in systems consisting of elements that interact in a nonlinear fashion. Even if the elements are relatively simple, nonlinearity in their interactions may lead to highly complex dynamic behavior, such as self-organization and pattern formation (see Haken, 1978; Kelso, 1995). The emergence of both order and chaos, for example, has been documented in neural networks (Amit, 1989) and cellular automata (Wolfram, 1986), where the elements are essentially binary.

This notion has clear implications for long-standing issues concerning the achievement of mental, behavioral, social, and societal structure. The nature of emergence is illustrated, for example, in the personal understanding of action, as depicted in action identification theory (Vallacher & Wegner, 1985, 1987). This theory holds that any action can be identified in many different ways and that these act identities can be scaled hierarchically, from lower level identities describing the more molecular and mechanical features of the action, to higher level identities describing the more comprehensive aspects of the action (e.g., its effects and self-evaluative implications). When an action can be identified in both relatively low- and high-level terms, people tend to show a marked preference for the higher level identity because of the more comprehensive understanding it provides—a notion that is somewhat reminiscent of pattern generation in Gestalt psychology (cf. Köhler, 1947). This tendency to embrace comprehensive high level identities when one is in a lower-level state is referred to as the emergence process. Empirical support for action emergence has been obtained in a variety of personal and interpersonal domains (cf. Vallacher, 1993). In the context of self-understanding, for example, there is evidence that people who are induced to think about the details of their behavior in a recent social interaction tend to accept subsequent feedback regarding their trait-like qualities in social settings (Wegner, Vallacher, Kiersted, & Dizadji, 1986).

We should note that emergence can, and often does, occur in the absence of external cues or influences. This point was made many years ago by Durkheim (1938), who noted the emergence of new properties at the level of groups and social systems as a result of the coordination of individual actions and desires. In the context of collective behavior such as crowd interactions, Turner and Killian (1957) discussed the emergence of group norms from the spontaneous coordination of individual impulses and actions. More recently, computer simulations and empirical research on social influence and interdependence (e.g., Nowak et al., 1990), described in Chapters 7 and 8, have revealed the emergence of group-level properties from simple social interactions. The spontaneous self-organization of basic elements into higher order structures within the individual, meanwhile, has been revealed in experimental work on social judgment (e.g., Vallacher et al., 1994), described in Chapter 3, and action identification (Vallacher et al., 1998), described in Chapter 4.

STABILITY AND CHANGE

Stability in social psychology is commonly assumed to mean the achievement of an equilibrium state, with forces operating to prevent changes in the state. Thus, judgments, feelings, and behavioral tendencies are said to be stable if they do not show noteworthy change on their own and tend to resist forces toward change. From the perspective of nonlinear dynamical systems theory, this view of stability is very limited and has the effect of confusing sustained dynamics with instability. A system may show constant evolution, but as long as these changes conform to a reliable pattern, the system may be considered every bit as stable as a system that has settled on a single value. This broadened conception of change and stability has considerable relevance for the understanding of phenomena in social psychology. In this section, then, we discuss how change and stability are conceptualized and measured in dynamical systems and illustrate how these ideas relate to topics and issues in social psychology.

Phase Space and Trajectories

As noted in Chapter 1, once the dynamical variables of a dynamical system have been identified, it is common to treat these variables as coordinates in an n-dimensional phase space. If the behavior of a system can be described with respect to two order parameters, for example, the phase space for the system would be two-dimensional, with each dimension representing possible values of one of the order parameters. Each point in the phase space, representing the intersection of the values of the dynamical variables defining each dimension, uniquely describes the state of the system. Temporal changes of the system, then, correspond to the motion of this point over time. This motion draws a curve in the phase space. This trajectory describes the set of points "visited" sequentially by the system during its temporal evolution.

For social psychology, a less demanding concept—*state space*—may prove to be more appropriate. State space is generally equivalent to phase space, in that its coordinates correspond to dynamical variables and each point describes a state of the system. But unlike phase space, there is no requirement that the description of the state of the system be complete. Some dynamical variables may not be represented, and different trajectories can have common points. This means that knowledge of the system at a given time does not allow for unique prediction of its successive states. Because a state space contains all the possible states a system can adopt, the evolution of the system may be described in terms of a rule specifying the succession of states. This rule may be deterministic in nature, with a well-defined order of transitions, or stochastic, such that the transitions between states are probabilistic.

To illustrate how the notion of state space may be applied to social psychology, consider Miller's (1944) depiction of approach–avoid conflict. Miller demonstrated that an object or location with both rewarding and aversive qualities elicits incompatible response tendencies reflecting approach and avoidance, respectively. Both the tendencies to approach and to avoid grow with increasing proximity to the mixed valence stimulus, but the avoid tendency grows more rapidly than does the approach tendency. So although the approach tendency may be stronger than the avoid tendency when the stimulus is relatively distant, the avoid tendency becomes dominant when this distance is reduced beyond a certain point. According to Miller, an individual faced with an approach–avoid conflict should oscillate around the equilibrium specified by the point at which the approach and avoid tendencies are equal in strength.

Imagine, for example, a person on a diet and his or her movement vis-à-vis the refrigerator. There are two conflicting tendencies at work: a desire to reward oneself with food, which motivates approach toward the refrigerator, and a desire to maintain the diet, which motivates avoidance of the refrigerator. In a room other than the kitchen, images of last night's pizza are highly salient and powerfully attractive. A strong approach tendency causes the person to start moving with increasing vigor toward the refrigerator. As the refrigerator comes into view, however, thoughts centering on poor self-control, weight gain, and the like come to dominate the person's mental state. A growing avoid tendency causes the speed of approach to slow considerably, and within arm's reach of the refrigerator handle, the person begins to re-verse the direction of his or her movement. After reaching a safe dis-tance from the source of temptation, the aversive images vanish rapid-ly and are gradually replaced by the irresistibly positive images, pro-ducing yet another change in direction. Let's suppose such oscillations are sustained for some time. The critical variables in constructing a state space are distance from the refrigerator, D, and the velocity of approach, V, which is positive when approaching and negative when avoiding the refrigerator. These variables provide the coordinates in Figure 2.3.

The idealized trajectory depicted in Figure 2.3 forms a circle. The force changing the movement is dictated by the difference between approach and avoid tendencies. Whenever the approach tendency is dominant, it will serve to accelerate movement toward the stimulus and to decelerate movement away from the stimulus. Whenever the avoid tendency is dominant, movement toward the stimulus slows down, and movement away from the stimulus increases. When the two tendencies are equal, there is no change in movement. At the maximal distance from the refrigerator, the velocity is 0 and increases gradually as the person approaches it. Just past the equilibrium dis-

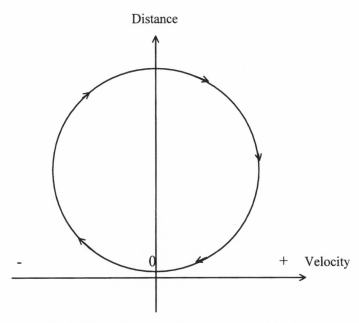

FIGURE 2.3. State space for approach–avoid conflict.

tance, the approach velocity decreases and reaches 0 before the refrigerator is contacted. The velocity then takes on an increasing value, but in the opposite direction, corresponding to a negative value in the figure. The escape from the refrigerator slows down at the equilibrium point and, finally, the person stops at a point beyond the equilibrium, only to reverse direction again and start the approach sequence. It is this oscillatory quality of approach and avoidance that is represented by the repeated traversing of the circle in Figure 2.3.

To construct a state space, it is necessary to choose the appropriate dynamical variables for describing the system's dynamics. Although a theory will sometimes specify these variables, a state space may also be reconstructed in an empirical manner. If the observed variables of the system are in fact dynamical variables, and the system undergoes nonrandom evolution, then empirically derived trajectories will be well formed and form a clear pattern. If, however, the observed variables are irrelevant to the determination of the system's evolution, the resultant trajectories will form a shapeless blob. One can, therefore, try to plot different sets of variables, looking for the emergence of a clear pattern. It is also possible to reconstruct the state space on the basis of a series of measurements of a single variable. This requires the use of more sophisticated methods, however, such as those developed by Takens (1981), Grassberger and Procaccia (1983), and Kaplan and Glass (1992). Nowak and Lewenstein (1994) provide a detailed description of these and other dynamical tools and methods.

Attractors

The trajectory of a dynamical system can visit points corresponding to many combinations of coordinates early in its evolution. After a period of time referred to as the transient regime, however, the trajectory of a *dissipative* system comes to occupy less volume of the phase space, visiting only a subset of points during its subsequent evolution. This subset of points is referred to as the system's *attractor*. In effect, the attractor "attracts" all the trajectories in a phase space, in that the trajectories eventually converge on the attractor, regardless of the system's initial conditions (i.e., its starting point). It is common to distinguish among four classes of attractors (Eckmann & Ruelle, 1985; Schuster, 1984): fixed-point, periodic, quasiperiodic, and chaotic.

A *fixed-point attractor* describes a system in which all trajectories tend to a single point in phase space, regardless of the system's initial conditions. This means that the set of all dynamical variables converges on some set of time-independent constant values corresponding to an equilibrium point for the system. Fixed-point attractors may prove useful in describing thoughts and behaviors that tend to a particular set of values over time. Such directionality despite differences in initial conditions and the influence of external factors is reminiscent of teleological explanations, which seem to suggest a reversal of customary cause–effect relations. This notion seems particularly well suited, for example, to capture the widely recognized phenomenon of goal-directed behavior. If we know that a person is pursuing a goal, it may be more feasible to predict the final outcome of a behavioral sequence than to predict the features of the sequence itself. Because of the teleological nature of the action, in fact, changing the sequence may have no effect on the final outcome.

A system's phase space may have more than one fixed-point attractor, each corresponding to an equilibrium for the system. The particular attractor that is reached depends on the initial conditions (the values of the system's variables). The task in such situations is to describe all the initial conditions leading to each of the system's stable points. The initial conditions leading to an attractor represent the *basin of attraction* for that attractor. If a system has multiple attractors, a strong influence on the system can throw the system into the basin of attraction of a different attractor, resulting in movement toward an entirely different equilibrium state. With respect to goal-directed behavior, this reasoning provides the basis for predicting when a given goal will be maintained in the face of obstacles and when it, instead, will be relinquished in favor of a different goal—perhaps one that is diametrically opposed to the original goal.

There are two general methods for establishing the existence of fixed-point attractors. The first involves observing changes in the distribution of the system's variables over time. In particular, diminishing change in the system's behavior over time (in the absence of external constraint) is a strong indication that the system is approaching a fixed-point attractor. Such a scenario is commonly observed when people contemplate a course of action (e.g., Gollwitzer, 1996; Vallacher & Kaufman, 1996) or when they judge someone with a preponderance of either good or bad qualities (Vallacher et al., 1994). In both cases, there is a period of vacillation among different (often conflicting) perspectives, followed by convergence on a stable value (e.g., an action plan or a global evaluation). In the second method, one actively perturbs the system and observes the resultant behavior. If a single, fixed-point attractor exists, the system will always return to the same state after some time, regardless of how strongly it was influenced. In the case of multiple fixed points, small perturbations will result in the system returning to its original state, but strong influences will result in the system moving toward a different equilibrium. The strength of a given fixed point, in fact, can be characterized by the magnitude of the influence required to move the system out of the basin of attraction for that point. If a given equilibrium is relatively unstable, even very small influences can have dramatic effects on the system's behavior.

This method seems particularly well suited for assessing the stability of psychological states, such as opinions, self-concepts, and relationships. An individual may express a flattering self-appraisal, for example, but if he or she experiences self-doubt when confronted with discrepant social feedback, one may conclude that his or her positive evaluation reflects a relatively unstable equilibrium. It can be noted in this regard that the certainty of people's beliefs, particularly beliefs about the self, has been accorded theoretical significance in recent years (e.g., Baumgardner, 1990; Campbell, 1990; Kernis, 1993; Swann & Ely, 1984; Vallacher, 1980). In view of the importance of stability in dynamical models, it may prove fruitful to explore this dimension with respect to a host of other social psychological phenomena, including close relationships, attitudes, and group morale.

The behavior of a system may repeat a particular sequence of values rather than converge on a single value. For such *periodic attractors*, each state of the system repeats after some time *t*, representing the period of motion. A single phase space can contain periodic attractors with different periods of motion. Which period the system is likely to display will depend on the system's initial conditions. As noted in Chapter 1, periodicity may be a fairly ubiquitous feature of social psychological phenomena, reflecting cyclic variation in people's thoughts, feelings, and actions. The temporal evolution of a system may also be governed by the superimposition of different periods (e.g., weekly and seasonal rhythms in addition to daily rhythms). This form of periodicity is referred to as *multiperiodic* evolution. The most complex case of multiperiodic evolution is *quasiperiodic evolution*, in which each of the system's variables exhibits different periods, and these periods are incommensurable (i.e., they are not multiples of a single basic period). In such instances, the values of all the variables repeat with some period, but the system as a whole never returns to exactly the same value. Fourier analysis is a mathematical technique designed to identify different periods and their relative importance in a system's behavior (see Schroeck, 1994). Newtson (1994), for instance, has used this approach to expose periods in seemingly aperiodic human movement.

Before the development of nonlinear dynamical systems theory, it was believed that all dissipative systems had to converge on either a fixed point, periodic, or quasiperiodic attractor. The excitement in science associated with nonlinear dynamics is due in large part to the discovery that the long-term behavior of a nonlinear dynamical system may exhibit yet another type of behavior, referred to as *chaotic evolution* (discussed in the next section). The temporal trajectories of systems undergoing chaotic evolution have very complex geometric structure and are commonly referred to as *strange attractors*. Observations of systems evolving on chaotic attractors have provided many seminal insights into the sources of complexity, unpredictability, and diverse phenomena involving intrinsic dynamics. In fact, a new science of complexity has emerged in recent years to focus specifically on these observations and insights (see, e.g., Casti, 1994; Cohen & Stewart, 1994; Davies, 1988; Kauffman, 1995; Pagels, 1988).

Bifurcations

In nonlinear dynamical systems, small incremental changes in the value of control parameters may lead to dramatic, qualitative changes in behavior, such as a change in the number and type of attractors. Radical changes in a pattern of behavior are usually called *bifurcations*, although they are sometimes referred to as dynamical phase transitions and critical phenomena. Bifurcations represent qualitative changes in a system's dynamics and thus are revealed by noteworthy changes in the values of the system's order parameters. Examples of bifurcations include change from periodic to chaotic evolution in the logistic equation, discussed earlier, and change from a single, fixed-point attractor to a multistable system characterized by two or more fixed-point attractors. Qualitative changes in patterns usually follow a small set of well-defined rules. The classification of bifurcations is the focus of catastrophe theory (Poston & Stewart, 1978; Thom, 1975; Zeeman, 1976) and the theoretical underpinnings of bifurcations represent a very advanced branch of mathematics (Ruelle, 1989). Bifurcation is a central concept in synergetics (Haken, 1978) and has been elaborated in psychology by Kelso and his colleagues (e.g., Kelso, 1984, 1995; Kelso et al., 1991; Schöner & Kelso, 1988).

There are several well-documented types of bifurcations (cf. Nowak & Lewenstein, 1994). The pitchfork bifurcation, for instance, occurs when a change in a control parameter causes a single fixed-point attractor to divide into two fixed points, which subsequently diverge. There is reason to think, for example, that the level of personal involvement regarding some issue operates as a control parameter to produce a pitchfork bifurcation in attitudes. Under low personal involvement, the person may have a single attitude reflecting the average value of information relevant to the attitude, even if the information is highly conflicting. At some value of involvement, however, the person may be no longer available to integrate all the relevant information, and his or her attitude may become tied to a progressively smaller subset of evaluatively congruent information. As a result, the person's attitude becomes polarized in either a positive or negative direction (see, e.g., Latané & Nowak, 1994). The saddle-node bifurcation is also a bifurcation from one fixed-point attractor to two fixed-point attractors. At some critical value of the control parameter, a new fixed-point attractor appears before the original fixed-point attractor has lost its stability. This bifurcation, which corresponds to the cusp catastrophe described by Thom (1975), has been used by Tesser and Achee (1994) to model the development and breakdown of close relationships and is described in detail in Chapter 6.

The Hopf bifurcation, meanwhile, is a change from a fixed-point into a periodic attractor. Such bifurcations are believed to be responsible for starting and stopping various biological rhythms (Bassingthwaighte, Liebovitch, & West, 1994; Kaplan & Glass, 1992). As a social psychological example, consider a married couple that displays the ability to reestablish equilibrium in their relationship following disagreements and conflict. This equilibrium corresponds to a fixed-point attractor. Conceivably, however, tension due to outside forces and circumstances might increase to the point where the maintenance of a stable equilibrium is no longer possible. Unable to maintain a single equilibrium, the couple may begin to display regularly alternating sequences of love and hate, corresponding to evolution on a periodic attractor.

Finally, period-doubling bifurcations occur when a periodic attractor of period t becomes unstable and is replaced by a new limit cycle of period 2t. A whole series of period-doubling bifurcations is characteristic of the dynamics resulting from iterations of the logistic equation under certain values (2.95 to 3.56) of the control parameter. In the restaurant example provided in our earlier discussion of the logistic equation, for example, the attendance at the restaurant alternates between two values when R was equal to 2.3. At somewhat higher values of R, the attendance begins to alternate between four values of attendance (i.e., the same attendance should be observed every fourth week instead of every other week)—hence, the period has doubled. By extension, attendance alternates between 8 values, then 16 values, and so forth, as the value of R is progressively increased. As the period tends toward infinity when R has a value of 3.56, another bifurcation occurs that brings the system into a chaotic motion.

The notion of bifurcations thus offers the important insight that qualitative changes in a system's behavior occur in only a limited number of well-specified scenarios (period-doubling, etc.). Such scenarios, moreover, are often accompanied by specific phenomena. In systems containing some amount of randomness (e.g., most biological systems), for example, as the bifurcation point is reached, one can usually observe moments during which both the old and new behaviors are displayed interchangeably. This realization has proven useful in studying the nature and dynamics of motor coordination (e.g., Kelso et al., 1991). There is evidence that this phenomenon also characterizes certain social psychological phenomena. In Chapter 8, for example, we describe research demonstrating that during social transitions (e.g., from a socialist to a free market economy), clusters or "bubbles" of the old and new realities coexist in varying degrees (Nowak et al., 1993).

DETERMINISM AND UNPREDICTABILITY

Perhaps the most popular insight concerning the emergence of complexity in simple systems involves deterministic chaos. This phenomenon is so important that quite often researchers, especially those outside of mathematics and physics, discuss the main insights from nonlinear dynamical systems as the theory of chaos. As the name indicates, the evolution of a chaotic system may be very irregular and seemingly random. The trajectory of such systems tends to visit a set of points in phase space that has a very complex structure, commonly referred to as a strange attractor because of its unusual and complex shape (Pietgen & Richter, 1986). Only nonlinear dynamical systems are capable of displaying such trajectories.

Deterministic Chaos

The fascination with chaotic systems is tied to the fact that although such systems are deterministic, they may be totally unpredictable in practice. This seeming paradox reflects the sensitivity to initial conditions (STIC) of nonlinear systems. In modeling weather fronts, for example, Lorenz (1963) found that the slightest changes in initial conditions, such as rounding the initial ambient temperature and humidity to the third decimal point, eventually led to entirely different patterns in his weather systems. More generally, anything short of infinite precision in one's knowledge of a system at one time can undermine knowledge of future states of the system. This is because all initial inaccuracies are amplified by the systems' intrinsic dynamics, such that the inaccuracies grow exponentially with time (e.g., doubling with each iteration). Exponential growth guarantees that after some finite (and relatively short) time, the size of the error will be greater than the possible range of states of the system's behavior. In practice, one can never specify completely the initial conditions for any real system, because there is always some error of measurement. Regardless of how precisely we know the initial conditions, then, it does not take long for any initial imprecision to grow to values that make prediction of future states of the system impossible. In addition to measurement error, slight and momentary perturbation of the dynamics can cause arbitrarily large effects after some time. In the popular literature, this aspect of STIC is referred to as the "butterfly effect." This colorful phrase is attributed to Lorenz, who suggested that the flapping of a butterfly's wings in, say, Brazil could produce a cascade of events culminating in a tornado sometime later in Texas.

Psychologists do not need to be reminded that human behavior is often unpredictable. The source of unpredictability in chaotic systems, however, is different from that in random systems. When unpredictability is due to randomness, either no deterministic rules exist for establishing the behavior of the system, or so many factors influence the system that it is impossible to account for all of them except by treating their joint effects as random influences. In a chaotic system, however, unpredictability results from the nonlinear interactions among a small number of variables. The system's behavior, then, is fully deterministic despite being unpredictable.

A system is capable of displaying both predictable time evolution and chaotic behavior, depending on the value of the system's control parameters. Below a certain value, for example, the system may be characterized by a fixed-point or periodic attractor, but beyond that value, the system will become chaotic. Several distinct scenarios by which systems become chaotic have been identified (see Nowak & Lewenstein, 1994). In a period-doubling scenario, for example, chaos is reached through a sequence of period-doubling bifurcations. The system makes a transition from a periodic attractor of period 2 to one of period 4, then 8, 16, and so on. The period goes to infinity at some finite value of the control parameter. Above this value, the motion of the system is chaotic. There are relatively few scenarios by which systems can approach chaos, and we use knowledge of them to make predictions regarding a system's behavior. If one observed, for example, that a change in a control parameter doubled the period of a system's evolution, and that further changes in the same parameter again resulted in a doubling of the period, one would expect that further changes would lead to the onset of chaos.

Fractals

In traditional geometry, the number of dimensions necessary to characterize an entity is an integer value. Thus, a point has a dimension value of 0, a line a dimension value of 1, a surface a dimension value of 2, a volume a dimension value of 3, and so on. Fractal geometry (Mandelbrot, 1982), however, specifies a new class of objects that have fractional dimension values (e.g., 1.78). Fractal objects have some of the properties corresponding to the higher dimension value (e.g., 2) and some corresponding to the lower value (e.g., 1). A fractal curve, for example, has properties of both a line (one dimension) and a surface (two dimensions), but cannot be adequately characterized by either. Length, first of all, is an inadequate measure because it depends systematically on the precision with which it is measured, tending toward infinity with increased precision as increasingly finer structures reveal themselves with enhanced resolution. The area occupied by a fractal curve, meanwhile, is inadequate because although the curve tends to be space filling, it does not cover all regions of the space it occupies. As a result, the dimension of a fractal curve is a value somewhere between that of a line (1) and a surface (2). The best measure of the dimensionality of fractal objects is obtained by estimating the extent to which increased precision changes the value of the measurement. The logarithm of this dependency defines the object's fractal dimension (Pietgen & Richter, 1986).

Fractal objects have an especially interesting property known as *self-similarity*. This means that parts of the object have the same structure as the object as a whole, and thus look remarkably similar when observed under different levels of magnification. Self-similarity has been shown to characterize many objects in the real world, such as mountains, clouds, coastlines, and leaves. Fractal geometry thus is ideally suited for the description of such objects (Mandelbrot, 1982). Not long after the development of fractal geometry, research established that fractal structure is inherent in physiological structures (Bassingthwaighte et al., 1994) and physiological functions (Glass & Mackey, 1988; Skarda & Freeman, 1987).

Fractals may also provide a useful way of describing the structure of certain social psychological phenomena. Before one can claim that a particular individual or group-level process has a fractal structure, however, it is necessary to measure the dimensionality of the process at different levels of generality and show that the resultant values tend to converge. To date, this approach is quite rare in social psychology. A noteworthy exception is research by Newtson (1994; Newtson et al., 1987) on the structure of human action. Newtson's pioneering work has revealed that a specific action can be broken down into smaller movements, the structure of which are similar to that of the action as a whole. The smaller movements in turn can be broken down into even smaller movements with a similar structure. Newtson demonstrated that the estimates of dimensionality at different levels of action converge on the same value.

Fractal structure may also prove to be relevant to issues of prediction in social psychology. As noted earlier, establishing the basins of attraction in systems with more than one attractor enables one to predict which initial states will lead to each attractor. The boundaries between basins of attraction, however, often have a fractal quality to them (Pietgen & Richter, 1986). This means that within the boundary separating two attractors there will be a fine-grained subdivision of states corresponding to each attractor. Because this subdivision repeats itself on progressively smaller scales, the slightest change in initial conditions can produce a change from one attractor to another. Whenever an initial state is in such a boundary region, then, prediction may be virtually impossible. Thus, for a system with fractal boundary conditions separating basins of attraction, it may be possible to predict the system's fate under some conditions (i.e., when it is on an attractor) but impossible to do so under other circumstances (i.e., when it is in a boundary condition). It is also the case that in some deterministic systems, the basins of attraction are themselves fractal, with neighboring points leading to different attractors (Lam & Noris, 1990). When this is the case, prediction may be virtually impossible under most conditions. Although this perspective holds potential for defining the limits of prediction in social psychology, we hasten to add that the various mental, emotional, and behavioral processes defining the field have yet to be analyzed in terms of fractal properties such as self-similarity.

THE ELEMENTS OF DYNAMICAL RESEARCH

Social psychology has become quite adept at identifying the causal structure associated with various facets of interpersonal experience. Humans clearly are open systems that interact with the environment, and it is eminently reasonable to document the various linkages fostered by such openness. To do so, the typical research paradigm involves the manipulation of one or more external factors (the suspected causes) at time 1 and the assessment of some individual- or group-level phenomenon (the predicted effect) at time 2. If the process under investigation varies in the predicted manner as a function of variation in the independent variables, the investigator can claim support for the theory under investigation. Although this general research strategy has established an impressive array of discrete causal mechanisms, it is not well suited to capture the internally generated dynamics that define human interpersonal experience. External factors may well have an impact on individual- and group-level phenomena, but these influences are channeled through the system's intrinsic dynamics. And because there is no limit to the number of relevant external influences, the resultant theoretical landscape of social psychology is highly fragmented, with numerous and often conflicting minitheories substituting for comprehensive understanding (cf. Vallacher & Nowak, 1994b).

In contrast, the dynamical systems perspective is ideally suited to derive simple understanding of the complex dynamic phenomena defining social psychology, and it holds promise for integrating widely divergent phenomena and levels of analysis in terms of common principles. In this section, we describe the research strategies used to investigate nonlinear dynamical systems and discuss their relevance to social psychology. Although many methods, analytical tools, and formal models are available, our aim is simply to outline the distinguishing features of the dynamical approach. These include the identification of patterns, the probing of a system's dynamics, the development and testing of models of qualitative understanding, and the use of computers to simulate dynamic processes and the emergent phenomena to which such processes give rise. Several of these strategies surface in later chapters in greater detail, when we discuss various research programs devoted to the major topics in the field.

Identifying Patterns

Prediction is often difficult, if not impossible in the investigation of nonlinear dynamical systems. In such cases, empirical research attempts to find patterns in data. In view of the complexity and unpredictability of human thought and behavior, the identification of patterns is an appropriate strategy for investigating social psychological phenomena at different levels of analysis (see Schroeck, 1994). Some patterns may express a causal relation, in which one event reliably follows another. Other patterns may express a linear correlation, wherein the values of one variable are directly and uniformly associated with the values of one or more other variables. Many other kinds of patterns are also possible, however, that cannot be subsumed by causation or linear correlation. Examples include the wave-like pattern in the movements of a person or the particular phase relations coordinating the behavior waves of two people (Newtson, 1994), the spatial distribution of attitudes in a society (Nowak et al., 1990), motor coordination (e.g., Kelso et al., 1991; Turvey, 1990), intermittent activity characterizing a person or a dyad (Baron et al., 1994), quasiperiodic oscillations in the evaluation of a target person (Vallacher & Nowak, 1994c), phase transitions in the evolution of a close relationship (Tesser & Achee, 1994), the distribution of values on a dimension of judgment (Latané & Nowak, 1994), and the complexity displayed in the sequence of binary choices (Selz & Mandell, 1994).

One of the most useful approaches for detecting a pattern in the relationships among variables or in the temporal evolution of a single variable is visual inspection of data in graphical form. The simplest procedure is to create a time series by plotting values of variables as a function of time. For a single variable, this approach may reveal such phenomena as periodicity, regions of stability versus change, smooth versus catastrophic changes, rapid versus slow time scales for the system's evolution, and tendencies toward stabilization versus increasing variance. When several variables are plotted against time on the same graph, meanwhile, inspection may reveal which of them tend to covary in time and which tend to evolve independently. One can also detect if changes in one variable tend to precede or follow changes in other variables. If several variables tend to change at the same point in time following a period of relative stability, one can try to identify what happened at that time (e.g., what, if any, external events occurred).

More systematic methods are available for identifying temporal patterns in a system. Some methods are based on linear assumptions, whereas others target the nonlinear domain. To detect linear patterns, the most widely used methods are autocorrelation, cross-correlation, and Fourier transforms (spectral analysis), all of which are contained in time series modules of major statistical packages. The autocorrelation method involves correlating the state of a system at time t with the state delayed by a certain interval, k. An autocorrelation function is obtained by increasing k and plotting the resultant correlation for each value of k. This function typically has a very high value (e.g., close to 1.0) for small values of k, but progressively smaller values for increased values of k. This method essentially characterizes how fast a system changes its states. Especially informative in this regard is relaxation time, which is the value of k for which the function reaches a value of 0. Roughly speaking, this is a measure of how quickly a system "forgets" its previous states. A related approach is cross-correlation, which measures the degree to which changes over time in one variable are related in a linear manner to changes over time in another variable. To obtain the cross-correlation function, one correlates the values of one variable at time t with the values of another variable at time $t + k$. This enables one to detect not only whether the time series of two variables are linearly related, but also whether changes in one variable precede changes in the other. With Fourier transforms, one tries to decompose temporal changes of a variable into waves of different frequencies. This method is ideal for detecting and describing all types of periodic evolution, even if the superimposition of waves of different frequences gives rise to nontrivial temporal trajectories. In general, this approach indicates the relative proportions of slow, intermediate, and fast components in a system.

Within the nonlinear approach, systematic means are available for reconstructing a system's state space and the trajectories within it. A common feature of these procedures is the identification of dynamical variables that are crucial for describing a system's dynamics. As noted earlier, variables that describe the system's dynamics on a global level represent the system's order parameters. In practical terms, the key dynamical variables may be known from previous work to be linked in important ways to the description of the phenomenon in question. Once these variables are identified, the investigator creates a state space by choosing different subsets of such variables and plotting the sequence of states through which the system passes. If the system's evolution follows a random pattern, or if the selected variables are irrelevant to the dynamics of the system, then no structure (a shapeless blob) appears, which is an indication that one should repeat this procedure with a different set of variables. The appearance of a well-defined pattern, on the other hand, is a clear indication that one's choice of variables is appropriate. The shape of this pattern, meanwhile, provides insight into the relationships among the chosen variables. A straight line in two dimensions or a plane in three dimensions, for example, indicates a linear relationship. More complex shapes (e.g., a parabola) are indicative of various types of nonlinear mechanisms underlying the dynamics (see Schroeck, 1994).

In social psychology, it is difficult to name all the appropriate variables, and even more difficult to measure their values precisely. Nonetheless, in nonlinear systems, one can reconstruct a phase space and identify basic properties of trajectories on the basis of measurements of a single variable on a time scale with equal intervals. This is because the value of each variable in a nonlinear dynamical system usually influences the values of all the other variables in the system, so that the effects of a system's variables can be inferred from the history of changes in any one variable. In a procedure developed by Takens (1981), consecutive measurements of the same variable serve as separate axes of a state space. That is, $t(1)$ serves as the first axis, $t(2)$ serves as the second axis, and so on. This results in current values of variables being plotted as a function of their past values. Each state of the system can thus be described as a point in such a space. Again, the idea is to see if the system's evolution produces a pattern in this space. One usually starts with a two-dimensional space in which two consecutive measurements define a single point. If no shapes appear, the next step is to assume a three-dimensional space by using three consecutive measurements to define a single point. This process of increasing the dimensionality may be continued further, although specific mathematical tools must be used to identify the appearance of patterns for the simple reason that patterns are opaque to visual inspection when they involve more than three dimensions (e.g., Grassberger & Procaccia, 1983). Based on similar principles, Kaplan and Glass (1992) have designed a specific method that allows one to reconstruct in a more precise way a system's trajectory from the observation of time series of a single variable (see Nowak & Lewenstein, 1994, for a detailed description of this procedure).

To illustrate this general approach, consider the phenomenon of empathy. One might define an empathic response as simply an emotional reaction that directly mirrors someone else's feelings. Linear methods are well suited to detect this form of empathy. It is possible, however, to envision forms of empathy that reflect more complex patterns. One can react with anger to sadness expressed by a friend who has been unjustly treated, with laughter to someone's expression of surprise, and so forth. The relation between one person's emotion and another's empathic reaction, moreover, may be nonlinear rather than linear. An expression of moderate sadness, for example, may elicit a corresponding expression of sadness from someone, but an expression of extreme sadness may produce little sadness but considerable anxiety and worry.

The methods we have outlined might uncover these forms of empathy. One could, for example, construct a state space with one axis corresponding to the emotional valence (positivity vs. negativity) expressed by one person and another axis corresponding to the emotional valence expressed by a second person. At specific time intervals (e.g., every several seconds), the valence of the two people could be assessed (e.g., from facial expressions) and plotted as a point in the space. An orderly distribution of points would be indicative of an empathic relationship between the individuals. To get a more detailed picture, the feelings of each individual could be displayed as two-dimensional (see Plutchik, 1980; Russell, 1991), resulting in a four-dimensional state space. Note that this approach enables one to describe not only patterns of relationships between variables, but also trajectories. Thus, one can draw a vector from each point to the next in the sequence of observations and note whether the resultant vector forms an orderly pattern. It is also possible that the reactions to someone's feelings might be delayed by a certain interval of time. An emotional reaction, for example, may need some time to become expressed. To assess this possibility, one could plot the emotions of one person at time t versus the emotions of the other person at time $t + k$, where k denotes the time lag.

The analysis of nonlinear patterns in the context of social psychology has been discussed in recent years. Mandell and Selz (1994; Selz & Mandell, 1994) introduce various measures of entropy that can be used to characterize complexity and randomness in a system's temporal evolution, and they develop psychological applications of these measures. Schroeck (1994) contrasts linear and nonlinear patterns and the methods for describing them, with special emphasis on coherent state analysis, of which wavelets are currently the most widely used manifestation. Nowak and Lewenstein (1994) discuss various methods for characterizing patterns, with special emphasis on the Grassberger–Procaccia (1983) algorithm and the Kaplan–Glass (1992) method. We hasten to add that most of the formal tools for analyzing nonlinear patterns have been developed quite recently and that new methods are currently being developed. Experience with these methods is thus somewhat limited, especially with respect to social psychological phenomena, so it is unclear which methods are likely to prove useful. Some are based on strong assumptions or impose conditions that are difficult to meet in experimental data (e.g., the Grassberger–Procaccia algorithm). Others seem to give results that are relatively robust (e.g., entropy measures). Perhaps diverse methods should be used to characterize the same data sets. If the results lead to similar conclusions, strong inferences may be drawn. If, however, the conclusions from one method are not substantiated by the results of other methods, caution should be exercised in interpreting results. It is our hope that as more experience is achieved in the application of these measures to social psychology, it will be possible to identify a subset of methods that has the greatest practical utility.

The identification of patterns differs from the traditional approach in social psychological research. In the typical experiment, participants' responses are averaged to obtain the the mean value of a dependent variable in each experimental condition. When dealing with a variable from a dynamical system evolving in time, however, averaging does not make much sense. If someone alternately hates and loves his or her parents, for example, it is misleading, at best, to suggest that this person on average mildly likes them. By averaging over time, one loses considerable information, perhaps the information that is most critical for understanding the phenomenon. Lacking this information, reconstruction of the temporal pattern may be impossible. Averaging is also likely to conceal meaningful patterns when dealing with an ensemble of different dynamical systems that have the same mechanisms. Imagine, for example, behavior in an approach–avoid conflict situation that may be described by a logistic equation. Every person may display the same qualitative pattern of behavior of approach and avoidance, but if there is no general mechanism for synchronization of individual actions, each person is likely to be at a unique point in the system's evolution with respect to this pattern at a given time. Because one person may be in an approach mode while someone else is demonstrating avoidance, the average behavior at each point in time would not show meaningful differences as a function of time, and the pattern of individual evolution would be concealed.

This does not mean that averaging is inappropriate when dealing with the information in nonlinear dynamical systems. It may be possible, for example, to classify each individual pattern and then compute statistics using the frequency of types of patterns as the dependent measure. Another approach is to characterize each individual pattern by a set of parameters and average the parameters rather than the raw data. Such parameters might include the regularity of each pattern, the complexity of each pattern, the speed with which each pattern changes over time, and so forth. Chapter 3 demonstrates this approach with respect to social judgment.

Stability Analysis

The dynamics of a system may be manifest as resistance to external influence. Conversely, a dynamical system at equilibrium may show an exaggerated response to external influence, so that even a small perturbation leads to a dramatic change. Analyzing the stability versus instability of a system thus provides another way of gaining insight into the system's dynamical properties. In effect, a system can be described not only in terms of the values of its various equilibria, but also in terms of the relative stability of these equilibria. In this approach, one attempts to perturb the system. By doing so in a systematic fashion, one can answer a number of questions: How quickly does the system return to its equilibrium state? How large does a perturbation need to be before the system adopts a new equilibrium? What is the time course of transition from one equilibrium to another? Are there specific phenomena associated with a change in equilibria?

Consider, for example, the nature of self-esteem. Research concerning this construct has typically focused on how positively or negatively people feel about themselves, either in general or in specific contexts or roles. In recent years, attention has shifted somewhat to the relative certainty and stability of self-esteem (e.g., Baumgardner, 1990; Campbell, 1990; Kernis, 1993; Vallacher, 1978, 1980; Vallacher & Wegner, 1989). For the most part, however, this research has investigated self-concept stability as a dimension of individual difference rather than as a dynamic property of the self-system. It is unclear, for example, how much disconfirming information is needed to change a person's self-evaluation. Does a person's self-evaluation return to its previous value after being destabilized, or does it move to a new value? What are the latent self-evaluations that will be adopted if one's current self-evaluation is destabilized? If it moves to a new value, what are the other possible values to which it can move? How fast does it return to its old value (if it does), or how long does it take before it stabilizes on a new value? Is the new value more or less stable than the previous value? Do changes in self-evaluation display hysteresis or rather an enhanced contrast effect? If both behaviors are possible, under what conditions are each displayed? Are changes in self-evaluation gradual or catastrophic in nature?

Similar questions can be posed with respect to virtually any phenomenon at different levels of social reality. Stability is a crucial factor, for example, when attempting to understand social relationships. A close relationship that appears positive and strong, for example, may rapidly dissolve in the face of apparently insignificant difficulties or small disagreements. Conversely, a relationship that seems relatively devoid of explicit affection or even characterized by negative sentiments may be able to sustain major difficulties and obstacles. A relationship may therefore be characterized in terms of the degree of perturbation necessary for changing its character or dissolving it altogether. Are changes in response to perturbation proportional to the magnitude of the perturbation, or are they catastrophic? What are the other possible equilibria values for the relationship? Can a broken love turn into friendship or indifference, or must it inevitably change to a hateful relationship? Can a small, positive experience in a relationship transform mild, positive feelings into romantic attraction? Or is it more likely that the same event will produce fascination and passion between those who dislike one another?

At a higher level of analysis, one can probe the stability of social groups or even entire societies. It is remarkable, for example, how small and seemingly insignificant the causes often are for revolutions within societies and for wars between nations. The collapse of communism in Eastern Europe and Asia in the 1980s, for example, began with the creation of the Solidarity union movement in Poland. This movement resulted from a wave of strikes along the Polish coast in 1981. The direct cause of these strikes was a 15% increase in the price of certain meat products in various shops. This does not mean that raising the cost of meat is a foolproof and reliable means of bringing down political empires. Rather, this disproportionality between cause and effect attests to the instability of the communist system at that point in time. This instability reflected such factors as economic inefficiency and the escalating cost of the arms race with the Western democracies. In principle, questions concerning equilibrium stability, other equilibria in the system, the abruptness of changes, and so on, can be posed for any social system.

Models of Qualitative Understanding

In mathematics and physics, nonlinear dynamical systems usually take the form of systems of interdependent equations. There is clearly an advantage to specifying a theory in terms of equations. We doubt, however, that social psychological phenomena can be described at present with such tools, and perhaps the problems inherent in the measurement of social psychological variables (e.g., the lack of ratio scales) make the development of precise mathematical descriptions impossible in principle. An alternative approach is to build *models of qualitative understanding*. Instead of trying to model a phenomenon in its natural complexity, one tries to isolate the most important features, which are often the qualitative aspects of the phenomenon. In physics, for example, qualitative aspects often refer to phase transitions, such as the change from liquid to gas or the emergence of macroscopic magnetic properties. In the social sciences, such qualitative changes represent the essence of understanding. The experience of sudden insight integrating diverse constraints in a problem, the change from an achievement mind-set to helplessness and depression, the switch from obedience to active resistance, the change from rejection to acceptance of a persuasive message, the switch from a readiness for aggression to a readiness for retreat, the emergence of coordination among strangers to push a car stuck in a snowdrift, and the loss of coordination in an army as it degenerates into a fleeing crowd of individual soldiers provide examples of qualitative effects in social psychology.

The first step in building a model of qualitative understanding is defining the most important characteristics of the system, which usually concern qualitative changes in the system's state or dynamics. Achieving precise description of these qualitative changes may require one to specify the order parameters of the system. One then tries to identify patterns both in the system's intrinsic dynamics and in the response of the system to external influence. Once such patterns are identified, the variables that promote qualitative changes in the patterns displayed by the system are isolated. The goal is to reproduce patterns and the change in patterns with the smallest number of these control parameters. Quite often, the systematic variation of control parameters across their entire range of values may be impossible, either because of technical reasons or perhaps because of ethical considerations.

A less demanding approach is to look for so-called signature phenomena that are known to exist in specific types of systems. The detection of hysteresis, for example, proves that the system is nonlinear. Sensitivity to initial conditions, in turn, is a signature of deterministic chaos in a system. And the detection of period-doubling specifies quite precisely how the behavior of the system changes from regular to chaotic dynamics with changes in the system's control parameters. Detection of signature phenomena may be an important step toward theoretical understanding. The discovery of hysteresis, for example, was an important development in the understanding of coordination in movement (Kelso, 1995). The demonstration of hysteresis in close relationships (Tesser & Achee, 1994), meanwhile, exposed the nonlinear dynamics underlying relationship formation, maintenance, and dissolution.

Models of qualitative understanding are clearly oversimplifications of natural phenomena. Indeed, the components of such models may seem unrealistically primitive. In simulating the emergence of public opinion, for example, Nowak et al. (1990) assumed that each individual could be characterized with respect to just three variables: his or her attitude on an issue, persuasive strength, and location in social space. This description obviously omits many personal qualities, such as the person's social identity, motives, and so forth. Although these characteristics are critical to the understanding of specific individuals, they may be disregarded when one's concern is the emergence of a group-level phenomenon such as public opinion.

In a sense, models of qualitative understanding are similar to the standard approach in social psychological research. Social psychology, after all, tries to discover the variables that most strongly influence a phenomenon of interest, and experiments rarely manipulate more than three variables at the same time. The levels of the these variables, in turn, are not chosen to mirror the likely values of these variables in real-world settings, but rather are set at values sufficient to produce salient changes in the values of the dependent variables. It is also the case, though, that models of social psychological phenomena are not designed to capture dynamics. As noted in Chapter 1, the system's operation is commonly reduced to a single pass and thus cannot expose the emergence of new properties, and the cause–effect nature of experimental procedures conceals the potential for bidirectional causality. The dynamic potential of social psychological theories is thus often unexplored. Commonsense considerations, for example, are often insufficient to predict the existence of signature phenomena, which in turn could be used to verify the theory, or to predict the emergence of patterns reflecting the nonlinear interactions among variables over time. Models of qualitative understanding, although quite simple and relating in only a qualitative way to real-world phenomena, are nonetheless quite precise in their specifications of the formal system modeling the phenomenon. Very specific predictions (usually of a qualitative nature) can be derived on the basis of such models.

Computer Simulations

In recent years, computer simulations have proven to be the tool of choice in developing models of social dynamics. Computers enable one to investigate a large number of interacting elements and to track the behavior generated by these interactions over many trials. There are many approaches to computer simulation in both the natural and social sciences (Hegselman, Troitzch, & Muller, 1996). In social psychology, the most popular approach models the emergence of global properties from the interactions of individual elements. Two levels of social reality are most often investigated in this manner. In models of social cognition, elements correspond to components of the cognitive system, and the global level refers to such macroscopic properties of the system as decisions and judgments (see Smith, 1996). At a higher level of social reality, elements correspond to individuals and the system-level properties refer to such group-level phenomena as the emergence of public opinion (Nowak et al., 1990) and cooperation in social dilemma situations (e.g., Messick & Liebrand, 1995).

Among the many advantages of computer simulation (see Nowak & Lewenstein, 1996), two are particularly noteworthy with respect to social psychology. Computer simulations, first of all, allow one to investigate the relationship between micro- and macrolevels of social reality. One can equip individual elements with established rules of behavior and observe how these rules give rise to global properties for the set of elements as a whole. In a reversal of this procedure, one can start with known global phenomena and trace backwards to discover what rules on the level of individual elements are necessary to produce the system-level phenomena. The second noteworthy advantage of computer simulations is their capacity to reveal temporal patterns. In social psychology, temporal aspects of interpersonal phenomena are largely unexplored. Yet, in many instances, it is unreasonable to expect the effects of a given cause to be revealed immediately. An insult may produce hate, for example, but the development of such a feeling may take a relatively long time to develop. And although love at first sight is a frequent subject of novels and movies, in reality, many interactions and prolonged contact may be necessary for a romantic attraction to develop. The very nature of computer simulations is ideal for studying the effects of multiple iterations of a given process. Decades of real time, and thousands of real interactions, may be compressed into seconds of computer time, revealing delayed consequences that simply cannot be observed in real time. Computer simulations, then, are ideal tools to investigate the dynamic consequences of a theory.

Computers are also the most potent tool for visualization of both experimental and simulation data. Computer visualization makes it possible to discover patterns existing in reality and predicted by theory. One can literally see the emergence of temporal and spatial patterns in a social psychological process, whether the spread of public opinion through social influence (Nowak et al., 1990) or the progressive differentiation of self-concept through socially provided feedback on one's qualities (Nowak, Vallacher, Tesser, & Borkowski, 1997). The comparison of patterns inherent in experimental data and produced by computer simulation of a model provides a new means of verifying a theory. We wish to stress that computer simulations are instrumental to all the elements of dynamical research we have described. It is noteworthy in this regard that the success of nonlinear dynamical systems theory in the physical sciences is due in large part to the widespread use of computer simulation and visualization.

THE RELEVANCE OF DYNAMICAL SOCIAL PSYCHOLOGY

The subject matter of social psychology, from individual-level function to group-level processes, is highly complex and dynamic. With the use of dynamical concepts and methods, it is now possible to discover and characterize the invariant aspects of complexity and dynamism that operate at different levels of analysis and for otherwise diverse topics. In establishing such commonality, the dynamical perspective redefines some of the most persistent and pressing issues in social psychology, and it provides new methods and analytical tools for resolving these issues. Thus, one can fashion research to explore the extent to which different phenomena (e.g., social judgment, self-evaluation, goal-directed action, intimate relationships, group dynamics) display intrinsic dynamics as opposed to changes brought about solely by external factors, and to characterize the nature of the observed temporal variation (e.g., convergence on a fixed point, periodicity, chaos). In identifying the intrinsic dynamics associated with an individual- or a group-level process, one can gain insight into the time scale on which such internally generated changes occur and how this time scale changes in response to variation in external factors.

The dynamical perspective also alerts us to possible nonlinearities in social psychological processes. One can specify the conditions under which a phenomenon of interest is likely to show gradual and incremental changes as opposed to sudden and catastrophic changes in response to external factors, for example, or predict when a seemingly minor change in an external factor will produce a disproportionately large change in the phenomenon. In like manner, dynamical concepts such as bifurcation and self-organization may prove useful in the investigation of a wide range of individual- and group-level processes, from goal-directed action to the development of group structure and the emergence of social norms. Because nonlinearity in dynamical systems conforms to a set of common rules, the identification of similar effects (e.g., hysteresis, pitchfork bifurcation) at different levels of social psychological inquiry (e.g., individuals, dyads, groups) provides an important precondition for integrative understanding of phenomena that are presently understood with recourse to wholly different theories.

This perspective also suggests that important regularities may be observed in areas that have yet to be examined. One particularly important class of regularities concerns the stability of social psychological phenomena. It is known, for example, that when a system is at an unstable equilibrium point, the state of the system may change dramatically in response to even a very slight influence. If a system is at a stable and strong attractor, however, even strong influences may have only short-lived effects. Knowing how a system reacts to external perturbation thus provides an important characterization of the system. Such a characterization could well have important practical consequences, providing a basis for knowing when and how to foster a change in individuals and groups.

The dynamical systems perspective is not necessarily in conflict with existing approaches in social psychology. Quite the contrary, this approach holds potential for enriching and expanding existing theories, particularly with respect to issues centering on the stability and dynamism of interpersonal processes. This benefit of the dynamical perspective is magnified by the theoretical coherence it might bring to an undeniably fragmented discipline (Vallacher & Nowak, 1994b). Assuming social psychological phenomena can be fruitfully investigated as nonlinear dynamical systems, we may not have to resign ourselves to explanations that are as complex and open to exception as the phenomena themselves. As has proven to be the case in other areas of science, we may discover that simple explanations exist for highly complex social phenomena. To the extent that dynamical principles are indeed invariant across different domains, it may prove possible to develop a general theory that integrates phenomena that are widely divergent in their surface features and associated causal mechanisms. As we enter the 21st century, then, the dynamical systems perspective may do for social psychology what it did for other areas of science in the final decades of the 20th century.

NOTES

1. In continuous time models, as described by differential equations, the rate of change of each variable is expressed as a function of the values of the other system variables. For both kinds of equations, however, knowledge of the states of all the system's variables at a given time enables prediction of the state of the system at succeeding points in time.

2. In more precise terms, in the point of transition between qualitatively different states, either order parameters or one of their derivatives must change in a noncontinuous manner (Schuster, 1984). If the discontinuity concerns order parameters, then we call the change of state a phase transition of the first order. If one of the derivatives changes in a nonlinear manner, however, the change of state is called a phase transition of the second order.

3

♺

Dynamics of Social Judgment

OF ALL THE PSYCHOLOGICAL phenomena identified over the years, none is more dynamic in nature than mental process. The mind represents a sustained flow of sensations, images, episodic memories, momentary concerns, and inferences, and this flow never stops for want of external stimulation. Even during sleep (Hobson, 1988) and under conditions of sensory deprivation (Zubek, 1969), the mind remains highly active, producing a rapid turnover in thought despite the lack of new input from the environment (see Wegner, 1996). The flow of thought, moreover, is irregular, with different cognitive and affective elements tumbling over each other in a manner that calls to mind James's (1890) stream of consciousness metaphor. Against this backdrop of mental turbulence, it is remarkable that people achieve coherent understanding of anything, let alone coherent understanding of objects as complex as their fellow human beings. Yet, somehow the flux of mental process gives rise to broad integrative frames with which people can understand and predict the behaviors of others, and which provide personal bases for social interaction. People clearly manage to relate to their social environment in a more or less coherent fashion, knowing whom to trust, whom to avoid, and whom to ignore.

In addition to the complex dynamism of mental process, the specific thoughts and representations that populate the stream of thought tend to be highly idiosyncratic in content, reflecting the particular experiences, hopes, and fears of each individual. This clearly poses difficulties for the scientific investigation of mental processes. If the content of each mind is unique, how can one hope to develop invariant principles that apply to people in general? One solution to this problem is simply to ignore the issue of content and focus instead on formal features of thought, in terms of which everyone can be characterized. Two people may well have non-overlapping thoughts and sentiments, but they may nonetheless be compared with respect to such yardsticks as hierarchical integration, cognitive complexity, category width, and differentiation (e.g., Bieri et al., 1966; Harvey, Hunt, & Schroder, 1961; Kelly, 1955; Pettigrew, 1958; Scott, Osgood, & Peterson, 1979; Witkin, Dyk, Faterson, Goodenough, & Karp, 1962).

Another approach is to find a common metric with which to scale otherwise idiosyncratic elements of mental content. This approach, which has a long tradition in social psychology, has consistently established that the most common dimension underlying thought in interpersonal contexts is evaluation (see Allport, 1935; Anderson, 1981; Osgood, Suci, & Tannenbaum, 1957; Rosenberg & Sedlak, 1972; Thorndike, 1920; Thurstone, 1928). So although two people may express entirely different characterizations of a third person (e.g., Dornbusch, Hastorf, Richardson, Muzzy, & Vreeland, 1965; Kelly, 1955; Rosenberg, Nelson, & Vivekananthan, 1968), the elements of each characterization can be scaled in terms of their evaluative connotations (see Anderson, 1968; Kim & Rosenberg, 1980). As it happens, shifting the emphasis from the flow of specific elements of thought to an undercurrent of evaluation not only solves a problem for social psychological research, but also helps explain how people can relate to one another in a coherent and meaningful way despite the mind's propensity for turbulence. Because individual thoughts regarding a person or group are all implicit, if not explicit, evaluations, they can achieve integration with respect to a common perspective and thus generate a consistent behavioral stance toward the person or group. On this view, people do not think about one another so much as they judge one another, and all the thoughts and feelings that arise in this enterprise press for a single-minded assessment. When all the elements of thought pertaining to a social entity have similar projections on the evaluative dimension, a stable unequivocal judgment of the target is likely to arise in little time.

Such uniformity of evaluation may be the exception rather than the rule, however. At least some of the information relevant to judgment is likely to be mutually inconsistent, making the achievement of a coherent judgment correspondingly difficult. This chapter is devoted to this issue. We begin by considering the means by which people integrate diverse elements of information into existing judgments. Emphasis is given to the stability of judgments and the potential for multiple equilibria in the judgment system. We then point out the potential for internally generated changes in judgment that can occur in the absence of incoming information and discuss the means by which the intrinsic dynamics of social judgment can be characterized and analyzed. We then introduce a distinction between two modes of integration in social judgment, each corresponding to a well-defined temporal trajectory in nonlinear dynamical systems. The chapter concludes with a consideration of the implications of the dynamical perspective for several perennial issues in social judgment.

DYNAMISM IN SOCIAL JUDGMENT

Judgment provides a basis for decision making, planning, and goal-directed behavior—functions predicated on the stability of people's thoughts and feelings regarding the target of judgment. In recognition of these functions, it is not surprising that social psychologists have commonly assumed judgments to be stable after their formation, thereby providing a consistent frame of reference for action. With this working assumption, temporal variation in social judgment is considered meaningful only if it occurs in response to some external source, such as new information or social pressure. In the absence of identifiable causes, variation over time in social judgment is commonly treated as noise obscuring an otherwise stable signal. From a dynamical perspective, however, the output of social judgment processes might display meaningful temporal variation in the absence of external influences. In this section, we explore both the external and internal sources of change in the global properties of social judgment.

Resistance to Change

The process of judgment formation is clearly dependent on external sources of information. In deciding whether a political candidate would make a good representative, for example, people attend to what they consider to be relevant sources of information—his or her voting record and stand on key issues, perhaps, or the opinions of other people about him or her. These separate pieces of information are combined in some fashion to reach a summary assessment, one that can provide a basis for deciding whether to vote for the candidate. Even after a provisional judgment is formed, people may remain open to further information that might modify this assessment and generate a different voting decision.

Once a judgment is fully formed, however, it can prove highly re-sistant to change. Whether the target of judgment is an individual or a social group, there are mechanisms that serve to stabilize the judg-ment and make it relatively impervious to substantial modification when new and potentially contradictory information is encountered. In effect, after compiling information to create an overall assessment of the target person or group, the resultant higher level unit of cogni-tion becomes self-sustaining and is stored in memory independently of the facts, behaviors, and other cognitive elements that generated it (e.g., Brewer, 1988; Brewer, Dull, & Lui, 1981; Cantor & Mischel, 1979; Dreben, Fiske, & Hastie, 1979; Fiske & Neuberg, 1990; Sher-man, 1996; Swann, Giuliano, & Wegner, 1982; Taylor & Crocker, 1981).

The inertia associated with social judgment is captured in a num-ber of prominent theoretical and research traditions in social psychol-ogy, including those centering on schema maintenance (e.g., Taylor & Crocker, 1981), reactance (Brehm & Brehm, 1981), belief persever-ance (e.g., Anderson, Lepper, & Ross, 1980; Wegner, Coulton, & Wenzlaff, 1985), and the tendency toward cognitive and affective consistency (e.g., Festinger, 1957; Heider, 1958). In these approaches, people are said to protect their impressions, beliefs, and stereotypes against potentially contradictory information through the selective processing of information and sometimes through outright distortion. Depending on which avenue provides the most effective strategy, peo-ple may discount or reinterpret contradictory information, attach dis-proportionate weight to confirmatory as opposed to disconfirmatory information, selectively remember confirmatory information, or dero-gate the source of the information.

What these perspectives have in common is a recognition that there are active mechanisms within a person that serve to maintain a given judgment, even in the face of contrary information and social pressures to change. Faced with seemingly overwhelming evidence that contradicts one's positive evaluation of a sports hero, politician, or best friend, a person will find ways to explain away, refute, deny, or trivialize the evidence so as to maintain his or her conviction. And intense social pressure to change the person's assessment may well backfire, not only strengthening the person's judgment, but also un-dermining his or her relationship with the source of influence as well. The mind, in other words, does not shut down and become dormant once a judgment is formed. To the contrary, it demonstrates intense and sustained activity that attests to the internal workings of the cog-nitive–affective system. The stability of social judgment, in short, is made possible by ongoing intrinsic dynamics of mind.

Incremental versus Catastrophic Change

It would be a mistake to assume that a judgment, once formed, is incapable of modification or change. After all, people have been known to switch political parties, become enemies with former friends, and fall out of love with those who matter most to them. It is tempting to see such changes as occurring in response to external influences. On this view, people's impressions, beliefs, and feelings are open to modification in the face of clear evidence that cannot be discounted or in response to especially effective social influence. Presumably, when exposed to such pressures for change, people adjust their judgments accordingly, with each new source of change having a corresponding impact on their thoughts and feelings regarding the target. The notion that judgment displays incremental and proportional changes in response to external influences is consistent with models holding that judgment represents a specified configuration of relevant information. Anderson's (1981) model of information integration, for example, assumes that a person's overall evaluation of a target represents a weighted average of the evaluative components associated with each element of available information.

Judgment may in fact change in an incremental and linear manner when the topic of judgment is of relatively minor importance to the person. Someone who has never been to France and is unlikely to do so, for example, may be easily convinced that his or her negative stereotypes about the French are unfair and unwarranted. Simply being told by a friend or an authority in such matters that the French are in fact a warm and friendly people might be sufficient to change the person's judgment from negative to neutral or even mildly positive. The extension of this possibility to judgments that are personally important would suggest that such judgments have somewhat more inertia, but that given sufficient information and social pressure, they too should change in response to external influence. After a particularly painful visit to Paris, for example, it may be hard to convince the traveler about the social niceties of Parisians, but in principle, such change could be induced if compelling evidence were assembled and presented by a credible source. From this perspective, judgments on important issues may be resistant to change, but if change does occur, the process is no different in principle than the process underlying change with respect to less personally relevant targets of judgment.

There is reason to believe, however, that the process of change for personally important topics is qualitatively different than the process of change for less important topics. Whereas change follows the receipt of information and influence for relatively uninvolving judgments, change in personally important judgments tends to occur in a categorical fashion, with abrupt shifts from one end of the judgmental dimension to the other. There are some classic, albeit exotic demonstrations of this potential for wholesale change in beliefs and feelings. Particularly compelling examples are provided by Rokeach (1964) in his depiction of the three Christs of Ypsilanti, and by Schein (1956) in his analysis of brainwashing in prisoner-of-war camps. The delusional figures in Rokeach's analysis went through a qualitative change in identity, from a conviction that they were Christ to an equally strong conviction that they were worthless. The victims of brainwashing, meanwhile, went from a firm belief in the value of democracy to an equally firm belief that democracy was evil and a primary source of misery.

A similar pattern of change is also observed in psychotherapy and in religious and political conversions. With respect to psychotherapy, for example, research on desensitization suggests that when someone overcomes a phobia, he or she does not simply become indifferent to the phobic object, but rather tends to become fascinated with it. With respect to ideological conversion, Hoffer (1951) described how converts typically switch from one firm set of convictions to another, rather than simply losing their faith in one of the systems of thought. Even scientists are not immune to this scenario of change. As Kuhn (1970) noted, theorists and researchers actively resist challenges to their preconceptions, even when such challenges are based on extensive and reliable evidence. When change does occur, it commonly involves the wholesale adoption of another theoretical perspective rather than movement toward a noncommittal, open-minded stance.

The propensity for wholesale change in evaluation of personally important topics is not limited to exotic examples. To the contrary, it may represent a basic and pervasive feature of the judgment process in everyday life. Consider, for example, how partners in an intimate (and hence important) relationship react to negative information about one another (Vallacher, 1995). Their very strong positive feelings about one another are not easily undermined by unflattering information. Indeed, the same sorts of information that might promote a slight adjustment in the overall evaluation of a casual acquaintance (e.g., a lowered evaluation upon seeing him or her overreact to a stressful event) is unlikely to promote any change at all in someone's overall judgment of his or her intimate partner. However, once a certain threshold is crossed, the feelings about the partner can switch dramatically from positive and loving to negative and even hateful—a switch far less likely to be observed in less important relationships.

Learning that one's partner has been unfaithful, for example, is likely to promote very strong condemnation of the partner, with the resultant feelings posing a threat to the continuation of the relationship.

The distinction between the catastrophic and incremental scenarios can be understood in terms of a model developed by Latané and Nowak (1994), which looks at attitudes and attitude change in terms of catastrophe theory (Thom, 1975). This model can be viewed in geometric terms as the interplay of three dimensions (see Figure 3.1). The balance of positive and negative arguments is represented as the x-axis of a graph, with higher values representing higher proportions of positive to negative arguments. The overall evaluation of the attitude topic or target is represented on the y-axis, with higher values representing more positive evaluations. The two dimensions, then, show evaluation as a function of positivity of arguments. There is additional dimension (z) in this model, however, corresponding to the importance of the topic in question. In catastrophe theory, this dimension is described as a splitting parameter. The value of this parameter determines whether attitude change follows a gradual, incremental scenario or a sudden, catastrophic scenario.

As Figure 3.1 illustrates, when judgments involve topics of low importance, the relationship between positivity and evaluation is a

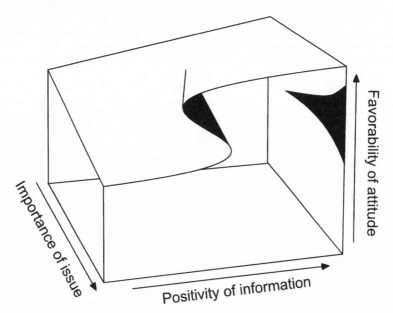

FIGURE 3.1. Attitude favorability as a catastrophe.

straight line, and for every degree of relative positivity, there is only one resultant evaluation. Under low importance, then, judgment tends to be incremental and linear in nature. With increasing importance, however, the relationship between relative positivity and evaluation becomes increasingly curvilinear. For very important issues, the relationship corresponds to an S-shaped curve, so that the same degree of positivity can be reflected in two very different evaluations. Which of these evaluations is actually observed depends on the history of the system up to that point. If relative positivity starts from a low value, subsequent increases in positivity are only slightly reflected in the resultant evaluation; only at high values of positivity does evaluation suddenly change to a highly positive assessment. The opposite scenario is observed when positivity starts at a high value and gradually becomes more negative. In this case, the overall evaluation remains positive past the point at which judgment was still negative under increasing positivity in the other scenario. Note that in both scenarios, when change does occur, it tends to be rapid and dramatic. For intermediate values of positivity, there is a region of hysteresis, such that two very different values are possible for evaluation, depending on the history of the system up to that point. As noted in Chapter 2, the observation of hysteresis is a signature phenomenon for nonlinearity.

Support for this model is provided by empirical evidence showing that although attitudes on unimportant topics are typically normally distributed, attitudes on personally important topics tend to be bimodally distributed, with intermediate values of favorability being psychologically unavailable (Latané & Nowak, 1994). Presumably, when a change in attitude occurs for an important topic, the resultant attitude avoids the unavailable regions of the distribution, gravitating instead toward the regions that are available, that is, toward highly favorable or highly unfavorable positions regarding the topic at issue.

Dynamics of Stability and Change

Catastrophe theory provides a highly restricted view of dynamics and thus may not provide a complete depiction of stability and change with respect to such an inherently dynamic phenomenon as social judgment. The catastrophe model is well suited, of course, to describe the points of equilibrium in a system, but it is not equipped to deal with the behavior of a system outside of equilibrium. Nonlinear dynamical systems theory, in contrast, provides insight into the nature of nonequilibrium as well as equilibrium states. Specifically, it depicts the forces and trajectories bringing a system back to equilibrium, and it provides conceptual and analytical tools for analyzing the stability of the system's equilibria (i.e., attractors).

From a dynamical perspective, social judgment can be characterized not only in terms of currently held evaluations, but also in terms of latent or potential values to which the system can jump if current values become destabilized. Thus, one can analyze the degree to which evaluation is free to wander as a result of incoming information versus being confined to a small number of predefined values. As noted in Chapter 2, a common approach to stability analysis is to perturb the system and observe whether it returns to its previous state, gradually changes in response to the perturbation, or jumps to a new attractor. With respect to social judgment, one can investigate which of these possible behaviors is expressed when a person is exposed to information or social influence that contradicts his or her current evaluation of someone.

It is noteworthy in this regard that recent research has explored the idea that people may hold two (or more) incompatible judgments of the same entity. With respect to racial stereotypes, for instance, there is evidence that many white people have conflicting images of African Americans (e.g., Katz & Hass, 1988; Lepore & Brown, 1997; McConahay, 1986; Smith, Fazio, & Cejka, 1996; Wittenbrink, Judd, & Park, 1997). Both judgments, however, may coexist in memory as relatively autonomous schemas. The research on this topic suggests that which schema is prepotent in a given instance depends on the presence of cues activating one or the other. The priming of particular prototypes or categories, for example, can call to mind one internalized assessment rather than the other (e.g., Lepore & Brown, 1997; McConahay, 1986; Wittenbrink et al., 1997). To the extent that these schematas are associated with qualitatively different affect (i.e., positive vs. negative feelings), it is plausible that mood congruence (e.g., Bower, 1981) could activate one global assessment, while suppressing the other. Following the induction of a positive mood, the person might evaluate a black target person in accordance with his or her positive stereotype of African Americans, but following the induction of a negative mood, the same person might evaluate the same target in accordance with a far less flattering stereotype.

The dynamical systems perspective suggests another way to explore the dual nature of social stereotypes, and of social judgment generally. Assuming that each global assessment functions as an attractor for the judgment system, one could perform stability analysis along the lines suggested in Chapter 2. Thus, each judgment in turn could be perturbed with increasing degrees of contradictory information or social pressure. This approach, first of all, would reveal the respective stability of the two judgmental attractors. It may be, for example, that positive impressions, beliefs, and stereotypes are easier to destabilize than are negative assessments. Or perhaps asymmetry in positive–negative judgments depends on the type of judgment (e.g., personality impression of an individual, stereotype of an ethnic group), the context in which the judgmental system is probed, or idiosyncratic features of the judge.

Beyond that, this approach enables one to track the output of the judgment system in nonequilibrium states. What happens to the judgment system when it is destabilized? Does it return to its original attractor, switch to an alternative attractor, or go through a process of disassembly and self-organization that leads to the emergence of a new attractor? What is the time frame for these scenarios? When a system is destabilized, does it become particularly open to external influences that can shape its subsequent evolution (Vallacher, 1993; Vallacher et al., 1998)? By framing social judgment in explicitly dynamical terms, such possibilities can be developed in terms of testable hypotheses and systematically investigated.

INTRINSIC DYNAMICS OF SOCIAL JUDGMENT

Thus far, it has been assumed that if judgments change, they do so in response to incoming information. In this on-line mode of judgment formation (Hastie & Park, 1986), new information is considered in light of the judgment formed up to that point. The person either maintains the existing judgment despite the new information, updates the judgment to accommodate the information as it is encountered, or changes his or her judgment in a catastrophic manner. In each case, the fate of the judgment process is governed to a large degree by the person's reaction to incoming information. This scenario can be referred to as *extrinsic dynamics*. The exact course of extrinsic dynamics, of course, is not entirely governed by incoming information, since this information interacts with other beliefs, attitudes, and temporary moods of the person. An element that may be meaningful for one person, for example, may be irrelevant for another. Nonetheless, the pattern of changes in general is driven from outside, so changes in judgment are informative about the meaning of incoming information.

Although social judgment is clearly responsive to new information and external influence, there is reason to believe that judgment may also display meaningful temporal variation due to the internal workings of the cognitive–affective system, even in the absence of external influences. Such internally generated temporal variation reflects the intrinsic dynamics of social judgment (Vallacher & Nowak, 1994c; Vallacher et al., 1994). Whereas extrinsic dynamics are informative about the evaluative structure of incoming information, intrinsic dynamics may provide a window into the workings of the cognitive–affective system producing judgment. In this section, we discuss the nature of intrinsic dynamics in social judgment, the means by which internally generated changes can be tracked, and the interdependency between intrinsic dynamics and the structure of the underlying set of elements relevant to judgment.

Internally Generated Change

The information relevant to any judgment is likely to encompass a wide range of cognitive and affective elements, including specific facts, fantasies, feelings, and images. The potential for temporal variation in social judgment reflects the fact that all these elements are rarely activated at the same time. Instead, because of the well-established limitations of working memory (Baddeley, 1986; Miller, 1956), only subsets of elements can be active concurrently. This means that as new elements enter working memory, they displace existing elements. It is the successive activation of such subsets of elements that gives rise to internally generated changes in social judgment. Hence, by characterizing the set of elements and the rules that give rise to their successive activation, one can achieve insight into the intrinsic dynamics of judgment. The dynamical perspective can therefore offer a framework within which specific cognitive mechanisms may be integrated and rendered amenable to dynamical predictions.

Attempting to reconstruct the exact trajectory of specific thoughts and feelings in social judgment may prove to be an impossible task. Each cognitive and affective element, after all, is necessarily unique, capturing perhaps a particular memory or a transitory feeling. Some elements, moreover, may be recalled repeatedly, while others may enter consciousness once and never reappear. Even if one could somehow manage to track the rise and fall in salience of individual elements of thought, then, it is unlikely that reliable and meaningful patterns in the judgment process would be observed. From the perspective of dynamical systems, however, what may appear as idiosyncratic, feeble, and impossible to describe on the level of individual elements may prove to be regular, meaningful, and organized on the level of the system as a whole, as reflected in the dynamics of the system's order parameter (Haken, 1982; Landau & Liftshitz, 1964; Nowak & Lewenstein, 1994).

With respect to the social judgment system, it is reasonable to view evaluation as a basic order parameter. Evaluation, after all, is commonly considered the most important aspect of social judgment (Anderson, 1981; Asch, 1946; Wegner & Vallacher, 1977), providing a "bottom line" assessment of social stimuli. A target of judgment clearly can be considered with respect to a variety of specific cognitive elements, of course, but each of these elements has a projection on an evaluative dimension (see Anderson, 1981; Kim & Rosenberg, 1980). These projections, in turn, tend to be combined in some fashion to promote an overall evaluation of the target, although there is disagreement concerning the specific combinatorial function involved (cf. Eiser, 1990; Fiske & Taylor, 1991; Ostrom et al., 1994). The single variable of evaluation thus provides a global description of the state of the system.

To capture the intrinsic dynamics of social judgment, then, it may not be necessary to track the rise and fall in salience of individual cognitive elements. In fact, the attempt to track a particular element of thought may prove fruitless, because it may disappear from thought altogether as one subset of elements gives way to another subset. Of course, a particular element of thought may have clear theoretical or clinical significance (e.g., memory of a traumatic event from childhood, an unwanted thought), and one may therefore have good reasons to track its appearance over time in consciousness (e.g., Pennebaker, 1988; Pope & Singer, 1978; Uleman & Bargh, 1989; Wegner, 1989). But if one's concern is with the dynamics of the social judgment system as a whole, it may be necessary to track the global output of the system over time. The stream of social judgment, in short, can be characterized in terms of the variation over time in some index of overall evaluation of the target of judgment.

To be more precise, the intrinsic dynamics of judgment represent the successive activation of subsets of elements, each representing a unique configuration that can be characterized in terms of a summary evaluation. On a macrolevel, then, the temporal trajectory of social judgment may be described as a succession of evaluations. This means that the current value of evaluation may determine, according to the rules of the system's dynamics, the value of this parameter at the next moment.[1] A system's dynamics are therefore reflected in patterns of changes in evaluation. Of course, if the cognitive elements are all positive or all negative in valence, the temporal changes in evaluation should be minimal. Even here, however, judgment may display polarization, with evaluation becoming progressively more extreme during the course of judgment as the valences associated with elements reinforce one another and lingering inconsistencies are dampened (Tesser, 1978).

More commonly, though, the cognitive elements concerning a target vary in their respective valence and thus do not promote an evaluatively consistent judgment of the target. Mixed valence and differentiation are in fact defining features of cognitive structure (e.g., Bartlett, 1932; Haken & Stadler, 1990; Harvey et al., 1961; Linville, 1985; Piaget, 1971; van Geert, 1991; Werner, 1957). When a representation of a target elicits conflicting assessments, or when the judge lacks a well-integrated schema concerning the target, polarization is unlikely to be observed (e.g., Liberman & Chaiken, 1991; Tesser & Leone, 1977). This does not mean, however, that mixed valence representations promote stability in evaluation. Stability would be expected only if both the positive and negative elements of a mixed valence representation were activated simultaneously, giving rise to a relatively neutral evaluation (i.e., an average of the positive and negative elements) each time the judgment is assessed.

It is possible, however, to envision more elaborate scenarios for mixed valence representations than simultaneous activation. If, for example, each positive element calls to mind a negative element and vice versa, one would expect regular oscillations in the overall evaluation. If we assume further that all the elements in the representation can be activated, one would expect decreasing amplitude in these oscillations, because each new element would reflect a correspondingly smaller percentage of the overall evaluation. On the other hand, if only a relatively small subset of elements can be held in working memory and thus contribute to the overall evaluation, one would not necessarily expect decreasing amplitude in the oscillation of evaluation. Of course, more complex rules of activation could lead to considerably more irregular temporal trajectories of judgment. Even a few elements linked in a nonlinear fashion, for example, could produce very complex patterns of change characteristic of deterministic chaos (cf. Schuster, 1984).

Without monitoring evaluation over small units of time, it is impossible to discriminate among these possibilities. Thus, if no change in overall evaluation is observed for a mixed valence representation over a 6-week or even a 10-minute interval, this could mean that no change has occurred on any time scale, or alternatively, that more complex temporal trajectories of evaluation (e.g., high-frequency oscillations) have occurred on a shorter time scale, but are not recorded. More generally, if only the central tendency of judgment, averaged over time, is assessed, or if the judgment is assessed at only two points in time, one cannot gauge the intrinsic dynamics of the judgment system (Nowak, Lewenstein, & Vallacher, 1994). Someone about whom we feel ambivalent, for example, may promote relatively rapid (frequent) and dramatic (high-amplitude) oscillations in our overall evaluation of him or her, but if our evaluation is averaged over time, it would appear that we have neutral feelings toward the person.

To an extent, the distinction between intrinsic and extrinsic dynamics maps onto the distinction between on-line and memory-based judgment (Hastie & Park, 1986). On-line judgment refers to the formation of judgment during the receipt of information concerning a target; such judgment likely shows temporal variation in accordance with the nature of the incoming information and thus corresponds to extrinsic dynamics. Memory-based judgment, meanwhile, refers to the generation of judgments based on information stored in memory; any temporal variation here should reflect the workings of the cognitive–affective system rather than incoming information (or other external factors) and thus correspond to intrinsic dynamics. This simple mapping is somewhat misleading, however. As Hastie and Park (1986) point out, it is natural to form a judgment when receiving information about a person, even without explicit instructions to do so. Special procedures, in fact, are sometimes necessary to suppress the formation of judgments on-line (e.g., presenting the task as a memory test).

In the absence of such procedures, there is a strong potential for the dynamics of judgment to become decoupled from incoming information. This could happen, for instance, when higher order frames emerge early on and override the processing of subsequent information. If only one such frame were generated (perhaps because the early information is highly consistent), there would be little or no temporal variation, despite the continued exposure to new information. On the other hand, if more than one frame were generated (perhaps because the early information is highly inconsistent), temporal variation in judgment would reflect the internal workings of the judgment system in its attempt to move from dynamic integration to static integration. In this case, the dynamics would reflect a mixture of intrinsic and extrinsic factors.

Characterizing Intrinsic Dynamics

In both the formative and integrative stages of judgment, then, the temporal trajectory of judgment may provide insight into the workings of the cognitive–affective system that generates judgment. Little in the way of such insight, unfortunately, has been produced in empirical research on social judgment. For the most part, research on judgment dynamics assesses judgment at only two points in time (e.g., before and after new information or a social influence attempt) and thus cannot reveal the temporal evolution of the judgment. Attitude polarization (Tesser, 1978), for instance, is assumed to reflect the rearrangement of cognitions in the service of evaluative consistency, but the measurement of evaluation at two widely spaced points in time precludes a direct test of this possibility. To explore the nature of dynamics and their role in social judgment requires assessing the output of judgment in a fairly continuous manner so as to observe the moment-to-moment trajectory of judgment.

Tracking the ebb and flow of people's stream of social judgment would seem to be a straightforward matter. People have a well-documented capacity for self-reflection, after all, and thus should be able to verbalize the contents of mind as they occur. Indeed, there is a strong tradition for just this approach to gaining insight into people's minds as they think about topics and events (e.g., Klinger, Barta, & Maxeiner, 1980; Pennebaker, 1988; Pope & Singer, 1978; Singer, 1988; Singer & Bonnano, 1990; Wegner, 1994). There are difficulties associated with this approach, however, that raise serious questions regarding its suitability for capturing the precise nature of the trajectories of judgment. To begin with, reflecting on one's thoughts as they unfold is a well-documented paradox (e.g., Hofstadter, 1979; James, 1890; Polanyi, 1969; Ryle, 1949; Wegner & Vallacher, 1981). The nature of the paradox is simple: To track what is going on mentally as one thinks about, say, a casual acquaintance is tantamount to changing what one is thinking about. Instead of thinking about the acquaintance, one is now thinking about one's thinking. If one then decided to reflect on *that* set of thoughts, the focus of thought would again change—from how one is thinking about the acquaintance to how one is thinking about thinking about him or her. There is clearly a potential for infinite regress in trying to report on one's thoughts as they unfold, with the likelihood of success no greater than that associated with trying to catch one's own shadow. One cannot both *be* in a mental state and *know* what it is like to be in that state, any more than one can simultaneously sleep and know what it is like to be asleep. This is what we expect of people, however, when we ask them to report on their thoughts as they occur.

An obvious solution to this problem is to let the thought process unfold naturally, and then ask participants to report from memory what their intervening thoughts and feelings were. There are problems here as well, however. For one thing, there is a danger that once an overall attitude or sentiment has been expressed, participants will be inclined to reconstruct their intervening thoughts to make them appear evaluatively consistent with the expressed attitude (e.g., Lingle & Ostrom, 1979). Considerations of cognitive consistency aside, there is reason to think that people simply are not very insightful into the workings of their own minds (e.g., Mandler, 1975; Nisbett & Ross, 1980; Nisbett & Wilson, 1977). A person may readily report his or her feelings about a target person, for example, but draw a blank or provide a rationalization when probed for the intervening steps leading to the resultant feeling. Even if people were fairly cognizant of the moment-to-moment feelings associated with their evaluation of some target person, they might not provide a faithful account of these feelings, preferring instead to describe their thoughts in personally flattering or socially desirable terms (Crowne & Marlowe, 1964; Edwards, 1957). Self-presentation considerations are particularly likely when it is apparent how various accounts are likely to be evaluated by the inquisitor (Rosenberg, 1965).

Finally, there is a very practical issue concerning limitations in the timing associated with traditional assessment techniques. The temporal patterns associated with social judgment can operate on different time scales, perhaps even those involving milliseconds. Tracking self-reports on such time scales is obviously out of the question. One can assess an attitude on a questionnaire at one point in time and do so again perhaps a few minutes later. But it is simply impossible to assess judgments in this way every few seconds, let alone several times a second.

There seems to be fundamental restrictions, therefore, on what one can hope to learn about the flow of thought from people's self-reports. They may tell you what they think, but when probed for the intervening thoughts on their way to their current state, they may provide answers that are fraught with paradox and lack genuine insight, revealing more about their intuitive theories of cognitive process, or perhaps their particular concerns over personal evaluation, than about the process that actually transpired (Ajzen, 1977; Nisbett & Ross, 1980). In view of these considerations, the stream of consciousness makes for a poor reflecting pool.

Gaining access to the flow of social judgment without perturbing it in the process is clearly not a simple task. The trick is to provide a means by which people can express their feelings continuously, but can do so without reporting on them. In an attempt to accomplish this goal, we developed a procedure that enables us to capture the dynamics of evaluative processes at a high degree of temporal resolution (Vallacher & Nowak, 1994c). This approach centers on a computer mouse used to control a cursor on a computer screen. Two symbols are presented on the screen: a small circle positioned in the middle of the screen and an arrow showing the position of the cursor. The circle is said to represent a particular target of judgment, and the arrow is said to represent the subject. The instructions follow from the suggestion that evaluation is an implicit approach–avoid response (Hovland, Janis, & Kelley, 1953). This idea implies that a judge's preferred proximity to a target represents an expression of his or her current feeling about the target. The closer the judge's preferred distance from the target, the more positive his or her feeling. By extension, movement toward or away from the target represents changes in the judge's feelings about the target.

In research employing the mouse paradigm, participants read a description of someone, or of an event involving themselves and a target person, and then are asked to think about and evaluate the target person. As they do so, they adjust the arrow in relation to the target circle by moving the mouse so as to express their moment-to-moment feelings of the target over a period of several minutes. The experimenter informs participants that if they feel positive about the target, they should move the arrow toward the circle by moving the mouse. By the same token, if participants feel negative about the target, they should move the arrow away from the target. Their placement of the cursor in relation to the target circle, in other words, represents their global evaluation at each point in time; the closer the cursor is placed to the circle, the more positive the evaluation. If their feelings about the target change, meanwhile, they are instructed to move the arrow toward or away from the target to express these changes. Participants are free to adjust their position relative to the target as often and as much as is necessary to reflect their feelings about the target as they continue to think about him or her. Movement of the cursor, then, signals instability in global evaluation; the more movement in a given period of time, the greater the instability in judgment.

A 20-second practice session is typically provided, during which participants move the mouse and observe the corresponding movement on the screen. The screen then clears, a description of the target person appears, and they begin the mouse procedure. The location of the arrow is assessed 10 times per second, so that for even a 2-minute judgment period, there are 1,200 potential data points. The program preserves the Cartesian coordinates of each data point, although for purposes of our research thus far, only the absolute distance (in pixels) from the target has been considered. This distance provides a measure of participants' moment-to-moment feelings about the target. Changes in this distance, in turn, reveal the volatility in participants' feelings. Special emphasis is given to the variance in distance, the speed (pixels per 0.1 second) and acceleration (change in speed) of mouse movements, and the time at rest (number of seconds without movement), as these measures provide intuitive and direct assessments of the turnover in participants' feelings. The greater the variance in distance, the greater the range in evaluation; the greater the speed, the more rapid the turnover; the greater the acceleration, the more unstable the rate of turnover; and the greater the time at rest, the greater the stability in evaluation.

Figure 3.2 presents representative temporal trajectories of evaluation in the mouse paradigm. Participants in this study (Vallacher & Nowak, 1994c) were asked to think about several hypothetical situations that were anticipated to engender some ambivalence on their part. Participants who were married, for example, were asked to imagine that they had just had a heated discussion with their spouse concerning their relative contributions to the household. In another scenario, participants imagined that a close friend had stolen money from another of his or her friends, and had never admitted to the theft or tried to make amends. In thinking about each description, participants used the mouse to indicate their moment-to-moment feelings about the target person (e.g., the spouse or friend). The four trajectories in Figure 3.2 each portray a different participant's continuous evaluation of the target in a particular scenario. The x-axis in these trajectories represents time (over a 2-minute period), and the y-axis represents absolute distance from the target (in pixels). Each trajectory was investigated with Fourier analysis and autocorrelations to gain insight into features of the time scale underlying judgment.

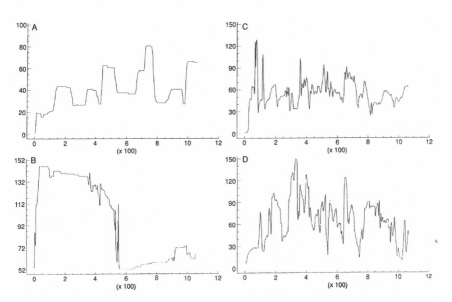

FIGURE 3.2. Trajectories of evaluation From Nowak & Vallacher (1994c). Copyright 1994 by Academic Press. Reprinted by permission.

Intrinsic dynamics were observed for all of the situations, with judgment in each case corresponding to one of several distinct temporal patterns. Inspection of panel A suggests that the participant's judgments alternated between positive and negative assessments of the target in a periodic manner. The autocorrelations gradually decreased in value, becoming negative after about 80 lags, a pattern indicative of simple low-frequency periodicity. The Fourier analysis revealed one dominant low frequency period in the trajectory. Panel B, in contrast, shows gradual change (increasing positivity) for the first minute, followed by a catastrophic change (sudden positivity), and finally some slight correction toward negativity by the end of the judgment period. The autocorrelations decreased only slightly over 120 time lags, a pattern indicative of slow dynamics, so that a judgment at one point in time is predictive of judgments at a later time. The Fourier transforms of this trajectory confirmed the lack of periodicity in this participant's judgments. The trajectory in panel C shows irregular oscillations with decreasing amplitude, suggestive of judgment converging on a stable attractor. The associated autocorrelations dropped rapidly to 0, became slightly negative, and then became slightly positive with increasing lags. This inability to predict far in the future suggests the operation of dynamics on a short time scale. The Fourier transforms, in turn, revealed many frequencies in this participant's judgments, none of which were dominant. The trajectory in panel D is similar to that in panel C in demonstrating irregular oscillations, but the variance in these oscillations did not decrease as much over time. The autocorrelations associated with this trajectory remained positive for close to 120 lags. The Fourier transforms revealed the presence of many periodic components in the participant's judgments, a pattern suggestive of chaotic dynamics.

These results confirm the importance of characterizing the temporal patterns in people's judgments of one another. One could, of course, determine the average assessment of a target by collapsing across time. This approach, however, would fail to characterize the person's stream of thought as he or she considered the target. Such characterization may provide important information about the judgment process. It is conceivable, for example, that this approach would reveal a new taxonomy of social judgment reflecting identifiable patterns of intrinsic dynamics. Thus, depending on the setting of a number of factors (the characteristics of the judge, the judge's relationship to the target, the target's behavior, the context surrounding the judgment, etc.), the temporal pattern of judgment might correspond to a fixed-point attractor, periods of different frequencies, deterministic chaos, or randomness. The identification of such patterns, in turn, may prove essential to prediction of judgment in the future. Knowing that judgment has a periodic structure in a particular context, for example, enables one to predict that in similar contexts, a positive evaluation will likely be followed by a negative judgment. In short, variation in judgment over time is not simply noise obscuring a "true" signal, but rather represents the essence of the judgment process itself. On this view, thoughts unfold in accordance with temporal patterns that suggest the operation of an underlying dynamical system.

System Coherence and Intrinsic Dynamics

Research utilizing the mouse paradigm suggests that this approach provides a window into the structure of the system producing social judgment (Vallacher & Nowak, 1994c; Vallacher et al., 1994, 1998). A pair of studies by Vallacher et al. (1994), for instance, exposed the differential dynamics underlying evaluatively consistent (univalent) and inconsistent (mixed valence) representations in social judgment. In each study, participants read descriptions intended to generate positive, negative, or ambivalent feelings about someone they knew. To foster ambivalence, for example, we asked participants in one study to think about someone they liked a great deal and then imagine that this person had done something morally wrong (stealing money from a mutual friend).

Participants performed the mouse procedure while thinking about the target person, and subsequently completed self-report questions with respect to him or her. Each dynamic measure (variance in distance, etc.) was calculated separately for the first 40 seconds and the last 40 seconds of the mouse period, so that we could assess changes over time in the dynamic properties of their judgments. We also developed software (written in C++) to assess the dimensionality of the system generating participants' temporal trajectories, as determined by the Grassberger–Procaccia (1983) method (see, e.g., Skarda & Freeman, 1987). This method uses the time series of a single variable (in this case, distance) to reconstruct the original phase space and trajectories corresponding to the temporal evolution of a system (see Chapter 2). The algorithm determines the dimensionality of the attractor drawn by the trajectory and hence the dimensionality of the original phase space. Dimensionality of the phase space corresponds to the number of dynamical variables needed to describe the evolution of the system. Fractal dimension values indicate a chaotic system, whereas integer values indicate a nonchaotic (e.g., periodic) system (see Nowak & Lewenstein, 1994, for a more detailed description of this algorithm in the context of social psychology).

Dimension scores were calculated separately for the early and late periods.

Because evaluatively consistent representations (whether positive or negative) consist of elements that are well integrated, we expected that whatever temporal variation existed during the initial phases of judgment would dissipate over time, giving way to a stable evaluation of the target. The dimensionality of participants' judgments was also expected to decline over time, reflecting the elimination of whatever interelement inconsistencies characterized their initial feelings about the target. The value of their judgment, meanwhile, was expected to become more extreme over time, in line with research demonstrating polarization in judgments of stimuli for which one has an internally consistent representation (Tesser, 1978). Mixed valence representations, on the other hand, are unintegrated and thus are likely to promote sustained instability in judgment. We therefore expected participants in this condition to display relatively high temporal variation in their evaluation of the target that would not dissipate over the judgment period. The unintegrated nature of their judgments was expected to be reflected in relatively high dimensionality and the maintenance of judgmental complexity throughout the judgment period. Despite the volatility and complexity of their judgments, however, participants were not expected to show changes in their mean evaluation of the target from the beginning to the end of the judgment period.

Results provided support for the hypotheses. Thus, participants judging a positive target showed moderate initial volatility (as indexed by variance in distance, speed, and acceleration) but stabilized at a point close to the target by the end of the judgment period, indicating positive polarization. Participants judging a negative target, meanwhile, showed somewhat higher initial volatility and then stabilized at a point farther from the target, indicating negative polarization. Participants judging mixed valence targets displayed a considerably different temporal pattern. Their judgments displayed a high degree of volatility, and this turnover in thought persisted throughout the judgment period, with no signs of stabilization (reflecting the lack of a stable equilibrium for such targets). And unlike participants judging a positive or a negative target, those evaluating a mixed valence target did not demonstrate polarization—their mean evaluation of the target did not differ from the initial to the final judgment period. Finally, there was a loss of dimension over time for the positive and negative targets, but not for the mixed valence targets. Dimension values in all cases were less than 8, suggesting the operation of a low-dimensional system (Grassberger & Procaccia, 1983). Thus, social judgment was generated by a system whose temporal evolution may be described by a small number of variables.

These results suggest that social judgment displays qualitatively different temporal trajectories, depending on the internal coherence of the cognitive–affective system generating judgments. When the elements relevant to judgment have the same valence (whether positive or negative) and thus form a well-integrated system, the resultant judgments tend toward stability during their formation and maintain their stability once formed. This occurs because the feedback mechanisms among the elements promote increased coherence with each iteration of the judgment process. In consequence, the cognitive–affective system loses dimensionality and the global evaluation becomes more extreme. In contrast, when the elements of the system differ in their valence and form an initially unintegrated system, the resultant judgments reflect this lack of coherence. The judgment system displays variability in evaluation that does not diminish substantially over time. Because of this sustained volatility in evaluation, the evaluation does not converge on either a highly positive or highly negative value, but rather retains its original (moderate) value. The lack of integration in the system is reflected in the relatively high number of independent dimensions underlying judgment and the maintenance of this dimensionality throughout the judgment period.

These distinct temporal patterns have clear implications for how one should assess people's judgments of social stimuli (e.g., other people, themselves, social issues). When the target of judgment is associated with a well-integrated representation, it may be reasonable to measure evaluation in a traditional manner with self-report instruments, looking for changes in the mean value over time. However, when the target is associated with a poorly integrated representation, it may be considerably more informative to identify dynamic properties of the judgment and assess the fate of these properties over time. By simply looking at the endpoints of the judgment process (i.e., the initial and final states), one might conclude that the judgment was stable rather than dynamic, reflecting a compromise among the diverse elements rather than a pattern of movement between conflicting evaluative frames.[2]

Ambivalence in Social Judgment

Assessing the dynamic aspects of judgment is particularly useful in gaining insight into the nature of ambivalence. Although ambivalence is commonly considered to be an unpleasant state, particularly if extended for long periods of time, it may be a necessary precondition

for cognitive growth. Moment-to-moment variation in global evaluation of a social stimulus (e.g., a new acquaintance, a political figure,
an unusual event) represents a condition in which the cognitive system is not ready to settle down on a stable equilibrium (i.e., fixed-
point attractor) but rather samples different evaluative states. In effect, the judgment system does not possess sufficient integration to
produce a judgment that could serve as a basis for action. In this light,
the pattern of temporal change in judgment can be seen as reflecting a
succession of changing frames (Minsky, 1985) or schemata (Rumelhart & Ortony, 1977) within which existing information about a target is given provisional integration. In this sense, the present perspective provides an extension of the schema concept to patterns of temporal evolution in the global properties of judgment.

Temporal variation in evaluation may also be the most adaptive
way for new information to be absorbed and considered within different and sometimes conflicting frames of reference (Kelso & DeGuzman, 1991; Mandell & Selz, 1994; Skarda & Freeman, 1987). In other words, when people are uncertain, the mind might generate a succession of different Gestalts with which to integrate old as well as new
information, in a search for a dominant perspective that could serve as
a basis for judgment and possible action. If the various states can be
integrated, or if one of the states becomes locked in by some environmental influence (e.g., social feedback, new information), movement
between different evaluative states sets the stage for the evolution of a
representation that provides coherent and stable understanding.

STATIC VERSUS DYNAMIC INTEGRATION

Despite the potential for shifting evaluations inherent in the stream of
consciousness, there is a press to achieve an integrated judgment that
can provide a stable frame of reference for action (Vallacher, 1993).
This press for judgmental integration and stability is a basic feature of
social judgment, although it can vary in accordance with contextual
factors, such as time constraints, as well as personality variables, such
as need for closure (Webster & Kruglanski, 1994). Social judgment
can also vary in its subjective importance (e.g., Boninger, Krosnick, &
Berent, 1995); some judgments are of trivial concern, whereas others
may have monumental significance. There is reason to think that the
way in which the press for judgmental integration is satisfied depends
on the subjective importance of the judgment (Vallacher & Nowak,
1997; Vallacher et al., 1998). In particular, variation in importance
may play a critical role in determining whether judgment will display

diminishing temporal variation and attain *static integration* or instead display sustained temporal variation and attain what we call *dynamic integration*.

The Basis for Dynamic Integration

Static integration is likely when the judgment at issue is relatively unimportant to the judge. This occurs, for example, when the consequences of judgment are trivial or when the target lacks personal relevance for the judge. Under such conditions, different subsets of elements become activated over time, each associated with a particular valence. The greater the variability in the respective valences associated with the succession of subset configurations, the more pronounced the moment-to-moment variation in evaluation. Without a strong investment in the judgment, each judgmental state is relinquished upon activation of the succeeding subset of elements. Eventually, however, judgment begins to stabilize as the various states become integrated via some combinatorial rule, such as the algebraic weighting of information (Anderson, 1981; Ostrom et al., 1994). In phenomenological terms, the judge may be said to find a compromise that effectively balances the pros and cons associated with the target, perhaps by simply averaging the most salient pieces of information. The convergence on a fixed-point attractor for judgment captures the essence of static integration.

By way of contrast, consider the judgment scenario when the judgment is highly important for the judge. This occurs, for example, when the consequences of judgment are significant or when the target holds personal relevance for the judge. Importance has two key features that have implications for the manner in which information is integrated in the judgment process. Importance, first of all, tends to increase the press for judgmental integration (e.g., Webster & Kruglanski, 1994). This makes it likely that each activated subset of cognitive and affective elements in social judgment will give rise to a provisional higher order frame that provides integration for these elements. Second, higher order frames for important judgments tend to have a relatively narrow latitude of acceptance (Sherif & Hovland, 1961). Hence, if the elements in an activated subset are even somewhat diverse or evaluatively inconsistent, a single frame may not be sufficient to provide integration. Elements that cannot be integrated into a provisional frame become especially salient—and thus perhaps better remembered (Hastie, 1980)—and set the stage for the emergence of a new integrative frame. With successive activation of diverse subsets of cognitive and affective elements, then, a set of inter-

pretive frames are generated from the stream of thought, each supplanting the lower level elements that gave rise to it. In effect, judgment becomes detached from lower level information concerning the
target, reflecting instead a set of higher order cognitive units.

If the emergent higher order frames are sufficiently consistent or
otherwise easy to reconcile, they become progressively integrated into
yet higher order frames, eventually leading to a stable, integrated
judgment. In this case, judgment is generated in a manner similar to
that purported to occur for less important judgments (e.g., simple averaging of the valences associated with each frame). If, however, the
higher order frames have mutually conflicting valences or are otherwise irreconcilable, it may be impossible to maintain such frames in
mind at the same time, particularly if there is overlap in their respective elements. Intrinsic dynamics in this case are not limited to judgment formation, but rather represent an alternation among emergent
higher order frames that may be sustained for a considerable period of
time. As each frame assumes prepotence, it provides distinct integration for the respective lower level elements and hence may generate a
correspondingly distinct judgment. The movement between two (or
more) different attractors for judgment is referred to as dynamic integration.

Whereas static integration may be achieved via some combinatorial rule that allows lower level elements to be integrated with respect
to a stable judgment, dynamic integration is achieved through the al-
location of time for the prepotence of each of the conflicting higher
order judgment frames. Because higher order units of cognition are
not easily relinquished in favor of other units at the same level (Festinger, 1957; Vallacher & Wegner, 1985), it is possible for the oscillation among the emergent frames to be sustained over time (Miller,
1944). In effect, the judge cannot settle on a single interpretive
scheme, in much the same way that someone viewing a Necker cube
continuously alternates between conflicting figure–ground interpretations. Ironically, then, under conditions of conflicting information,
the more important the judgment, the less likely it is that stable integration will be attained. Of course, at some point even conflicting
frames can give rise to static integration. Judgments provide the basis
for decisions and courses of action, and in the face of such pressures
for integration, vacillation among conflicting frames will eventually
cease. When this occurs, stable integration may be achieved by the ascendance of one interpretive frame at the expense of the other (or
others). Judgment here does not reflect a compromise between different evaluative states, but rather becomes linked to the most prepotent
higher order frame.

These two modes of integration are interesting to consider in light of an ongoing debate concerning the nature of person perception and social judgment (Eiser, 1990; Hastorf, Schneider, & Zebrowitz, 1977; Zebrowitz, 1990). The issue essentially is whether a global judgment represents a linear combination of relevant information (e.g., Anderson, 1981) or instead represents a configuration of information that cannot be decomposed into separate additive components (e.g., Asch, 1946). From a dynamical systems point of view, this issue can be reframed in terms of linearity versus nonlinearity in information integration. Static integration clearly falls in the linear camp, in that the process represents some linear combination of elements. Thus, elements may easily compensate for one another, the grouping of elements does not affect the resultant judgment, and such nonlinear phenomena as chaos are impossible. The model of information integration proposed by Anderson (1981) provides a well-documented exemplar of linearity in social judgment and may provide the underpinnings for static integration. Dynamic integration, on the other hand, clearly belongs to the nonlinear domain of models. Here, the resultant judgment is not a linear combination of individual elements, the meaning of each element depends on the other elements with which it is grouped, and complex dynamical phenomena are possible. In social psychology, an early appreciation of the dynamic nature of social judgment was provided by Asch's (1946) work on impression formation.

It is not necessary to declare a winner in this debate. Both linearity (static integration) and nonlinearity (dynamic integration) provide adequate characterizations of social judgment under different circumstances. Each mode of integration has counterparts in prominent models of social judgment. As already noted, the static integration of information associated with unimportant or uninvolving judgments may conform to a weighted averaging model (Anderson, 1981), although there are other models emphasizing different algebraic weighting of information (Ostrom et al., 1994). Dynamic integration, in turn, is reminiscent of the Gestalt perspective on perception and judgment, as epitomized by the classic configurational model proposed by Asch (1946). Various features of dynamic integration can be found in other research traditions as well. The oscillation among conflicting integrative frames, for example, has counterparts in the deliberative phase of decision making (e.g., Gollwitzer, 1990, 1996; Jones & Gerard, 1967; Kaplowitz & Fink, 1992). Postchoice dissonance reduction can also be viewed as oscillation between conflicting interpretive frames, prior to stabilization on a single frame. The detachment of higher level frames from lower level elements, meanwhile, is consistent with work showing the persistence of beliefs even after the informational base for these beliefs has been discredited (e.g., Ross, Lepper, Strack, & Steinmetz, 1977; Wegner et al., 1985).

Finally, the idea that dynamic integration promotes the ascendance of one higher order frame at the expense of others is consistent with the potential for catastrophic change in attitudes, as proposed by Latané and Nowak (1994). In this model, attitudes on unimportant issues are typically distributed normally, whereas attitudes on personally important issues tend to be bimodal, with the midpoint of the scale being psychologically unavailable. This suggests that achieving stable integration for personally important judgments involves choosing between conflicting interpretations rather than finding an intermediate position representing the weighting of irreconcilable perspectives. This possibility is also consistent with depictions of successful dissonance reduction and of thought-induced polarization of attitudes (Tesser, 1978). In both of these models, the respective effects are observed only when the judgment is important by some criterion. Research on the preconditions for dissonance has established that the inconsistent action must be freely chosen and associated with significant consequences (Wicklund & Brehm, 1976). Research in the polarization paradigm, in turn, has revealed that the object or topic being evaluated must be schematic (i.e., personally important) in order for extremification of valence to occur (e.g., Liberman & Chaiken, 1991; Tesser & Leone, 1977).

Dynamic Integration and Stereotypes

Stereotypical thinking is not as simple as it seems. On the surface, maintaining a stereotyped view seems easy enough. One simply applies a sweeping generalization to everyone that fits a certain category, whether it reflects race, ethnicity, gender, occupation, social status, age, country of origin, or some other basis for dividing up humanity (Allport, 1954). The maintenance of such generalizations requires the suppression of within-group variance (e.g., Linville, Fischer, & Salovey, 1989; Quattrone, 1986), however, and this is where things become more tricky for the person. Unless the person manages somehow to avoid exposure to information that undermines the stereotype (e.g., by avoiding contact with members of the stereotyped group), he or she must engage in a host of cognitive mechanisms to persist in his or her global assessments. Upon learning that a young African American male from an inner city has performed a noble deed requiring self-sacrifice, for example, a confirmed racist must find ways of explaining away the act, discounting its importance, or convincing him- or herself that it was simply the "exception that proves the rule." Ironically, then, it is the very simplemindedness of stereotypical judgments that creates the potential for complex intrinsic dynamics in thinking about members of stereotyped groups.

With the advent in the 20th century of mass communication and technology enabling the rapid, far-ranging spread of information, the difficulty of maintaining simple stereotypes has become correspondingly magnified. For every Willie Horton, there is an equally salient Bill Cosby or Thurgood Marshall brought to everyone's attention through information technology. Despite the availability of various biases and other cognitive mechanisms to support people's preconceived notions (e.g., Bodenhausen, 1990; Duncan, 1976; Hamilton & Trolier, 1986), such evidence of within-group heterogeneity would seem to pose serious problems for stereotypical judgments. In an information-rich age, one might expect stereotypes to crumble altogether or at least undergo constant modification to accommodate new information. Even if a person had a negative stereotype about a particular social group, he or she might be expected to adjust his or her preconceptions to take into account inconsistent information that is not easily reinterpreted or discounted. Upon learning that an African American male has done a noble deed, for example, someone with an unflattering image of people in this social category should modify his or her overall assessment in a positive direction. Static integration of this kind may in fact be the mode of judgment when assessing the actions of others who fit psychologically unimportant categories. People who are not particularly wedded to racial stereotypes, for instance, may reach a judgment about an African American male that represents a weighted average of new and old information. The aforementioned person performing the noble deed thus might be judged less positively than a white male performing the same act, but more positively than an African American male about whom nothing is learned.

This scenario, however, may fail to capture the dynamics at work for personally relevant or otherwise important judgments. Category-based judgments represent an essential feature of social thinking for everyone (Fiske & Taylor, 1991) and the reliance on categories such as race and gender remains strong for many people in contemporary society (Dovidio & Gaertner, 1986). Assuming the sustained prepotence and importance of such categories in judgment, one might expect to observe dynamic rather than static integration when investigating people's response to information that is not easily assimilated to a stereotyped view. As the person considers incongruent information, the seeds of an alternative evaluative frame for accommodating the information may be established (e.g., Kunda & Oleson, 1995; Rothbart & Lewis, 1988; Weber & Crocker, 1983). Initially, the person may judge the person in terms of the stereotype but do so with considerable turnover in thoughts and feelings as the conflicting information vies for prepotence with the stereotype. Over time, the person may begin to reframe the inconsistent information in a qualitatively different manner, thereby providing an alternative basis for judgment. Because conflicting frames are not averaged for personally important judgments, the person's mode of integration involves oscillating between the two frames rather than combining them in some fashion.

It is interesting to consider the work on "modern racism" (e.g., McConahay, 1983, 1986) in terms of dynamic integration. According to this idea, people in contemporary society have both positive and negative attitudes toward members of racial and ethnic groups, either set of which can be activated at different times or under different circumstances. This enables people to accommodate the heterogeneity within a given group and yet maintain highly valenced attitudes and opinions regarding the group as a whole. This suggests that exposure to diverse information regarding a group does not promote averaging to achieve a single (and relatively neutral) perspective on the group. Rather, in line with dynamic integration, opposing frames are established that provide integration for separate sets of information and considerations. On this view, contemporary stereotypes are often characterized by a diversity of thoughts and feelings that are segregated into internally homogeneous perspectives, each of which can be prepotent under certain conditions (e.g., Lepore & Brown, 1997; Macrae, Bodenhausen, & Milne, 1995; McConahay, 1986; Wittenbrink et al., 1997). Presumably, when cues favoring one perspective over another are lacking, the person's judgment will display intrinsic dynamics reflecting alternation among the competing frames.

The extension of dynamic integration to issues in stereotyping was investigated by Sussman, Vallacher, Nowak, and Wade (1997). At an initial session, white college students of both sexes completed a questionnaire assessing the extent to which they had conflicting perspectives on issues of race in American society. Each of the 20 items in this questionnaire presented a statement describing a racially relevant social issue (e.g., affirmative action, the fairness of the legal system, individual vs. societal responsibility for poverty). Participants used a 7-point scale to indicate the extent to which they had *very mixed feelings* versus *not at all mixed feelings* regarding each issue. Responses to these items were averaged to create an index of racial ambivalence. Several days later, the students returned individually to participate in the experiment. They were asked to think about a college-aged male (William), who committed either an admirable act (returning a wallet full of money to its owner) or a morally reprehensible act (stealing money from someone and never confessing to anyone). For half the participants, William was a 24-year-old white male; for the remainder, William was a 24-year-old black male.

Participants then indicated their moment-to-moment feelings about William by means of the mouse procedure (Vallacher & Nowak, 1994c). They used the computer mouse to adjust the position of the cursor in relation to a small circle representing William. The closer they positioned the cursor to the circle, the more positive their current feeling about William. The absolute distance from the circle was assessed 10 times per second over a 2-minute interval. We divided the judgment period into three 40-second intervals, and for each we calculated the average distance, the variance in distance, the average speed of mouse movements, the average acceleration (change in speed) of mouse movements, and the amount of time without mouse movements (time at rest). The distance measure provided an index of global evaluation, while the variance, speed, acceleration, and time at rest measures provided indices of judgmental volatility. By tracking these variables over time, we could assess changes in evaluation and dynamism and the emergence of new frames for integrating the information provided.

Results revealed interesting temporal patterns consistent with the distinction between static and dynamic integration. For evaluation (average distance from the target circle), there was a behavior valence effect, such that negative as opposed to positive behavior by either target generated relatively negative evaluation. For the measures of dynamism, however, results revealed a change over time suggesting the increased salience of stereotype-based expectancies. Figure 3.3 presents the results for variance in distance during the first and third time periods for each combination of target and behavior. During the first 40 seconds, there was only a behavior valence effect, such that negative as opposed to positive behavior by either target generated relatively high volatility in judgment, with movement among different evaluative states (distances from the target circle). By the third (final) 40-second period, however, dynamism reflected the interaction of race and behavior. For the white target, dynamism was greater if he acted negatively as opposed to positively. The opposite was observed for the black target: dynamism was greater if he acted positively (returning a wallet) than if he acted negatively (stealing money). Note that the two cases associated with dynamism at the end of the judgment period were those that represent stereotype inconsistency

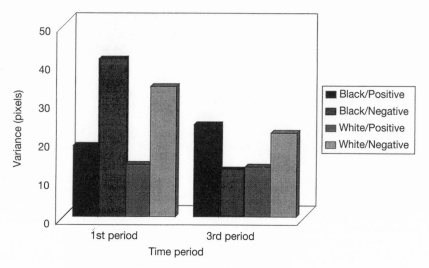

FIGURE 3.3. Variance in evaluation by race and behavior.

for white judges: criminal behavior on the part of a young white male and moral behavior on the part of a young black male.

Apparently, participants' initial focus on the behavior broadened to consider the behavior in light of expectancies for the target's social category. Behavior consistent with these expectancies promoted static integration and hence little sustained dynamism, whereas behavior inconsistent with expectancies served to destabilize participants' judgments. Looking only at the distance measure, one would conclude that only behavior mattered: Distance was greater for the negative act than for the positive act at both the beginning and final periods of the judgment task. But the behavior was also judged in terms of its fit with existing stereotypes. Behavior that could not easily be assimilated to a stereotype spawned moment-to-moment volatility in judgment, as conflicting frames vied for prepotence, with neither one capable of providing a stable equilibrium in evaluation. Had participants been asked only to provide an overall judgment, we would have concluded that they had disregarded race and judged the person only on the quality of his deeds. This summary assessment, however, belied the experience of judgmental volatility when the behavior was inconsistent with stereotypical expectations.

This interpretation is supported by the results of correlational analyses involving the measure of racial ambivalence. During the first 40-second period, scores on this measure were not associated with evaluation (distance) or any of the dynamic measures. By the final 40-second period, however, racial ambivalence was reliably correlated with judgmental dynamism. Compared to participants who scored as nonambivalent, those with mixed feelings regarding racially relevant social issues displayed greater variability in evaluation (variance in distance) and less stability (time at rest) when evaluating positive behavior on the part of the black target. For these participants especially, a simple consideration of the behavior in question gave way to considerations reflecting conflicting perspectives regarding race and behavior.

Models of Dynamic Integration

It is possible to state more formally the conditions under which static versus dynamic integration is likely to be observed (Vallacher & Nowak, 1997). Two control parameters are crucial in this model: the evaluative consistency versus inconsistency of the elements to be integrated and the personal importance of the judgment. As noted earlier, evaluative inconsistency is a precondition for dynamic integration—in the absence of inconsistency, static integration is to be expected regardless of the judgment's importance. The role of importance is to establish the threshold of inconsistency for changing integration from the static to the dynamic mode. When importance is relatively low (e.g., when the target of judgment has little significance for the judge), the threshold is relatively high, so that even fairly diverse elements are likely to be integrated with respect to a single higher level frame. With enhanced importance (e.g., when the target can affect the judge's outcomes), the threshold is correspondingly lower, so that even moderate inconsistency can promote the emergence of irreconcilable higher order frames. In summary, the same degree of inconsistency can promote either static or dynamic integration depending on factors that influence the importance of the judgment to the judge.

Both evaluative consistency and manifestations of judgment importance (e.g., personal involvement, self-relevance, vested interests, etc.) are recognized as crucial in the formation and maintenance of social judgments (Fiske & Taylor, 1991). For its part, inconsistent information has been shown to trigger a host of mechanisms aimed at restoring cognitive and affective consistency (Abelson et al., 1968). The importance of the judgment, meanwhile, has been shown to affect the manner in which relevant information is processed (Chaiken, 1980; Petty & Cacioppo, 1986). Generally speaking, information relevant to important judgments is said to be processed in a systematic manner involving controlled processes, whereas information relevant to less important judgments is said to be processed to in a heuristic manner involving peripheral or automatic mechanisms. These variables are thus not novel to judgmental phenomena, and they are certainly not unique to the present model. The dynamical consequences of these variables, however, have yet to be explored. It is not clear, then, how the established mechanisms associated with evaluative consistency versus inconsistency and judgmental importance relate to dynamical patterns of global judgment.

In static integration, the system has a single equilibrium that corresponds to the weighted average of the valences associated with the elements forming the judgment. This equilibrium may drift as new elements come into play. In dynamic integration, there are two (or more) equilibria, each corresponding to a respective integrative frame, and the system moves between these equilibria. The time spent in each equilibrium is proportional to the strength or stability of the equilibrium. The transition between static and dynamic integration can be represented as a pitchfork bifurcation, where a single attractor becomes unstable and divides into two new attractors (see Figure 3.4). The dotted line shows the unstable equilibrium (i.e., the repellor) to which the original equilibrium changed. Figure 3.5 shows the energy surface corresponding to this scenario. The system's dynamics may be visualized as a ball rolling down the energy surface. A single energy minimum changes into two gradually divergent minima with change in the control parameter's value. Eventually, with continued change in the control parameter, each attractor becomes more stable and the attractors are better separated. At some point, the frequency of switching should decrease, and the system should settle on one of the attractors.

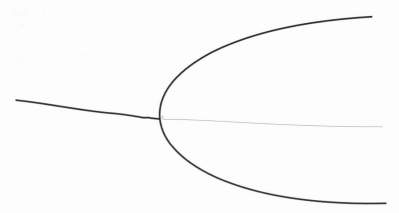

FIGURE 3.4. Pitchfork bifurcation.

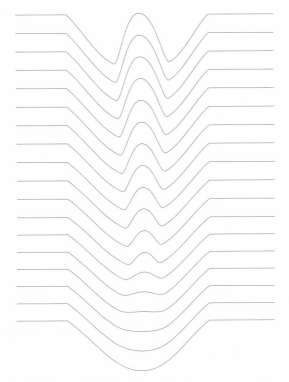

FIGURE 3.5. Energy landscape for dynamic integration.

In the case of static integration, the final state of the system is determined by a weighted average of the evaluative components and thus is highly predictable. In the case of dynamic integration, however, prediction of the final state of the system is more complex and less predictable. After a period of instability, a stable judgment may well emerge, but its value may be difficult to anticipate. The judgment may represent a yet higher order integrative frame that resolves the conflict between the two existing frames, or it may simply represent the prepotence of one frame at the expense of the other. In the latter case, items of information contained in the rejected frame will not influence the judgment, unless these elements are also contained in the prepotent frame. Random or unpredictable factors may dictate which frame is ultimately adopted, making it difficult to predict not only the final state of the system but also which elements will be rejected in service of integration. In this case, the final value of a judgment may have to some degree the characteristic of a "frozen accident" (Gell-Mann, 1994). The person may seek out and interact with others, for example, in order to determine the validity of each integrative frame. Whoever happens to be the interaction partner at the critical moment for social influence may serve to lock in one of the frames as the judgment for the person.

Prediction for final evaluation in the dynamic integration mode is complicated further by the potential for any element of information to have different values. The same element may enter into both configurations, and in each of them it may have a different meaning and value, which is determined by other elements in the configuration (Asch, 1946). Information suggesting that the target is intelligent is likely to have a positive value when it is considered in the context of other information suggesting that the target is warm and trustworthy, for instance, but it is likely to have a negative value in the context of information suggesting that the target is cold and manipulative. For the system as a whole, then, the consistency versus inconsistency of any element of information will depend on which integrative frame is currently prepotent—an element that is highly consistent with one frame may well be inconsistent with the other frame. Because the prepotence of these frames changes over time, the degree of conflict associated with each element necessarily shows temporal dependency as well. This means that no information is likely to be permanently suppressed in a system characterized by dynamic integration.

The logic of this model suggests that the judgment system may achieve considerable stability under both low and high levels of importance, but the nature of this stability will be markedly different for these two values of the control parameter. For unimportant judgments, the system's stability is due to its ability to absorb incoming information and adjust its equilibrium accordingly. For highly important judgments, on the other hand, the system's stability is due to the strength of the attractor that ultimately provides integration. Even if inconsistent information is subsequently encountered or retrieved from memory, it is likely to be rejected and thus will not adjust the system's equilibrium. Only when the accumulated weight of such information reaches a critical value will it destabilize the system's equilibrium, producing a rapid shift to one of the other attractors for the system. In this case, the evolution of the system will follow a catastrophe model and display hysteresis (see Latané & Nowak, 1994).

As noted, this depiction of dynamic integration corresponds to a pitchfork bifurcation, in which one stable attractor develops into two stable attractors, which then diverge. There is nothing inside the system that makes the movement between the two attractors inevitable. Rather, the movement is caused by incoming or retrieved information or by such factors as mood, stress, distraction, priming, or introspection. It is possible, however, to envision a very different model of dynamic integration in which the observed dynamism is intrinsic to the system, corresponding to a periodic or chaotic attractor. For a judgment that evolves with period 2, for instance, there is regular switching between two values, neither of which has any degree of stability. Quite the opposite in fact—adopting one frame immediately produces movement to the other frame. It is unclear at this point whether dynamic integration represents movement between two stable attractors or whether it corresponds instead to evolution on a periodic attractor. The resolution of this issue may prove to be important, since different psychological mechanisms may underlie these contrasting models.[3] Regardless of which model ultimately provides the best fit to social judgment data, however, the fundamental features of the process are the same. When faced with an important judgment task and inconsistent information relevant to this task, an individual is likely to develop alternative frames for integrating this information. As these frames vie for prepotence, the individual will move between them and render correspondingly different judgments at different times.

JUDGMENT DYNAMISM IN PERSPECTIVE

Like dynamical systems in other areas of science, social judgment can be described in terms of multiple lower level elements (thoughts, memories, images) that interact in some fashion (e.g., averaging, spreading activation, and inhibition) to produce macrolevel behavior (e.g., evaluation). Dynamical systems also commonly display internally generated changes over time in their macrolevel behavior, and there is reason to think that social judgment fits this criterion as well. Within the mouse paradigm, changes in evaluation—the proposed macrolevel behavior for social judgment—can be characterized in the same manner that the changes in any dynamical system's behavior can be characterized (e.g., speed, periodicity, proximity to an equilibrium state, dimensionality). These properties, moreover, have been shown to vary in accordance with principles at work in a wide variety of dynamical systems (e.g., the dampening of dynamics in the vicinity of an equilibrium state).

In the research to date, we have limited our focus to very basic properties of temporal dynamics (e.g., rate of change in evaluation). A wide variety of other tools and methods are available for analyzing the properties of dynamical systems, however, many of which may have application to psychological data (Nowak & Lewenstein, 1994), including the type of data obtained within the mouse paradigm. In addition to assessing the dimensionality of judgment with the Grassberger–Procaccia (1983) algorithm, it is possible to identify temporal patterns through coherent state analysis and Fourier analysis (Schroeck, 1994), to test for determinism with an algorithm developed by Kaplan and Glass (1992), and to assess the complexity of temporal trajectories with measures of topological and metric entropy (Mandell & Selz, 1994). An overview of these and other relevant methods is provided in Chapter 2. Their application to social judgment data is a priority for future research.

It is encouraging in this regard that several lines of research have begun to emphasize and assess dynamism in social judgment. Perhaps the most noteworthy approach is the attempt to model social cognitive dynamics within a connectionist or neural network framework (e.g., Eiser, 1994a; Kunda & Thagard, 1996; Read et al., 1997; Shultz & Lepper, 1996; Smith, 1996). As noted in Chapter 1, connectionist models are defined in terms of nodes (corresponding to neurons) and connections (corresponding to synapses). With respect to social judgment, nodes represent the features of an object or event and connections represent relationships between these features.[4] The connections are established in the process of learning and can assume either positive (excitatory) or negative (inhibitory) values. Presenting a stimulus to a network is equivalent to selectively activating those nodes that correspond to features inherent in the stimulus. In the process of recognition (or reasoning), nodes change their level of activation depending on the total input received from other nodes. An input from an activated node along an excitatory connection contributes to activation, whereas an input from an activated node along a negative connection has an inhibitory effect. Such networks are multistable, in that they tend to stabilize on one of many network configurations, each of which corresponds to a unique cognitive representation. Beyond its ability to explain a multitude of specific empirical data concerning social judgment (see, e.g., Smith, 1996), this approach allows one to capture in precise ways a set of important concepts stemming from the early dynamic period of social psychology, as described in Chapter 1. Thus, such notions as emergence, pattern formation, balance, and forces toward equilibrium play a central role in this line of research, as do more contemporary concepts such as schema, cognitive consistency, and priming.

Models of decision making have also been considered from a dynamical perspective. Kaplowitz and Fink (1992), for example, have used a computer mouse to observe how people decide between two courses of action. The two alternatives are represented as points at different positions on the screen, and participants are asked to move the mouse toward the alternative they favor at the moment. Following Newtonian assumptions, arguments for a particular decision may be modeled as forces pulling the decision in the direction of that decision, whereas arguments against the decision are modeled as forces pushing the decision away from that decision. The process of decision-making is analogous to the dampening motion of a pendulum in the presence of friction. As one set of arguments is given greater consideration, the system overshoots its equilibrium, so that the second spring pulls stronger. If no new information enters the system, the oscillations become increasingly smaller and the system settles on an equilibrium. In a somewhat more complex theory of decision-making dynamics (Busemeyer & Townsend, 1993), the outcomes of each decision are represented as sets of consequences. For instance, the decision to locate a factory in a particular region has consequences for the region's economy, the environment, health hazards, employment, esthetic effects, and so forth. The momentary value of the decision is achieved by multiplying the evaluative value of each aspect by some weight and summing these weighted values. Those weights are not constant, but rather reflect the amount of attention given to each aspect at a given moment in time. As the salience of each aspect changes due to changes in attention, so does the resultant evaluation.

An emphasis on dynamics is also reflected in models emphasizing the narrative nature of social thought (e.g., Zukier, 1986, 1990). In this view, representations of social objects and events are not static schemata or categories, but rather correspond to stories that unfold in time. Well-defined regularities can be discerned in a given story. Thus, there may be a happy solution after a period of suspense or a near catastrophe, or conversely, everything may collapse for a person just when things begin to look optimistic. This perspective on social judgment is consistent with research on jury deliberations (Hastie, Penrod, & Pennington, 1983). The outcome of such deliberations does not reflect a logical weighting of arguments but rather competition between the respective stories provided by the prosecution and defense. It is interesting to consider certain high-profile court cases (e.g., the O. J. Simpson criminal and civil trials) in these terms.

A focus on the dynamics of social judgment cannot substitute for more traditional approaches emphasizing content and meaning. In exploring likely order parameters (such as evaluation and static vs. dynamic interaction), one gains insight into the intrinsic dynamics and structural complexity of a social judgment system, but in doing so, one necessarily sacrifices information about the content of specific cognitive elements. On the other hand, a focus on the temporal sequence of specific elements of thought (e.g., memories of traumatic events) is appropriate for highlighting idiosyncratic features of mental content and process (e.g., Pope & Singer, 1978; Uleman & Bargh, 1989), but this very idiosyncrasy may pose problems for establishing general rules governing the social judgment system. To provide a complete characterization of social judgment, then, approaches emphasizing dynamics and those emphasizing content are both essential and should be considered complementary.

The dynamical systems perspective provides an extremely rich set of heuristics and has gone far toward integrating a host of diverse topics in science in terms of a coherent set of principles. We suspect that this perspective will serve a similar function for the various domains of social judgment. Approaches that track the evolution of social judgment on various time scales, for example, could be extended to topics beyond those discussed in the present chapter, including such basic phenomena as attitude formation, moral judgment, action identification, and causal attribution. Beyond establishing new insights into the mental dynamics associated with each of these phenomena, research of this kind might also establish basic commonalties among them (e.g., the dynamics associated with transitions from one state to another). In short, the investigation of different phenomena from an explicitly dynamical perspective provides a means of identifying both what is unique about each and what is invariant across them and thus representative of social thinking generally.

NOTES

1. Note that this holds only for a specific set of values of control parameters. If the control parameters change in value, then the temporal pattern of dynamics may be dramatically different. Even if the control parameters do not change in value, prediction of the future states of the system requires knowledge of all relevant order parameters. Although evaluation is a likely order parameter of social judgment, there may well be others that are necessary for full description of the system. Such integrative factors as activity and potency (Osgood et al., 1957), for example, may be needed to provide complete description of the social judgment system at any point in time and thus allow for prediction of the system's future state. Thus, a characterization of an object as highly positive but relatively weak will lead to a different subsequent judgment than will a characterization reflecting both high evaluation and high potency.

2. We should note that the two studies reported by Vallacher et al. (1994) employed slightly different procedures. In the first study, mouse movement in any direction was displayed on the screen and recorded for subsequent analyses. In the second study, movement was constrained to a hori-

zontal axis extending from the target circle to the edge of the screen corresponding to subjects' dominant hand. Only the horizontal component of movement was displayed on the screen and any vertical movement left the position of the cursor unchanged (except for any associated horizontal movement). The results associated with each procedure showed the same pattern of effects, although there were indications that constraining subjects to the horizontal axis tended to reduce the complexity and dynamism of their judgments. We therefore conducted a subsequent study that directly compared the results obtained with these procedures in a common experimental design (Kaufman, Vallacher, & Nowak, 1993).

The results revealed that the unconstrained procedure produced greater dynamics (e.g., more variation in distance, higher acceleration) than the constrained procedure when judging mixed valence targets. We also found that the dynamic measures were correlated more strongly with relevant self-report measures among subjects using the unconstrained as opposed to the horizontally constrained procedure. For example, acceleration, which reflects instability in evaluation, was highly correlated with both self-reported uncertainty and ambivalence in the unconstrained condition, but only marginally correlated with these measures in the constrained condition. These data suggest that allowing subjects unconstrained movement provides better access to their moment-to-moment feelings. Perhaps asking subjects to restrict mouse movements to a single dimension introduces a theoretically irrelevant controlled process into the situation and thus disrupts the spontaneous flow of judgment.

3. With respect to perception, there is evidence that the model assuming the existence of two stable attractors better accounts for switching between different interpretations of visual stimuli (Hock et al., 1997).

4. This interpretation applies to models in which localist representations are assumed and thus is closely related to models of associative networks. In many connectionist models, only patterns of activation across all the neurons may be meaningfully represented, and single neurons have no semantic representation.

4

⮎

Mental Dynamics in Action

IN PSYCHOLOGY, BEHAVIOR HAS provided the primary focus for theory and research fashioned within a dynamical systems perspective (e.g., Beek & Hopkins, 1992; Newtson, 1994; Saltzman & Kelso, 1987; Turvey, 1990). There is good reason for this. No aspect of human experience lends itself so readily to direct and quantifiable observation as behavior. Thoughts and feelings may well be inherently dynamic, but characterizing these phenomena in dynamic terms requires special techniques and tools that ultimately require an article of faith on the part of investigators. Behavior, on the other hand, can be defined objectively in terms of geometric coordinates, effort expenditure, and time. The dynamic approach to behavior has proven highly successful, generating rich insights into the microstructure of individual acts, the self-organization of limb movements to produce coordinated action, and the patterns of movement that define the interaction between two or more individuals (see Kelso et al., 1991; Newtson et al., 1987; Rosenblum & Turvey, 1988; Schmidt et al., 1991).

Despite the readily quantifiable nature of behavior, and although behavior is said to be the ultimate concern of theory and research, social psychology rarely focuses on "mere behavior," preferring instead to concentrate on the somewhat more abstract notion of "action" (see Wegner & Vallacher, 1987). The thinking here is that the things people do cannot be understood apart from the mental underpinnings that give rise to overt behavior. In this view, in fact, people's physical movements are not only secondary but also ultimately misleading because of the equifinality or functional equivalence of goal-directed action. Thus, when people help or harm others, conform to majority opinion, or obey legitimate authority, the physical means by which these broad actions are performed are immaterial. Indeed, the use of operational definitions in social psychological research essentially guarantees that the important categories of human action are decoupled from issues of motor control, interlimb coordination, patterns of movement, and so on. In investigating obedience to authority, after all, one is hardly interested in the dynamics of toggle pushing, nor does research on altruism concern itself with the physical movements involved in sharing pennies or picking up objects from a broken shopping bag.

With social psychology's emphasis on abstract behavioral categories, mental processes are understandably accorded considerable importance, seemingly in direct proportion to the loss of concern with how these categories are physically instantiated. It is as though the processes of movement were of a different realm than the processes of mind, with each conforming to fundamentally different mechanisms. The dynamical systems perspective challenges the logic of this implicit dualism. A primary value of this approach is its emphasis on basic principles that transcend not only topical boundaries, but also levels of analysis. In principle, then, the dynamics of movement coordination may have much in common with the dynamics of categorically defined action, despite the substantial gulf separating the level of limbs and the level of minds. Both levels of analysis can be understood in terms of the mutual influence among basic elements, the emergence of macrolevel behavior from such influences, and the reciprocal causality between macro- and microproperties of the system.

This perspective on human action provides the point of departure for this chapter. We suggest that mind and behavior together form a system, with feedback loops linking these levels of human function. This system, like any other dynamical system, is self-organizing, with increasingly higher order representations of behavior (e.g., plans and goals) developing from the interplay of lower level representations (e.g., representations of movement). Once higher order representations emerge, they come to control the lower level elements from which they developed, thus lending stability and direction to behavior. Although the reciprocal feedback between different levels of action representation promotes reasonably effective mind–action coordination, a variety of factors can introduce dysfunction into the system. We discuss possible sources of such faulty coordination and the role of emotion in signaling the overall coherence of the mind–action system. In a concluding section, we suggest how the dynamical perspective provides a new way to classify the basic forms of human action.

THE SELF-ORGANIZATION OF ACTION

Models of human action all agree that action is organized hierarchically (see Carver & Scheier, 1999; Gallistel, 1980; Goldman, 1970; Newtson, 1973; Powers, 1973; Schank & Abelson, 1977; Vallacher & Wegner, 1985). Essentially, this means that anything a person does can be broken down into increasingly smaller elements—or built up into increasingly larger units. The elements at each level provide integration for those at the next lower level, so that the hierarchy is functional as well as simply structural. In cleaning the house, for instance, one does several things at a lower level, such as vacuuming the floors, taking out the trash, and discretely moving a lamp to hide a glass stain. Each of these seemingly basic aspects of the action is itself superordinate to yet more basic elements; vacuuming, for instance, involves moving the vacuum back and forth, progressing across the room, and so on. The hierarchy can also be extended in the other direction. The superordinate action of cleaning the house may be but one action element with respect to any number of yet higher level units of action, such as preparing for company, setting an example for the kids, or getting the house in shape to sell. In dynamical terms, the hierarchical organization of action reflects a hierarchy of systems, in which an action system at one level effectively becomes an element in a higher level system.

The Emergence Process

Perhaps the model of human action that comes closest to casting the hierarchical nature of action in dynamical terms is the theory of action identification proposed by Vallacher and Wegner (1985). This theory holds that actions do not have fixed meanings, but rather can be mentally represented or identified in many different ways. Even something as seemingly straightforward as "turning on the lights," for example, can be identified as "providing illumination," "causing people to squint," "preparing for an activity," or "using up electricity," depending on the context in which the act occurs. The available identities for a given action differ to a large extent with respect to their level in an overall act-identity structure for the action. Thus, "turning on the lights" can be identified in lower level terms as "flipping a switch," which in turn can be identified in yet more basic terms as "moving a finger," and so on. Moving in the other direction, "turning on the lights" can be identified in terms of the higher level identities noted earlier ("causing people to squint," etc.), and these in turn can be seen as basic elements for even higher level identities (e.g., "getting people angry").

Whenever more than one identity is available for representing and guiding one's action, there is a tendency to prefer the identity that provides the most comprehensive and meaningful depiction of what one is doing (or has done). This means that higher level identities are likely to assume prepotence at the expense of lower level, more mechanical identities. In "turning on the lights," for instance, the person may be inclined to think of this act in terms of its effects or consequences, such as "causing people to squint" or "preparing for an activity," rather than as simply "flipping a switch"—or "turning on the lights," for that matter. This preference for higher level identities, because of the more comprehensive understanding they provide, is reminiscent of pattern generation in Gestalt psychology (e.g., Köhler, 1947). In looking at a visual display, for example, people tend to identify patterns and overlook the perceptual elements upon which the patterns are based. And as in Gestalt psychology, it is possible for the same basic elements, that is, the same lower level identities, to become organized into qualitatively different higher level patterns, and for different sets of elements to be identified in terms of the same higher level pattern. The meaning of action, in other words, does not reflect a linear combination of basic action elements, but rather a Gestalt-like configuration of such elements.

In this view, the lower level identities of an action may change without any corresponding change in the action's higher level identity. Whether one flips a switch with one's hand or one's elbow—or whether one uses a clapper rather than a switch—one is still turning on the lights. By the same token, when the meaning of action undergoes change, this does not necessarily mean that the underlying lower level identities have changed at all. Thus, one may perform the same physical movements on two occasions and come away with vastly different notions of what one has done. People in a low-level state, in fact, are highly vulnerable to alternative meanings for what they are doing or have done. The tendency to re-identify one's action so as to provide more integrative understanding is referred to as the *emergence process*. Research has shown that people in a low level state display heightened sensitivity to cues to higher level identities in the action context, even when these identities have a seemingly arbitrary connection to the lower level elements (Vallacher, 1993). When people focus on the details of their behavior in social interaction, for example, they tend to accept whatever feedback they receive regarding their trait-like qualities in social settings (Wegner, Vallacher, Kiersted, & Dizadji, 1986).

Intrinsic Dynamics of Action Emergence

Research on the emergence process typically provides the higher level identities with which participants can integrate their lower level identities in service of comprehensive understanding. This tack reflects the reasonable assumption that salient cues to higher level meaning are common in everyday contexts. However, one can envision circumstances in which such cues are lacking or perhaps mutually contradictory, thus requiring people to generate their own higher level identities for their behavior. When engaged in a conversation with a new acquaintance, for instance, it may be difficult to discern whether one is coming across as charming or flippant, constructive or critical, interesting or self-absorbed. All one knows for sure is that one is talking, gesturing, maintaining eye contact, and so forth. Lacking clear avenues of action emergence, people are left to their own devices to generate higher level meaning for their behavior.

Because the same set of lower level identities can be reidentified with respect to quite different meanings and implications, the emergence process in this case may be characterized by the generation of several potential higher level identities for the act in question. Each of these high level identities represents the self-organization of lower level identities. If these high-level identities are not easily reconciled and compete for prepotence, people will demonstrate dynamic as opposed to static integration in their mental representation of their behavior. The oscillation between the conflicting high-level frames should be relatively short-lived, however, because of the press toward a single frame for action. At this point, one of the higher level identities, or perhaps some integration of two or more of them, is likely to assume prepotence.

We employed the mouse paradigm to provide insight into this form of emergence (Vallacher, Markus, Nowak, & Strauss, 1996). We asked participants to think about their behavior in a recent social interaction with an opposite-sex person. Half were induced to think about their behavior in low-level, mechanistic terms (e.g., "spoke rapidly") and half were induced to think about their behavior in high-level, comprehensive terms (e.g., "offered support," "gave criticism"). In both cases, participants generated five act identities for their behavior and entered these into the computer. We then asked all participants to reflect on how they felt about having performed the behavior they had just identified. They then used the mouse task to express these feelings for a 2-minute period. Specifically, they moved the cursor toward the circle, which represented themselves, if they felt good about their behavior and away from the circle if they felt bad about their behavior. Half the participants began the mouse procedure immediately after generating the act identities (no delay), whereas the other half thought about their behavior for 1 minute before beginning the procedure (delay).

We anticipated that low- and high-level participants would display different trajectories of self-evaluation and that the delay manipulation would enable us to capture different portions of these trajectories. Assuming that high-level participants begin the judgment process with a set of provisional higher order frames for their behavior, they should show pronounced temporal variation at the outset, reflecting the valences associated with these frames. For their part, low-level participants must generate higher-level identities before they can oscillate among them in service of integration. In the no-delay condition, then, we expected high-level participants to demonstrate greater temporal variation in their judgment at the beginning of the mouse task than their low-level counterparts. This difference should begin to diminish by the end of the 2-minute period as high-level participants move toward integration and low-level participants begin to generate high-level identities. In the delay condition, meanwhile, high-level participants are likely to have achieved a fair degree of integration prior to the mouse procedure, whereas low-level participants are likely to have begun generating and oscillating among provisional higher level identities by this time. Consequently, high-level participants were expected to demonstrate *less* temporal variation in their judgment than low-level participants, with this difference increasing from the beginning to the end of the mouse period.

To test these predictions, we computed the variance in participants' positioning of the cursor vis-à-vis the target circle, both early (initial 40 seconds) and late (final 40 seconds) in the mouse task. This measure reflects the degree of variability in participants' self-evaluation of their behavior and hence indicates the extent to which they are considering different higher level perspectives. As hypothesized, participants who provided lower level identities for their behavior tended to display increasing variance in their evaluation of the act over time (from the initial 40 seconds in the no-delay condition to the final 40 seconds in the delay condition). Presumably, in the absence of external cues to the action's higher level meanings, the set of low-level identities led to the emergence of different possible higher level frames, each associated with a somewhat different implication for self-evaluation (e.g., "I offered constructive criticism," "I demon-strated insensitivity"). The opposite temporal pattern was observed, however, among participants who identified their behavior in higher level terms prior to the mouse task. The variation in self-evaluation was greatest at the outset for these participants (the initial 40 seconds in the no-delay condition), and tended to diminish over time (by the final 40 seconds in the delay condition). This suggests that high level participants initially alternated among different high-level frames for their behavior, and that this evaluative dynamism gave way to a more or less stable judgment as they achieved integration of the conflicting identities. The contrasting temporal patterns of high- and low-level participants are presented in Figure 4.1.

As an additional test of the hypotheses, we asked another group

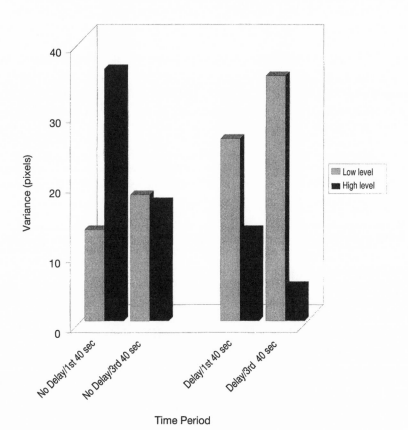

FIGURE 4.1. Variance in self-evaluation of action.

of participants to rate the self-evaluation implicit in each of the five identities generated by the original participants. Identities such as "demonstrated concern" and "complimented him (her)" were rated as highly positive, for instance, whereas identities such as "behaved rudely" and "showed insensitivity" were rated as highly negative. We then computed the variance in these ratings for each of the original participants and correlated this measure with the variance in their mouse movements during the early and late time intervals. As predicted, results revealed that the greater the evaluative variance in the identities generated by high-level participants, the greater the variance in their mouse movements in the initial period of the mouse task in the no-delay condition.

Taken together, these results suggest that participants for whom low-level cognitive elements were prepotent lagged behind participants for whom higher level integrative frames were prepotent. Presumably, participants in the high-level conditions began by considering the higher order frames they had generated for their behavior, oscillating among them to achieve integration, whereas participants in the low-level conditions had to generate such frames from more basic cognitive elements before they could begin the process of integration. In terms of the dynamic integration model, this interpretation assumes that participants' judgment tasks were personally important. Although this seems like a quite reasonable assumption in light of the self-relevance of participants' tasks, it nonetheless warrants explicit examination in future work.

Both scenarios in this study are consistent with the self-organization of basic action elements to create a unique configuration with emergent properties. The two scenarios, however, reflect different starting configurations experienced by people in everyday life. Sometimes, people have only a low-level understanding of what they are doing and must configure these basic elements to achieve integrated understanding. Without guiding cues from the environment, the elements can self-organize in different ways, each of which may have a different projection onto the evaluative dimension. To the extent that these resultant identities are distinct, the mental system attempts to reconcile them so as to achieve a single frame for the action. This point in the integration process may represent the starting point for people in other situations. If the act in question is fairly familiar, for example, people may have prepackaged high-level identities in mind rather than low-level identities that are devoid of inherent meaning. The task here remains one of integration, but the elements are not as elastic and thus not as easily reconciled as the elements in the other starting configuration. In this case, it may be difficult for the system to generate a yet higher level identity that provides organization for these elements. Rather than combining these frames in some fashion, then, integration may take the form of choosing one identity at the expense of the other (inconsistent) identities.

THE COORDINATION OF MIND AND ACTION

In principle, mental dynamics could exist in isolation, divorced from real-world contexts and constraints. In practice, however, autonomous thought is a rare occurrence. When people think, contemplate, and form judgments, it is usually for reasons that reflect very real concerns about how to behave in specific contexts and with respect to particular individuals. In the absence of such concerns, the mind can go horribly wrong. A person might conclude that he or she can win an argument with a lawyer or master calculus or carpentry in a week, for example, but unless the person attempts these acts, there is no basis for revising the original assessments or refining their means of implementation to accommodate reality. On its own, then, the mental system has the potential for becoming entangled in a self-reinforcing feedback loop in which a host of increasingly out-of-touch thoughts go unchallenged and hence uncorrected. By the same token, overt behavior is dependent on the mental system. Aside from personal mannerisms, reflexes, motor habits, and overlearned behavioral sequences (e.g., driving a car, answering a phone), the things people do are associated with higher order thought processes. Thus, people plan their actions, monitor their behavior, and reflect on the consequences and implications of what they have done. Mind and action, in other words, have a reciprocal connection, with judgments providing a basis for action and action providing information regarding the quality and utility of one's thoughts, decisions, and judgments.

The Self-Regulation of Action

The reciprocal relationship between mind and action can be discussed in terms of self-regulation. This topic has received considerable attention over the years, usually within the context of cybernetics (see Carver & Scheier, 1981, 1999; Miller, Galanter, & Pribram, 1960; Powers, 1973). The basic idea is that a feedback loop is established between a reference value (e.g., a goal) and the current state of the system. If a discrepancy is detected between the goal and the current state, appropriate action is generated to reduce the discrepancy. In this way, self-regulatory systems can achieve a prespecified equilibrium (i.e., the goal state) and maintain this equilibrium despite changes in the context surrounding the action. This basic idea is easily captured in dynamical terms (Vallacher & Nowak, in press). As discussed earlier, the dynamical properties of a system, and thus the system's attractors, depend on the setting of control parameters. In a self-regulatory system, a feedback loop is established in which the settings of control parameters not only dictate a system's dynamics but also depend on the system's current state or dynamics.[1] This dependence may take the form of a cybernetic loop in which discrepancies between the system's current state and its desired attractor (e.g., a goal) adjust the control parameters in such a way that the discrepancy is reduced. The familiar furnace thermostat metaphor in cybernetics provides a simple example of this form of feedback-based self-control. The control parameter here is the rate of fuel supplied to the furnace, and the state of the system is described by the temperature. The feedback loop is established by a thermostat, which adjusts a valve controlling the rate of fuel supplied, depending on the temperature inside the furnace. In fact, this is actually a dynamical system with a fixed-point attractor representing a single equilibrium for the system.

The dependence between control parameters and a system's state or dynamics, however, may also take forms that go beyond traditional cybernetic concerns. To begin with, the attractors in a dynamical system are not restricted to static reference values (i.e., fixed-point attractors) but can correspond as well to sustained patterns of evolution (e.g., periodic or chaotic). Even in the furnace thermostat example, the system's attractor may be periodic rather than fixed-point. This is because the system is likely to systematically overshoot its target value due to inertia in both the thermostat and the furnace, resulting in a time delay in the feedback loop. Thus, rather than settling on a fixed value, the temperature will oscillate around the equilibrium in a relatively regular manner. More generally, whereas feedback loops in cybernetics are designed to reinstate a system's equilibrium, feedback loops in dynamical systems can represent a wide variety of relationships—including, of course, restoration of equilibrium. Indeed, feedback loops in dynamical system can take the form of any linear or nonlinear relationship and establish highly complex patterns of evolution in such systems.

Insight into the nature of self-regulatory systems is provided by Lewenstein and Nowak (1989a, 1989b), who introduced self-control mechanisms in attractor neural networks (Hopfield, 1982). Attractor neural networks, a subclass of connectionist models, are programmable dynamical systems. They are often used to model cognitive processes such as recognition and learning (McClelland & Rumelhart, 1986). In this approach, memories are encoded as attractors of the network. Lewenstein and Nowak demonstrated that when a stimulus is presented, the network can determine whether it is familiar or novel in the first moments of processing, long before it recognizes it in detail. This "prerecognition" is accomplished in one of two ways, both of which provide an instant measure of the proximity of the network's state to its closest attractor. First, the system can monitor the volatility of its own dynamics. When the incoming stimulus approximates a well-known pattern in the network, corresponding to an attractor, the network is characterized by relatively slow dynamics (i.e., a small proportion of neurons changing their state). When the incoming pattern is novel and thus does not approximate one of the network's attractors, however, the network is characterized by more volatile dynamics. Second, the system can determine the coherence of the signals traveling in the network. In the vicinity of an attractor, the signals arriving at a given neuron from other neurons are consistent in dictating the state of the neuron. But when the network is far from an attractor, the system is characterized by incoherence—the signals arriving at a given neuron from other neurons dictate conflicting states of the neuron.

Both rate of neuronal change and network incoherence may be used to construct a self-control feedback loop. The control parameter is the level of noise in the network, corresponding to the random component of neuron firing. Self-control is established by making the noise level dependent on either the rate of neuronal change or the degree of network incoherence. With increasing levels of incoherence, for instance, the network increases its noise level, which in turn decreases the coherence of the network, and so on, in a self-perpetuating manner. This has the effect of making progressively stronger attractors inaccessible. In this way, the network avoids false recognition of novel patterns by raising the noise to a level where no attractor can capture a system's dynamics. The network, then, tentatively forgets progressively stronger memories, until at some level of noise the network is unable to recognize any incoming pattern. The dynamics of the network in effect become governed by noise (i.e., the dynamics become random), which may be interpreted as a "don't know" response. On the other hand, because familiar stimuli are coherent and hence produce only low levels of noise, the feedback loop results in their correct recognition. By means of this feedback loop, in summary, the network is able to regulate its own recognition process. The recognition process is maintained when the network is characterized by coherence (produced by familiar patterns), but is interrupted by strong noise when the network detects its own incoherence (produced by novel patterns).[2]

The general mechanism offered in this model can be interpreted in the context of action systems. Thus, in a malfunctioning system or in one that is destabilized by external influences, the action elements are no longer coherent (i.e., they provide one another conflicting signals) and thus cannot be coordinated into a congruent pattern. When cues to action are ambiguous or conflicting, or when novel circumstances arise that disrupt the normal course of action, the action elements lose their coordination. Upon detection of incoherence, the self-regulation feedback loop adjusts the system's control parameter to disrupt the dynamics of the system. This has the effect of disassembling the system into its lower level elements, which can then be reassembled in a different configuration that restores coherence to the action system.

This perspective can be extended to incorporate the hierarchical nature of action systems. Such a hierarchy is established when the control parameters dictating the attractors in one system become dynamical variables in another system. The temporal evolution of the higher level system is thus tantamount to continual adjustment of the control parameters in the lower level systems. After a relatively short time, the higher order system is likely to evolve (or stabilize) on one of its attractors. Its evolution on the attractor will be reflected in the systematic pattern of changes in the attractors of the lower level system. The control parameters of the higher order system, in turn, may become dynamical variables in a yet higher order system, and so on, resulting in a multilevel, hierarchically organized dynamical system. Each action system in effect becomes an element in the resultant higher order action system. In learning to drive, for example, a number of separate acts (e.g., braking, steering, parking) become integrated into a higher order system of driving, which in turn may be part of a yet higher order system (e.g., getting to work, going for a vacation). In summary, in a hierarchically organized action system, a higher order system adjusts the control parameters of lower level systems, initiating and shaping the dynamics of these systems, thereby organizing them into coherent action patterns.

Because of the feedback loops and resultant interdependence among levels, the image of firmly entrenched hierarchies of self-regulatory action systems is somewhat misleading. Action systems rarely maintain a fixed organization, but rather evolve and otherwise change in response to changing conditions. As noted earlier, the relations among system elements change in response to adjustments of the system's control parameters. Systems may also be assembled and disassembled, with new elements added or old elements eliminated, and with new self-control feedback loops supplanting existing feedback loops. It is also the case that two or more systems with different (or conflicting) goals may try to organize overlapping lower level elements. In short, the nature of self-control feedback loops in human self-regulation may get very complex, linking several levels and not readily organized in a well-defined hierarchical arrangement. A more appropriate image of human self-regulation is one of constantly evolving systems punctuated by periods of disorder and the emergence of new patterns, in a manner reminiscent of gestalt notions of pattern formation and reorganization (Vallacher et al., 1998).

The Role of Consciousness

Consciousness is not simply awareness of ongoing processes of action, but rather plays a vital role in the system generating action. The basic notion is that consciousness is called upon whenever a system of automatic self-regulation is insufficient to perform an action. Although many systems may be hardwired by genetic and other biological mechanisms, others may require active assembly on the person's part. Quite often, it is far from trivial how to assemble elements and establish self-control feedback loops into a system that will produce desired patterns. In such instances, consciousness may be required to select elements and establish basic connections among them and thus construct a dynamical system. Consciousness, in effect, plays the role of an outside agent that controls the system's dynamics by adjusting the control parameters on-line. The suggestion that conscious attention is necessary to establish a workable dynamical system is consistent with theory and research on the nature and function of controlled processing (Bargh, 1997; Schneider & Shiffrin, 1977).

Conscious control is especially likely when there is little direct experience with putting together elements for an unfamiliar or difficult task. In learning to ski, for example, consider the amount of conscious attention devoted to such basic elements as the position of one's legs and the distribution of one's body weight over the skis. With repeated activation of a system, the control parameters become directly linked to the system's dynamics, enabling the system to become increasingly capable of self-regulation and hence relatively autonomous in its operation. When a system becomes firmly established with feedback loops controlling its evolution, its dynamics follow a well-defined attractor. Overlearned acts thus become very rigid and follow the same pattern each time they are performed. The progressive automaticity in patterns of thought and behavior is consistent in broad form with the literature on both automaticity (Wegner & Bargh, 1998) and skills acquisition (Anderson, 1990).

The transition to automatic self-regulation in a system through the establishment of self-control feedback loops obviates the need for consciousness to micromanage the dynamics of the system. Once consciousness is relieved of the task of adjusting control parameters, it becomes available to assemble the system with other autonomous systems to create a higher order system. After a budding skiier has established an efficient system for making left and right turns on a ski slope, for example, this system becomes an element that is integrated with other elements (e.g., dealing with moguls) into a complex pattern of downhill skiing. In principle, there is no limit to the progressive integration of separate subsystems and the concomitant upward mobility of consciousness. Unconstrained, the content of conscious thought could become increasingly bereft of the details of self-regulation, defined instead in terms of increasingly comprehensive goals, plans, and the like (Vallacher et al., 1998).

Reality, of course, is not so accommodating. There are clear constraints on the progressive integration of systems that keep consciousness firmly tethered to lower levels of action regulation. For one thing, it may be difficult to assemble systems with overlapping elements but incompatible dynamics into a higher order system. Walking and talking, for example, are easily integrated, but talking and singing make conflicting demands on the same vocal elements and thus are poor candidates for integration. The progressive integration of systems is also constrained by the difficulty of the component systems. Some acts involve complex patterns of temporal coordination among basic movements and never achieve complete automaticity. No matter how experienced one is with skiing or raising a child, a considerable degree of conscious attention is required to maintain a desired pattern of thought and behavior for these action domains. A related constraint concerns environmental instability. Even simple, overlearned action patterns require adjustment to accommodate novelty in the action context from one occasion to another. No matter how routine the trip from work to home has become, for example, situations may arise (e.g., a cow crossing the road) that the autonomous driving system is not prepared to handle. In short, the conscious regulation of action systems diminishes greatly with automatization but does not evaporate entirely.

Consciousness is also critical in the resetting and repair of systems of self-regulation that become dysfunctional. If a system's elements do not cohere into a pattern that is instrumental in achieving a goal, it is necessary to change the relations among elements or the dynamics of any specific set of elements in order to establish the desired pattern. As depicted in the Lewenstein and Nowak (1989a, 1989b) model, a system can detect its own dysfunction by assessing the coherence of its own dynamics. If functionality cannot be restored by the system's self-control feedback loops, consciousness is directed to the system's elements in an attempt to reassemble them so as to achieve and maintain a desired pattern. A person experiencing awkwardness in a social encounter, for instance, may consciously consider the specific things he or she is doing and make adjustments accordingly in an attempt to achieve the desired coherence.

From this perspective, the level at which an action is consciously identified represents an order parameter describing the basic features of coordination in the system. Actions identified at different levels engage qualitatively different types of self-regulatory loops and thus display different dynamic properties. When an act is identified in low-level terms, different subsets of coordinated elements have yet to achieve integration, and there is little coordination in the action system as a whole. Each of these subsystems may have its own control parameters and thus behave in accordance with different dynamics. The separate components of a skilled action such as tennis, for example, each have their own criteria of effectiveness (e.g., hitting the ball, running to a shot) and are defined in terms of distinct patterns of motor movement. On the other hand, once an action achieves higher level coordination, the act as a whole becomes an entity with emergent properties. The lower level systems become enslaved by the higher level system and thus are no longer regulated with respect to independent feedback loops. This makes the lower level systems less reactive to factors that might otherwise change their form of enactment. So while physical fatigue might bring about a cessation of running and hitting on a tennis court, these component actions are likely to be maintained if they are coordinated in service of a higher level system (e.g., winning a tennis match).[3] As an order parameter for action, then, level of action identification specifies qualitatively different modes of self-regulation.

Considered together, the progressive assembly of lower order systems into higher order systems and the repair of disrupted systems impart a dynamic pattern to conscious experience. Each time one's attention is diverted from a higher order system to lower level elements and systems, there is a tendency for consciousness to reassemble the elements into a higher order system and reestablish consciousness in more comprehensive and abstract terms. This sequence of disassembly and self-organization is consistent with the emergence process specified in action identification theory (Vallacher & Wegner, 1987). Thus, whenever consciousness is redirected to lower level identities for an action, there is readiness to embrace higher level identities that provide coordination for the lower level identities (e.g., Wegner, Vallacher, Macomber, Wood, & Arps, 1984). To the extent that the resultant coordination differs from the earlier pattern of interelement connections, the emergent high-level identities may be qualitatively different from the antecedent high-level identities as well. With each enactment of the disruption–repair pattern, then, there is potential for the creation of a new higher order system of self-regulation. From this perspective, the content of consciousness is open-ended and ever-changing, representing a constructive process that fosters adaptation to changing task demands.

DYSFUNCTION IN ACTION SYSTEMS

Systems incapable of automatic self-regulation cannot function effectively in the absence of conscious attention. On the other hand, if conscious attention is focused on an autonomous self-regulating system, it switches the system's operation from automatic to "manual" control, disrupting the flow and slowing the system down by substituting serial for parallel processing (Schneider & Shiffrin, 1977). It follows that for every process, there is an optimal level in the hierarchy of self-regulation to which consciousness should be directed. Action identification theory describes how the optimal level of conscious attention depends on the characteristics of the system and task demands (Vallacher & Wegner, 1987). Research has established that people's conscious attention centers on high-level identities for tasks that are easy, familiar, or undisturbed, but moves to lower level subsystems and elements in order to perform actions that are personally difficult, unfamiliar, or disrupted in some manner (Vallacher, 1993). In short, the level at which an action is identified is indicative of the level at which consciousness assembles the self-regulation system for human action or intervenes in its operation.

Nonoptimality in Mind–Action Coordination

The feedback processes underlying self-regulation are hardly foolproof. Despite the general tendency toward mind–action coordination, conscious attention can be drawn to nonoptimal levels of identification that undermine efficiency in the action system. This occurs for the simple reason that actions are enacted in real-world contexts, replete with factors that can strongly influence the level at which action will be consciously represented (Vallacher & Wegner, 1985, 1987; Wegner & Vallacher, 1986). Most of the contexts defining everyday life provide cues to an action's causal effects, socially labeled meanings, and potential for self-evaluation, and thus are stacked in favor of relatively high-level identities. When offered a reward or threatened with punishment for engaging in a particular act, for instance, it may prove impossible for a person not to define what he or she is doing in these terms. In similar fashion, situations involving audience evaluation, competition, or other pressures to do well may keep the person mindful of high-level identities of a self-evaluative nature (e.g., "demonstrating my skill," "trying to win," "impressing others") at the expense of the action's more basic representations. If the action at stake is personally difficult and thus best regulated with respect to low level subsystems, the context-induced high-level identities lack sufficient detail and explicit coordination of components to enable the person to conduct the action effectively.

In addition to the relevant research on optimality in action identification (e.g., Vallacher, Wegner, & Somoza, 1989), evidence in support of this reasoning is provided by several lines of research demonstrating that performance of a complex or unfamiliar action is adversely affected by factors that charge the action with significance. Performance on a complex task has been shown to suffer, for example, when salient rewards are made contingent on the task (e.g., Condry, 1977; McGraw, 1978; Schwartz, 1982), when the task is performed under conditions emphasizing competition (e.g., Baumeister, 1984; Sanders, Baron, & Moore, 1978), and when the task is performed in the presence of an evaluative audience (e.g., Cottrell, 1972; Innes & Young, 1975). These factors all impart a fairly high-level representation to the task (earning a reward, demonstrating one's skill, impressing an audience), so it is not surprising that they impair performance when the task is difficult or unfamiliar and hence best undertaken with respect to more molecular representations. In effect, the basic action elements are discharged without the degree of conscious control necessary to assure their moment-to-moment coordination.

By the same token, one can imagine contexts that induce a level of conscious attention that is too *low* for effective action. This is likely to occur when the situation contains distractions, obstacles, or other sources of disruption that call attention to the details of one's action (e.g., Vallacher et al., 1989; Wegner et al., 1984). A bandaged finger, for instance, can reduce "preparing a chapter" to an agonizingly long sequence of discrete keystrokes. The lower level aspects of action tend to become prepotent as well when one is doing something in a novel setting lacking familiar cues to higher level meaning. In yet other contexts, a person may be asked or required to monitor the details of his or her behavior as it is being enacted and in this way experience a lower level of identification than would normally be the case (e.g., Wegner et al., 1984, 1986). When the action is personally easy for the person and thus best performed with respect to relatively high-level identities, the prepotence of lower level identities resulting from disruption, novelty, or instruction can undermine the quality of the person's performance. This conclusion is consistent with research showing that performance can be disrupted when attention is drawn to the overlearned details of an action (e.g., Kimble & Perlmuter, 1970; Langer & Imber, 1979; Marten & Landers, 1972). In effect, consciousness is trying to micromanage a problem that is best left to lower level echelons to work out among themselves.

We have emphasized the role played by identification level, but there are no doubt other properties of act identities that can dictate the operation of the mind–action system. The valence (i.e., positivity vs. negativity) of high-level identities, for example, can clearly influence the likelihood of acting on the basis of the identities. The avoidance of reality checks seems especially likely for people whose act identities center on fear of failure, inadequacy, and other dimensions of negative mental content. Depressed people, for example, are notorious for not expending effort in situations where such effort could well make a difference (e.g., Abramson, Metalsky, & Alloy, 1989; Seligman, 1975). Extreme shyness, meanwhile, can promote avoidance of social situations and intimate relations for fear of embarrassment and rejection (Zimbardo, 1977). Yet other dimensions of individual variation (e.g., low self-esteem, external locus of control) can be considered in this manner. In each case, there is a breakdown in the feedback between mind and action, so that the person's system of thoughts is not brought into alignment with the world of likely effects and consequences.

Emotion and System Coherence

The tripartite distinction among action, cognition, and emotion is arguably the most widely accepted division of psychological processes. Thus far, we have focused on cognition and action, with only passing reference to emotion. This does not mean that emotion is irrelevant to self-regulation. To the contrary, emotions can qualitatively change the functioning of the self-regulatory system and establish attractors for the system's dynamics. Indeed, because of their global and encompassing nature (LeDoux, 1989), emotions can reset all elements of a self-regulatory system into a congruent mode, in which specific systems of self-regulation can be activated (Oatley & Johnson-Laird, 1987). The activation component of emotion, first of all, directly influences the rhythm of thought and behavior. When one is agitated, for example, there is a rapid turnover in thought and motor movements become rapid and erratic. The content of emotion, meanwhile, makes salient specific elements and dictates how they are connected. A feeling of happiness, for example, can promote connections among positively valenced cognitive elements, creating a pattern of thought in which the person recalls primarily positive events and encodes new events in optimistic terms. Emotion thus can function as a control parameter in action systems, entering into the feedback loops that define self-regulation.

Anxiety is of special interest because of its potential for disrupting dynamics and thus stopping ongoing action (see Berkowitz, 1988; Mandler, 1975; Simon, 1967). Anxiety is aroused by dysfunction in a system, reflecting either insufficient progress toward a goal or incoherence in system dynamics. It can stop action and bring consciousness to repair an existing action system or to assemble a new system capable of goal attainment. A special manifestation of anxiety is discussed in the context of self-conscious emotions, such as guilt and shame (Tangney & Fischer, 1995). Such emotions not only inhibit an ongoing pattern of action, but they also promote the salience of standards of regulation contained in the self-system (cf. Carver & Scheier, 1999; Higgins, 1996). Consciousness is then brought to bear in order to reassemble the system, in line with our earlier discussion. In effect, the arousal stemming from faulty coordination becomes manifest phenomenologically as a special form of anxious self-scrutiny.

It is interesting in this light to note the emphasis placed on self-focused attention in various models of task performance. There is reason to think that this state is associated with heightened arousal (e.g., Wegner & Giuliano, 1980) and that it tends to impair performance. Opinion is divided, however, regarding the means by which self-focused attention produces this effect. In some models, to be self-conscious is to be aware of the potential self-evaluative implications of one's behavior (e.g., Hull & Levy, 1979; Wicklund & Frey, 1980). Defined in this way, self-focused attention is said to impair performance by reducing attention to task-relevant features (e.g., Henchy & Glass, 1968; Sarason, 1972). Test anxiety, for instance, occurs when the test taker is preoccupied with self-evaluative thoughts (e.g., "I'm going to fail," "I'll be embarrassed") to the relative exclusion of attention to the subtleties of the task at hand (e.g., Wine, 1971). In other formulations (e.g., Kimble & Perlmuter, 1970; Langer, 1978), self-consciousness refers to heightened awareness of the processes or mechanics underlying the execution of behavior (e.g., the physical movements involved or the coordination of such movements). In this view, a con-

scious concern with the process of performance essentially disintegrates the action, robbing it of its normal fluidity and rhythm (e.g.,
Baumeister, 1984; Langer & Imber, 1979).

These contrasting views of self-consciousness can be understood
in terms of nonoptimality in action identification. The self-evaluative
implications of behavior constitute a special class of high-level action
identification (e.g., Wegner & Vallacher, 1986), whereas the mechanics of behavior reflect considerably lower levels of action identification. In the context of mind–action coordination, neither orientation
is inherently linked to self-consciousness; rather, both low and high
levels of identification can give rise to self-scrutiny depending on the
personal difficulty of the action. In particular, the experience of self-
consciousness arises when one's conscious level of action control is either too high or too low, given the action's personal difficulty. When
performing a simple act or a complex one that has become fairly auto-
mated, people feel self-conscious to the extent that they are conscious
of the molecular features of the action. But for a difficult act that is
best performed with such features in mind, self-consciousness is associated instead with sensitivity to the act's high-level meanings, effects,
and implications.

Empirical support for this perspective on self-consciousness and
its role in performance is provided in a study by Vallacher et al.
(1989). Participants were asked to deliver a prepared speech to either
an easy-to-persuade audience or a difficult-to-persuade audience. Half
the participants were induced to think about the action in high-level
terms (e.g., "Try to persuade the audience"), and half were induced to
focus on the lower level details of delivering the speech (e.g., their
voice quality). As predicted, participants were more effective in delivering the speech when their level of action identification was calibrat-
ed with the difficulty of the act. In particular, speech errors were relatively infrequent when the task was personally easy and identified at
high level, and when the task was personally difficult and identified at
low level. Participants also rated themselves with respect to their performance and feelings while delivering the speech. Results showed
that ratings of self-consciousness (as well as anxiety, tension, etc.) par-
alleled the pattern obtained for speech fluency: It was relatively high
when the easy task was identified in low level terms and when the difficult task was identified in high-level terms.

The arousal and negative emotion associated with incoherence
in an action system diminish as people bring their conscious representation of what they are doing into line with the action's difficulty.
This does not mean that a person's affective state is disengaged when
mind–action coordination is achieved. To the contrary, people experi-

ence a special kind of positive affect when there is a match between the demands of a task and their mental and behavioral readiness to perform the task. This experience of "flow" (Csikszentmihalyi, 1982, 1990) or "dynamic orientation" (Wicklund, 1986) is characterized by total absorption in the activity and a corresponding loss of self-consciousness. Because positive emotions provide signals of effective self-regulation at a given level, they allow consciousness to move upward to assemble higher order action systems. So whereas negative emotions serve to focus consciousness on the factors that produced them, positive emotions direct consciousness to higher levels of integration, including those centering on plans, goals, and meanings.

A DYNAMICAL TAXONOMY OF ACTION

The dynamical perspective provides a new way of classifying the basic types of human action. The usual tack for building taxonomies in social psychology is to identify the content of people's behavior. This approach has generated important insights into the themes underlying superficially different behaviors. Although every act is unique with respect to lower level identities, virtually everything a person does can be seen in service of such goals and concerns as achievement, affiliation, cooperation, competition, egotism, altruism, justice, self-enhancement, self-consistency, and self-assessment. The dynamical perspective complements this approach by introducing the dimension of time when attempting to identify invariant features of action. In particular, the myriad actions performed by people may sort themselves into three basic forms, each defined in terms of a particular type of temporal trajectory or attractor.

The most familiar temporal pattern is convergence on a single state. Such fixed-point attractors represent the default action pattern in social psychology. Goal-directed behavior is commonly understood in these terms (e.g., Carver & Scheier, 1990; Gollwitzer, 1996), as is behavior in the service of reducing guilt or other unpleasant affective states (e.g., Cialdini & Kenrick, 1976; Higgins, 1987; Wicklund & Frey, 1980). The dynamism associated with fixed-point behavior is typically confined to the consideration of possible options for accomplishing one's goals and thus dissipates quickly as lower level strategies are developed. Two general methods are often used to establish the existence of fixed-point attractors. The first involves observing changes over time in the distribution of the system's dynamical variables (e.g., order parameters). Diminishing variability in the system's behavior as it evolves (in the absence of external constraint) is a strong indication that the system is approaching a fixed-point attractor. As noted in Chapter 3, this method has proven useful in determining the conditions under which social judgment converges on a single evaluation (e.g., Vallacher et al., 1994).

The second method involves actively perturbing the system and observing its subsequent behavior. If a single fixed-point attractor exists, the system will return to its original state after some time, provided the disruption is not too great. This method is highly relevant to investigating goal-directed behavior. By perturbing a person's behavior, first of all, one can identify the strength of his or her goal orientation. If a person's goal is unstable, minor obstacles and distractions may be sufficient to derail the person's sense of direction with respect to his or her behavior. Second, stability analysis can determine whether the person's action system is characterized by multiple goals. If the system has multiple fixed points, small perturbations will result in the system returning to its original goal orientation, but strong influences can throw the system into the basin of attraction of an entirely different equilibrium state, with behavior directed toward a goal that may be diametrically opposed to the original goal.

Not all behavior, however, is so unequivocally tied to a single end state. Although there is a press for integration in thought and behavior, fixed-point stability may be hard to achieve under certain circumstances. When this is the case, the person's behavior may demonstrate periodicity, akin to periodic attractors in dynamical systems. A person's behavior toward certain people (e.g., an intimate partner), for example, may alternate between two extremes, such as affection and hostility, and this pattern rather than either of the endpoints, may provide the best characterization of what he or she does. Even goal-directed behavior, commonly discussed in terms of desired end states, may have a periodic structure rather than a fixed-point tendency. A person might be concerned with both safety and novelty, for instance, and alternate regularly between boring activities and thrill seeking. This broadened conception of goals allows goal-directed behavior to be investigated in the context of various dynamical methods and tools. One can make use of the laws of bifurcations, for example, to specify how the structure of goals may change in response to variables influencing the system. With increments in a relevant control parameter, for instance, a single goal may give way to two or more goals that alternate in prepotence, in accordance with one of the bifurcation scenarios discussed in Chapter 2.

The final temporal pattern looks like random behavior, with the person displaying unpredictable changes in his or her action. Random behavior is always a possibility, of course. This is likely when the action is driven by external stimuli rather than following patterns established by organized action systems. Behavior that appears to be random, however, may instead be an instantiation of deterministic chaos (Vallacher & Nowak, 1997). One might seek a life full of adventures and unexpected turns rather than even the most attractive stable realities, for example, or prefer relationships that are constantly evolving as opposed to stable and predictable. The potential for chaotic behavior reflects the nonlinear interactions among the forces at work. This is somewhat analogous to the idea of statistical interactions (Carver, 1997), where the effect of one variable depends on the level of the other variables at that time. In a complex system, of course, there are often numerous variables, so that the potential for interactions can easily exceed the "2 by 2" scheme that dominates theorizing and experimental designs in social psychology. It is also the case that the interactions themselves interact with the time dimension, producing a highly complex temporal trajectory as the action unfolds.

The complex interplay of forces giving rise to chaotic trajectories in action can be just as opaque to the actor as to an observer. Indeed, even isolated causes that are apparent to an observer (or an experimental psychologist) can be lost on an actor, leaving him or her to invent reasons for what he or she did (Nisbett & Wilson, 1977). As the web of determining factors becomes increasingly interconnected in nonlinear fashion, it is not surprising that people fail to see the causal underpinnings of their thought and behavior, investing themselves instead with a sense of self-determination and free will—or alternatively, with a sense of being at the whim of random forces they cannot hope to understand, let alone control (Vallacher, 1998). From a dynamical perspective, the sense of free will provides ironic testimony to people's connection with the multiplicity of forces and mechanisms defining their physical and social worlds.

NOTES

1. As discussed in Chapter 2, a system's state or dynamics is described by order parameters. In this light, the feedback loop described here usually links the control parameters and order parameters in a system. It is also possible, however, for the control parameters of a system to become linked to the dynamics of a single element in a system, in which case the system is likely to display erratic behavior.

2. This relatively simple self-control mechanism may be used as an element in a larger system capable of more complex self-regulatory functions. In a system composed of several networks in which each network encodes sepa-

rate memories, for example, the presentation of a stimulus will block the recognition process in all the networks that have not encoded the stimulus, so that recognition will take place only in the network that actually remembers the stimulus (Zochowski, Lewenstein, & Nowak, 1993). It is also possible for a neural network to switch dynamically between a recognition mode and a learning mode (Zochowski, Lewenstein, & Nowak, 1995). In this model, the network engages in a recognition process when presented with familiar stimuli. But upon detection of its own incoherence during recognition, the network will stop its own recognition process and initiate instead a process of learning. In this way, the network acquires memories for unknown patterns, which can be subsequently used in recognition. In short, the introduction of self-control mechanisms into attractor neural networks provides for richer dynamics and allows such networks to perform much more complex functions.

3. Of course, it is possible for a lower level system to reestablish its own self-regulatory dynamics and become independent of the higher order system. This scenario would seem to characterize behavior that is impulsive and open to temptation rather than deliberate and goal-oriented.

5

❧

Dynamics and Self-Organization

Of all the elements of thought that populate the stream of consciousness, it is fair to say that none surface more frequently, for longer duration, or in a wider variety of contexts than those having to do with one's sense of self. It's hard to imagine any setting that is immune to the sudden appearance in the mind's eye of memories, hopes, fears, and evaluations regarding the self. Once engaged, moreover, self-reflection is likely to produce at least some degree of variability in evaluation, with a mix of positive and negative self-assessments unfolding over time. The stream of consciousness, after all, is noted for its tangential associations, unwanted thoughts, and other features of uncontrolled mental process. It would be surprising indeed if every thought about the self that surfaced in this breeding ground for turbulence pointed in the same direction for self-evaluation. Even someone with the highest level of self-regard is no doubt plagued from time to time by sudden remembrances of events that were personally embarrassing or negatively judged by those whose opinions matter. Self-reflection, from this perspective, is a highly dynamic process that is driven and sustained by the internal workings of the cognitive–affective system, and that is capable of promoting noteworthy temporal variation in moment-to-moment self-evaluation.

It is also the case, however, that the self-concept is commonly viewed as providing an important reference point for personal and interpersonal action—a function better served by stability than instability in self-assessment. And indeed, there is reason to believe that people do manage to achieve a fair degree of coherence in self-understanding, enough that it qualifies as a cognitive structure (e.g., Markus, 1980). This structure is sufficiently stable and coherent to provide a platform for action and self-regulation (cf. Carver & Scheier, 1981; Duval & Wicklund, 1972; Higgins, 1987; Markus & Nurius, 1986; Sedikides & Skowronski, 1997; Swann, 1990). So although self-reflection creates the conditions for intrinsic dynamics in self-evaluation, over time, such dynamism is likely to give way to a coherent, evaluatively consistent perspective on the self. In this chapter, we discuss the dynamical basis of self-reflection and suggest how it can be reconciled with assumptions concerning self-concept stability. This reasoning is developed in the context of a cellular automata model that demonstrates the emergence of self-structure from dynamic processes within the self system. In a final section, we discuss the mechanisms by which self-structures provide bases for self-control beyond those provided by the feedback between mind and action discussed in the preceding chapter.

INTRINSIC DYNAMICS OF SELF-EVALUATION

There is clearly potential for intrinsic dynamics in self-reflection. People's knowledge structure concerning themselves, after all, is more extensive and diverse than their knowledge structure for any other social object. Given the number and variety of thoughts and feelings concerning the self, self-reflection would seem to be a breeding ground for moment-to-moment variability in self-evaluation. There are forces toward stability and coherence in self-concept, of course, but the mental processes involved in achieving such integration are likely to be associated with considerable dynamism as different elements relevant to the self rise and fall in salience over time. The nature and extent of moment-to-moment variation in self-evaluation may provide insight into the degree of evaluative diversity and inconsistency in the self system, in much the same way that dynamism in social judgment signals the coherence of mental representations of other people (e.g., Vallacher et al., 1994).

Self-Dynamics in Social Psychology

The potential for dynamism in self-evaluation has hardly been lost on social psychologists. Indeed, much of the contemporary work on the self is compatible in principle with this perspective on self-dynamics. In a broad sense, *all* models of the self imply an internally driven temporal trajectory of some sort, simply because a mental process, however minimally defined, is presumed to take place in real time between the instigation to self-scrutiny and the resultant self-evaluation. Some perspectives, however, lend themselves more readily than others to the potential for internally generated and sustained dynamism in self-evaluation once the self system is engaged. In some cases, this potential reflects a purported conflict within the self system. From the perspective of self-verification theory (Swann, 1990), for instance, it is plausible that social feedback inconsistent with one's prevailing self-concept sets in motion a chain of thought that oscillates in some fashion between acceptance and rejection of the feedback before the conflict is finally resolved. Especially for low self-esteem people who experience a "cognitive–affective" crossfire when provided positive feedback (e.g., Swann, Griffin, Predmore, & Gaines, 1987), one might reasonably expect a sustained pattern of thought characterized by vacillation between positive and negative self-assessment.

In other models, the potential for intrinsic dynamics reflects the availability of multiple perspectives for evaluating the self. Self-discrepancy theory (Higgins, 1987, 1996), for instance, suggests that multiple self-standards can be simultaneously salient for a person and that these standards may promote mutually incompatible self-feelings. Conceivably, the person under such conditions might oscillate among the various evoked sentiments, with the oscillation sustained by the interplay of the sentiments themselves rather than by their initial instigations. In a similar manner, models that emphasize possible selves (e.g., Markus & Nurius, 1986) or self-complexity and differentiation (e.g., Linville, 1985; Vallacher, 1980) could be extended to incorporate the potential for internally sustained dynamics in self-evaluation. Thus, with an increase in self-differentiation or the number of possible selves, there is a concomitant increase in the variety of ways in which self-relevant information can be integrated. Once this information enters the self system, then, it can generate a succession of different self-evaluative states as the various integrative frames alternate in prepotence. In yet other models, feedback processes among cognitive mechanisms suggest the potential for sustained volatility in self-evaluation, well after the external instigation to self-evaluation has subsided. The work on rumination (e.g., Martin & Tesser, 1989, 1996) and on the ironic effects of thought suppression (e.g., Wegner, 1994), for example, both imply (for different reasons) that once self-directed thought is initiated, it can acquire a rhythm of its own and become self-sustaining.

In view of the intuitive appeal of this view of self-dynamics and the ready fit it has with existing theories of the self, it is curious that it has not received much empirical attention. Of course, it could be that researchers have entertained the issue and simply decided it is not worth investigating. The stream of consciousness, after all, is full of stray, nonessential, and idiosyncratic elements of thought (see Wegner, 1996). Apart from the difficulty in trying to track the flow of such elements, one may wonder what is to be gained from taking a perspective that emphasizes fleeting change rather than stability. Adopting a fine-grained approach to the stream of consciousness is clearly essential to documenting the ebb and flow of particular thoughts and feelings (e.g., Csikszentmihalyi & Figurski, 1982; Klinger et al., 1980; Pennebaker, 1988; Pope & Singer, 1978; Singer, 1988; Singer & Bonanno, 1990), but if one's concern is with establishing basic principles of judgment that transcend the particular, it is tempting to dismiss such elements as noise obscuring an otherwise stable signal. Theories, after all, are based on regularities associated with invariant features, not on sequences of ever-changing idiosyncratic elements. It is perhaps not all that surprising, then, that theorists and researchers have tended to ignore the turbulent undercurrent of phenomenal experience, focusing instead on higher order features of thought that admit to stability and structure.

Intrinsic Dynamics and the Press for Integration

This implicit theoretical divide between dynamism and equilibrium in self-assessment is unnecessary at best and may prove to be misleading. From a dynamical perspective, in fact, it is precisely because of the press toward coherence in the self system that self-evaluation displays intrinsic dynamics. A person's sense of self, after all, is based on many elements of information derived from diverse sources, including reflected self-appraisals and feedback from others in social interaction, direct comparisons with others, self-perceived results of one's own actions, and the results of reasoning and interpretative processes. In view of the diversity of these sources, it is likely that the various elements of self-relevant information will vary a great deal with respect to both their respective valence and their respective importance. A person's sense of humor, for example, might be highly valued by some people but ridiculed by others. And others who provide positive feedback on one element of the self (e.g., sense of humor) may indicate their displeasure with another element (e.g., taste in computer games). Because of the general press to achieve integrative understanding when one is attentive to lower level components of one's experience (cf. Vallacher & Wegner, 1985), the inevitable conflict among elements of self-relevant information promotes efforts to maintain or achieve coherence. The processes associated with this concern are what give rise to intrinsic dynamics in self-evaluation.

Social interaction provides an especially potent and pervasive source of threat to the coherence of people's self-concept. Social encounters clearly have the potential for inducing reflection on one's self-defining qualities, and some encounters may be especially likely to render a host of diverse self-elements salient. To the extent that the valences associated with these elements are mutually inconsistent, cognitive operations are necessary to maintain or restore a coherent perspective on one's self. For a person with high self-esteem, for example, negative feedback on an important aspect of the self from a valued and credible source (e.g., a spouse or a professional psychologist) may prove difficult to reconcile with his or her preexisting self-assessment. The cognitive operations set in motion when people are exposed to destabilizing information is time-dependent and thus should be reflected in dynamic properties.

It is conceivable, of course, that in such cases the person will reconcile the conflicting frames by finding a compromise that integrates both. Research on people's reactions to social feedback, however, suggests that this form of integration is infrequent in everyday life. When people are exposed to an interpersonal assessment that contradicts their self-view, they tend either to experience affect in line with the assessment, thereby indicating implicit acceptance of the new self-view, or to reinterpret, reject, or otherwise discount the threatening perspective in favor of their preexisting self-concept (Baumeister, Smart, & Bowden, 1996; Jones, 1973; Shrauger, 1975). This idea is consistent with the notion of dynamic integration, introduced in Chapter 3. Thus, when judgment is personally relevant—as it clearly is for the self—conflict is unlikely to be resolved in a combinatorial manner. Rather, one pole of the conflict is likely to become ascendant at the expense of the other, following a period of dynamism driven by the successive prepotence of both. Which frame ultimately achieves prepotence is likely to depend on the relative stability and integrative value of each. From this perspective, the well-documented positivity bias in self-evaluation (e.g., Baumeister, 1982; Jones, 1964; Markus, Kitayama, & Heiman, 1996; Myers & Diener, 1995; Steele, 1988; Taylor & Brown, 1988; Tesser, 1988) suggests that for most people, positive frames are more stable than negative frames and have greater potential for integrating self-relevant information.

There is no guarantee, however, that positive internal frames— or internal frames of any valence, for that matter—provide stable and comprehensive integration for self-relevant information. People may think about themselves on a routine basis, but all this cognitive effort does not necessarily lead to a stable and coherent self-concept. Indeed, theory and research in recent years have identified self-concept certainty as a significant basis of individual variation in self-understanding, perhaps just as important as self-concept valence (e.g., Baumeister, 1993; Baumgardner, 1990; Campbell, 1990; Kernis, 1993; Pelham, 1991; Swann & Ely, 1984; Vallacher, 1980; Vallacher & Wegner, 1989). As it happens, there is a strong relationship between these two variables, such that people who view themselves negatively tend also to have an unclear sense of what they are like with respect to important attributes, whereas people with higher levels of self-esteem tend to express considerable confidence regarding their standing on such dimensions (e.g., Baumeister, 1993; Baumgardner, 1990; Vallacher, 1978). An uncertain self-concept is also an unstable self-concept. Lacking a firmly anchored sense of self, an uncertain person is routinely at the mercy of whatever opinions and perspectives he or she encounters in daily life (Baumeister, 1993; Swann & Ely, 1984; Vallacher & Wegner, 1989). Such a person may feel negative about him- or herself on the heels of an interaction with someone who provides criticism, for example, only to rebound to a positive view when later exposed to more sanguine communication from someone else.

Even in the absence of social contact, people with a poorly defined sense of what they are like may experience instability in self-evaluation during periods of self-scrutiny. In effect, when uncertain people reflect on themselves, they experience a succession of independent elements that have yet to form integrated subsets. To the extent that these elements have varying self-evaluative implications, the process of self-reflection for uncertain people is likely to be marked by noteworthy temporal variation in global self-evaluation. Someone with a poorly integrated image of him- or herself as a student, for example, is likely to experience a succession of different self-evaluations as he or she separately considers the various pieces of information relevant to this assessment (e.g., recent exams, feedback from instructors, enthusiasm for different courses, diligence in doing homework). Because none of these elements enjoys a privileged phenomenal position, and in light of the heightened importance of judgments regarding the self, the volatility in self-evaluation on the part of uncertain people is likely to be sustained for relatively long periods before dissipating in favor of a single perspective.

The Stream of Self-Consciousness

Unfortunately, this depiction of dynamism and integration in self-assessment remains largely unexamined, primarily for want of appropriate tools. If the flow of thought underlying self-evaluation shows meaningful temporal variation, it likely does so on very short time scales, with individual elements and subsets of elements changing on a moment-to-moment basis. It is clearly not feasible, even in principle, to track the turnover in thought at such levels of temporal resolution through standard self-report methodology. Recently, however, we adapted the mouse paradigm (Vallacher & Nowak, 1994c) in order to capture the intrinsic dynamics associated with the press for integration in self-evaluation (Vallacher, Nowak, Froehlich, & Borkowski, 1997). Beyond providing a means for characterizing the stream of self-directed thoughts and feelings, this study revealed that individual differences with respect to three basic self-variables—self-esteem, self-certainty, and self-stability—are associated with theoretically meaningful properties of intrinsic dynamics and with different degrees of success in achieving integration.

The participants in this study completed several self-report instruments, including a set designed to measure their global self-evaluation, self-concept stability, and self-concept certainty. Self-evaluation was assessed with Rosenberg's (1965) test of self-esteem. Using Likert-type scales, participants expressed their agreement versus disagreement with 10 statements tapping a sense of personal worth (e.g., "I feel that I have a number of good qualities"). Responses to these items were averaged to yield a measure of self-esteem. Self-concept stability was assessed with an additional four items developed by Rosenberg (1965) that assessed participants' agreement versus disagreement with statements expressing ambivalence and inconsistency in self-concept (e.g., "Some days I have a very good opinion of myself; other days I have a very poor opinion of myself," "I have noticed that my ideas about myself seem to change very quickly"). Like the self-esteem items, these items were highly intercorrelated and thus were averaged to generate an overall measure of self-stability. To measure self-concept certainty, we asked participants to use 7-point scales to indicate how certain versus uncertain they were of their standing with respect to 20 common personality traits (e.g., sincerity, sociability, independence). These ratings also formed a highly reliable scale and were averaged to yield an overall measure of self-certainty. Self-esteem was reliably correlated with self-certainty ($r = .57$), in line with previous research (e.g., Baumgardner, 1990; Vallacher, 1978), and both constructs were correlated with self-stability ($r = . 69$ for self-esteem, .59 for self-certainty).

Several days later, participants returned individually to take part in an ostensibly unrelated experiment involving memory and judgment. Two-thirds of them were asked to think about five past actions that reflected either positively or negatively on themselves. Participants entered brief (one- or two-sentence) descriptions of each of these acts into a computer. Participants in a control condition were not asked to think of past actions. After this priming manipulation, participants were instructed to describe themselves by speaking into a tape recorder positioned next to the computer. They were encouraged to describe themselves as fully and completely as possible with respect to personality traits, goals, plans, relationships, or whatever else came to mind (although they were advised not to mention their names or other information that might identify them). They were assured of anonymity and confidentiality, and were encouraged to be as frank and honest as possible in describing themselves. After answering questions about this procedure, they were left alone for up to 5 minutes to create the tape.

Upon completion of the tape, participants listened to the tape and indicated how positive versus negative their descriptions were by means of a computer mouse. They were instructed to move the mouse-controlled cursor vis-à-vis a target circle in the middle of the screen to indicate the valence of each element of their self-description as they listened to their narrative. Movement toward the circle conveyed positive feelings about the particular self-description they were hearing, whereas movement away from the circle conveyed negative feelings about the self-description. The tapes ranged from 1½ minutes to the allowable 5 minutes (M = 3 minutes), so the length of the corresponding mouse trajectories varied in the same manner. Each resultant trajectory was divided into three equal time intervals, and for each one, we derived the following measures: distance, variance in distance, speed, acceleration, and time at rest. This enabled us to assess self-evaluation and self-dynamism, and the changes in these properties over time.

Results revealed that both self-evaluation and self-dynamism initially varied in response to the priming manipulation. During the initial portion of their tape recordings, participants who had been induced to think about negative past actions displayed reliably greater distance (M = 108 pixels) from the target circle than did those induced to think about positive actions (M = 61 pixels) or not induced to think about past actions (M = 66 pixels). A similar effect was obtained for speed: participants in the negative priming condition demonstrated reliably faster turnover in self-evaluation (M = 26 pixels/second) than did those in the positive priming (M = 18.3 pixels/second) and no priming conditions (M = 14.7 pixels/second). Introducing negative elements into participants' self systems had the effect, then, of promoting relatively low self-evaluation (i.e., large distance from the circle) and frequent changes in self-evaluation (high speed). Presumably, calling to mind negative elements of the self served to destabilize participants' self-concept and set in motion cognitive mechanisms to reestablish equilibrium.

The effect of the priming manipulation tended to be short-lived, however, as the activated internal mechanisms worked to achieve organization in the self system. In a sense, participants' characteristic mode of self-reflection began to reassert itself during the second and third time periods. To reveal different manifestations of this general tendency, we split the sample into the upper and lower 40% on each self-variable (self-esteem, self-stability, and self-certainty) and considered the resultant constructs over time for each priming condition. It is worth noting that despite the shared variance among the self-variables, the dichotomous constructs we created demonstrated somewhat unique patterns of effects with respect to the dynamic measures.

Figures 5.1–5.3 display the change over time in self-evaluation on the part of low and high self-esteem participants in each of the priming conditions. It is apparent that participants with low self-esteem expressed lower self-evaluations in their taped descriptions than did those with high self-esteem (overall M = 98.8 vs. 61.7 pixels). A more intriguing difference between low and high self-esteem participants concerns the relative stability of their self-evaluation over the duration of their self-description narratives in each of the priming conditions. For low self-esteem participants, self-evaluation tended to become increasingly negative over time in the negative and no-prime conditions. This suggests that the process of self-reflection for such people is likely to produce polarization in a negative direction. Presumably, because there is a relatively high proportion of negative elements in their self system, the mutual influences among elements tend to promote coherence with respect to a negative frame. In the positive prime condition, self-evaluation tended to remain stable,

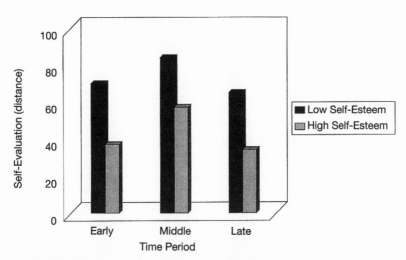

FIGURE 5.1. Change in self-evaluation by self-esteem (positive priming).

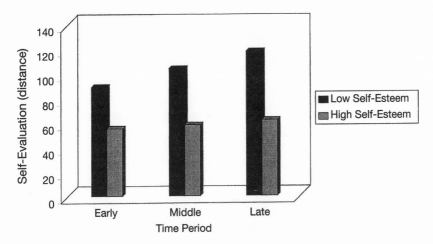

FIGURE 5.2. Change in self-evaluation by self-esteem (no priming).

suggesting that activating positive elements can inhibit the unfettered tendency toward negative polarization on the part of people with low self-esteem.

For high self-esteem participants, in contrast, self-evaluation tended to remain fairly stable across the three time periods for each of the conditions. This suggests that the mutual support among positive elements in a largely positive self system dampens the impact of negative elements and otherwise enables the person to resist changes in

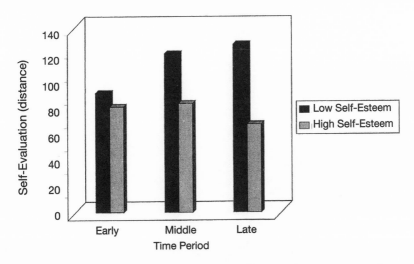

FIGURE 5.3. Change in self-evaluation by self-esteem (negative priming).

global self-regard. The fact that activation of positive elements did not produce positive polarization could signify the operation of a ceiling effect, a reasonable possibility in view of the positivity bias in self-concept (e.g., Baumeister, 1982; Steele, 1988; Taylor & Brown, 1988; Tesser, 1988). Alternatively, high self-esteem people may have a better structured self system (e.g., Kernis, 1993), a property that may lend coherence and stability to the output of their self-reflection processes.

Results also revealed divergent temporal patterns in self-evaluative dynamism on the part of participants with low versus high levels of self-stability. As Figure 5.4 reveals, both groups began their respective narratives with the same degree of irregular changes (as indexed by acceleration) in self-evaluation, presumably in response to the priming manipulations, but thereafter showed substantial differences. Participants with an unstable self-concept displayed heightened instability in self-evaluation in the middle portion of their self-descriptions and then stabilized somewhat during the final portion. In contrast, participants with a stable self-concept displayed progressively less instability in self-evaluation from the beginning to the end of their self-descriptions. This suggests that self-reflection on the part of people with stable self-concepts quickly converges on a stable self-evaluation equilibrium, whereas self-reflection on the part of people with unstable self-concepts promotes movement between different equilibria, each of which is insufficiently stable to provide a firm basis for self-evaluation.

Yet a third pattern was observed when the data were blocked on low versus high levels of self-certainty. Overall, participants with an

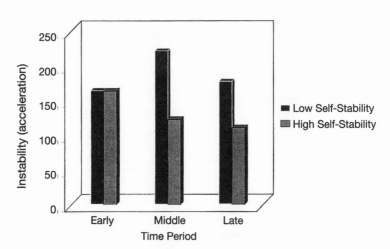

FIGURE 5.4. Instability in self-evaluation by self-stability.

uncertain self-concept displayed reliably greater volatility (as indexed by speed) in their self-evaluation than did their more certain counterparts (M = 23.7 vs. 15.0 pixels/second). Results also showed that both certain and uncertain participants tended to become more stable in their self-evaluations from the beginning to the end of their respective self-descriptions—with one intriguing exception. As Figure 5.5 reveals, participants with low self-certainty who were not induced to think about past acts, displayed increasing as opposed to decreasing volatility in self-evaluation from the beginning to the end of their self-description. This suggests that uncertain people are especially likely to experience conflicting self-evaluations when they are not prompted to think about themselves from one particular frame (positive or negative). Left to their own devices, as it were, uncertain people find it difficult to achieve coherence and stability in their sense of self. Perhaps this tendency underlies the tendency of uncertain people to modify their self-image to accommodate feedback from interaction partners (e.g., Swann & Ely, 1984). In essence, feedback (and other external sources of self-relevant information) provides structure and stability for self-evaluation among those who cannot supply these features for themselves.

The results also revealed an interesting (though unanticipated) pattern for the length of participants' self-description protocol. The longest self-descriptions were provided by participants with stable self-concepts who were induced to think about positive acts (M = 3 min-

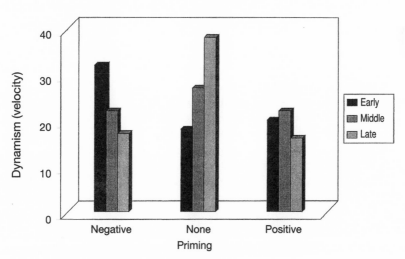

Note.   Data for participants with low self-certainty

FIGURE 5.5. Dynamism in self-evaluation by priming.

utes, 36 seconds), whereas the shortest self-descriptions were provided by those with uncertain self-concepts who were not induced to think about past acts (M = 2 minutes, 23 seconds). From a purely rational perspective, one might expect the opposite: Stable people have the fewest conflicts concerning their qualities to express and thus should have less to say, while uncertain people presumably have the largest set of unintegrated elements and thus should have a great deal to say. The fact that stability promoted lengthy self-descriptions and uncertainty promoted abbreviated self-descriptions suggests that verbalizing thoughts about oneself can be a pleasant and self-sustaining experience or an unpleasant and self-terminating experience, depending on how well this act allows one to maintain or achieve coherence in self-evaluation.

To illustrate the differential dynamism observed in this experiment, we present representative trajectories of self-evaluation (Figure 5.6). In each one, absolute distance from the target circle (in pixels) is plotted as a function of time. The first trajectory (A) was obtained from a participant with high self-esteem, high self-certainty, and high self-stability, who was asked to think about positive acts in the past. The second trajectory (B) was obtained from a participant with low self-esteem, low self-certainty, and low self-stability, who was not asked to think about past actions. Note the two clusters of negative self-evaluations in trajectory A, with convergence toward positive evaluation by the end of the self-description. This pattern suggests that this participant had well-integrated frames for integrating positive and negative elements of the self, and that over time, the positive frame became ascendant. By way of contrast, note the erratic dynamics of self-evaluation in trajectory B. If anything, this pattern reveals initial suppression of negative assessments of the self, followed by a rapid switch to a negative frame for thinking about the self. This general negativity, however, was punctuated frequently and erratically by small bursts of positive self-evaluations.

The results of this study serve as a reminder that attempts to manipulate people's level of self-regard may well produce reliable effects, but the nature of these effects must be understood in terms of their interaction with the intrinsic dynamics of the self system. Initially, everyone responds somewhat to the valence of influence attempts, with negative inputs to the system producing reduced self-evaluation and positive inputs enhancing global self-evaluation. As subsequent thoughts and feelings about the self unfold, however, there tends to be a restoration of preexisting levels of self-regard. This restoration is associated with considerable internally generated dynamism as the elements in the self-system influence each other to reestablish equilibrium. The extent of such dynamism, and the degree to which it suc-

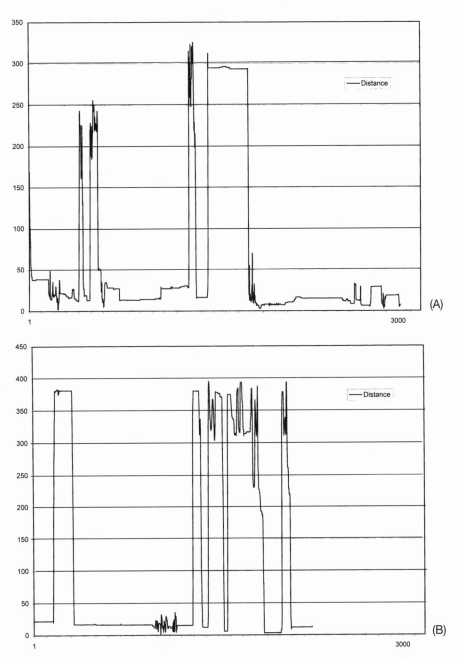

FIGURE 5.6. Trajectories of self-evaluation.

ceeds in restoring equilibrium, depend on the stability and internal coherence of the self system. Participants in this study who had an unstable as opposed to a stable sense of self showed increasingly rapid and irregular changes between different self-evaluative states during the second time period, and this dynamism was still evident toward the end of their self-descriptions. Participants with relatively low levels of self-stability and self-certainty also tended to end their self-descriptions sooner than did their more stable and certain counterparts, suggesting that the volatility in their self-reflection was not effective in achieving stable equilibrium in self-evaluation.

Indeed, there is reason to think that self-reflection in the absence of information inputs can be destabilizing rather than stabilizing for people who lack internal coherence in their self system. Thus, the participants in this study who had the least self-certainty experienced the most dynamism when they were induced to reflect on themselves without first being primed to think about evaluatively consistent elements of the self. This suggests that self-uncertainty reflects a disordered system that, left to its own internal mechanisms, produces disordered global output. On this view, the responsiveness of uncertain people to social feedback (e.g., Kernis, 1993; Swann & Ely, 1984) represents an attempt to achieve coherence by incorporating new insights around which existing information and considerations can become organized.

Taken together, the results of this experiment suggest that self-evaluation is an inherently dynamic process, driven by the internal workings of the cognitive–affective system. Engaging this system sets in motion a stream of self-reflection that is characterized by varying degrees of volatility as the system attempts to maintain or achieve coherence among various elements and subsets of elements. But while these data illuminate the dynamics of the self system, they do not provide a window into the structure of the system per se. An explicit concern with the relation between dynamics and structure provides the focus for the following section.

SELF-STRUCTURE AND DYNAMICS

The self is obviously a very special object of cognitive representation. It is the largest structure in the cognitive system, encompassing all personally relevant information derived throughout one's life (see Markus, 1983), and it has strong and pervasive effects on other psychological systems (social judgment, action, interpersonal relations, etc.). Self-relevance, for example, has been shown to produce the deepest levels of information processing (e.g., Craik & Lockhart,

1972; Rogers, Kuiper, & Kirker, 1977). The elements that populate the self system, meanwhile, are unique in that they represent thoughts and feelings derived in large part from real and imagined relationships with specific and generalized others (e.g., Cooley, 1902; Goffman, 1959; Mead, 1934; Rogers, 1961). In recognition of the unique and pervasive nature of the self, theorists and researchers have identified a number of processes that are specific to the self and make it unlike other psychological structures. Such phenomena as self-esteem maintenance (Tesser, Martin, & Cornell, 1996), self-verification (Swann, 1990), self-deception (Gur & Sackheim, 1979), self-conscious emotions (Tangney & Fischer, 1995), identity maintenance (Brewer & Kramer, 1985), and maintenance of personal standards (Carver & Scheier, 1981; Duval & Wicklund, 1972; Higgins, 1987) attest to the special nature of the self-structure.

Integration and Differentiation in the Self System

But while the self is clearly unique, it can also be viewed as a complex system composed of many interacting elements. As such, self-structure and process can be understood in terms of multiple feedback loops and the emergence of properties from the operation of such feedback loops over many iterations. Integration in the self system thus is not achieved through control by a higher order structure, but rather is an emergent property that derives from the local interactions among elements. In the process of integration, each element adjusts itself to the joint input coming from other relevant elements. Each element, of course, also reacts to incoming information. But without internal mechanisms working to achieve integration, the coherence of the self-structure would never exceed the coherence of incoming information.

For such a large structure as the self, these local mechanisms are unlikely to produce global integration. Instead, integration is achieved among specific subsets of elements, corresponding to roles, domain-specific self-images, self-schemata, and areas of personal competence or concern (see Biddle & Thomas, 1966; Gergen, 1971; Goffman, 1959; Linville, 1985; Sarbin & Allen, 1968; Vallacher, 1980). In view of the importance of evaluation to social judgment generally (Chapter 3) and to self-concept in particular (e.g., Duval & Wicklund, 1972; Tesser & Campbell, 1983), the various subsets of self are likely to achieve internal coherence with respect to a shared valence. When each region of the self system achieves such coherence and the various regions differ in their overall valence, the self system as a whole can be described as evaluatively differentiated. In a perfectly differentiated system, there is clear separation between those aspects of self that are viewed positively and those that are viewed negatively. In effect, the person knows in which realms he or she is good and in which realms he or she is bad.

The particular subsets that develop in a self system are likely to vary considerably from person to person and as a function of cultural and subcultural differences. This is because the evaluative dimension can provide integration for elements that are quite disparate with respect to cognitive content and means–end relations (see Vallacher & Nowak, 1994c, 1997). Resisting the temptation to cheat on one's taxes and helping a person in need are clearly distinct elements, for example, but both reflect positively on one's sense of self as a socially responsible person. By the same token, cognitive elements that form a logically consistent structure may be vastly different in their evaluative implications. Being helpful to a stranger in need, for example, has a conflicting evaluative connotation with being helpful to a criminal. Because evaluative consistency provides the ultimate basis for integration, these two elements may be hard to reconcile with respect to one's sense of self. In short, although elements can be related to one another in many ways, the degree to which they are effectively integrated is signaled by their evaluative consistency (Abelson et al., 1968).

By itself, any element of the self is vulnerable to incoming information that undermines its validity. The sense that one is a good test-taker, for example, can be shaken by a string of mediocre exam performances, or even poor performance on a particularly salient exam. When an element is integrated into a coherent subset, however, it receives supportive influence from the other elements in its local neighborhood. Test-taking ability, for instance, may be part of a larger self-domain involving one's overall competence as a student. Thus, in the face of negative feedback regarding test performance, one can maintain a positive self-view as a student because of other relevant self-as-student elements (instructor feedback, success in writing, performance on other types of tests). Even if incoming information causes an element in a well-integrated structure to change, the influence of the other elements in the structure is likely to restore its original value. The certainty associated with an integrated subset of elements, then, may be considerably higher than the certainty associated with any of the elements in isolation. A differentiated self system thus provides for self-certainty and a sense of personal integration.

Intrinsic Dynamics of Self-Organization

Nowak et al. (1997) developed a cellular automata model to illustrate the basic nature of integration processes in the self system. This model shares some of the general features of the cellular automata model of social influence proposed by Nowak et al. (1990), described in detail in Chapter 7. We assume that a self system is composed of *n* elements, each reflecting a specific aspect of the self. The elements are represented as cells arranged on a two-dimensional grid. The physical proximity between any two elements corresponds to their degree of relatedness. Each element is characterized with respect to its current evaluation. For sake of simplicity, an element can be either positive (denoted by light gray) or negative (dark gray). Some elements are more important than others and thus have greater weight. An element's importance is denoted by its height and does not change in the course of simulation. As a simplification, each element influences and is influenced by its eight neighboring elements (four on the adjacent sides and four on the connecting diagonals).

In the course of simulation, a randomly chosen element tries to adjust to its neighboring elements. It does this by checking how much influence it receives from the positive as opposed to the negative neighbors. This involves weighting the valence of each neighbor by the neighbor's importance. The resultant computation is the weighted sum of evaluations of the neighboring elements, reflecting a process similar to information integration (Anderson, 1981). This evaluative input from neighboring elements is then compared to the current state of the element. If the sign of the element agrees with the overall evaluation suggested by its neighbors, the element's evaluation does not change. If the sign of the element differs from the overall evaluation suggested by its neighbors, the element changes evaluation only if the combined weight of evaluation from other elements is higher than the element's own weighted evaluation. In other words, it is relatively easy for neighboring elements to change the evaluation of a relatively unimportant element, but it is difficult to change the evaluation of a more important aspect of self. After the element's state is adjusted, another element is randomly chosen and the process is repeated. This continues until each element has been chosen. In the next simulation step, each element has a chance to adjust its state again. This is repeated for several simulation steps until the state of the system reaches an asymptote, reflecting either no further change in the states of elements (static equilibrium) or a stable pattern of changes in the system (dynamic equilibrium). There are three basic measures derived in this model.

Self-Evaluation

Self-evaluation is the weighted average of all the elements in the structure (Anderson, 1981), with the weight of each element corresponding to its importance. It is computed according to the following formula:

$$Eval = \frac{\sum\limits_{i=1}^{n} (V_i * W_i)}{\sum\limits_{i=1}^{n} W_i},$$

where V_i is the valence for element i, with $+1$ denoting positivity and -1 denoting negativity, and W_i is the weight (importance) of element i. This index can range from -1 to $+1$, with a value of 0 corresponding to a balance between the weighted average of positive and negative elements.

Evaluative Differentiation

Evaluative differentiation reflects the degree to which the elements form clusters of similar valence. This measure reflects the proportion of neighbors sharing a common valence (as compared to the total number of possible links among neighbors).[1] It is computed according to the following formula:

$$Diff = \frac{(C_{obs} - C_{chance})}{(C_{max} - C_{chance})},$$

where C_{obs} is the number of existing links between neighboring elements of the same valence, C_{chance} is the number of links between neighboring elements of the same valence expected in a randomly ordered system, and C_{max} is the maximum number of links between neighboring elements of the same valence possible in a system where positive and negative elements form two compact clusters. By this measure, 0 reflects a random arrangement of elements, $+1$ reflects the separation of elements into two clusters, and intermediate values reflect varying degrees of spatial order. While C_{obs} is based on observation, C_{chance} and C_{max} are derived theoretically to reflect the number of positive and negative elements and the geometry of the matrix (see Latané, Nowak, & Liu, 1994). In a maximally clustered system, all the elements (except those on the border of a cluster) are surrounded by other elements of the same valence. In a system lacking evaluative differentiation, the probability of two neighboring elements having the same valence is dictated only by the overall proportions of positive and negative elements.

Self-Dynamism

Self-dynamism reflects the proportion of elements that change their state in a given simulation step. At each simulation step, it is computed according to the following formula:

$$Dyn = \frac{k}{n},$$

where k is the number of elements that change their value and n is the total number of elements (i.e., 400). The value of this measure varies between 0, reflecting no change, and 1, reflecting a change in all the sampled elements. When tracked over time, this measure characterizes the volatility of the system's temporal evolution. The value of this measure at the last simulation step (i.e., after the system has reached an asymptote), then, specifies whether the self system has reached a static equilibrium, or instead can be characterized in terms of a dynamic equilibrium with a specific value of volatility.

Figure 5.7 shows a typical course of simulation. In the starting configuration, the positive and negative elements are arranged randomly, corresponding to a self that is undifferentiated (lacking in structure). To capture the positivity bias in self-evaluation (e.g., Taylor & Brown, 1988), 60% of the elements are positive, and 40% are negative. Because some elements are more important than others, a weighted average is calculated to represent overall self-evaluation. Importance is assigned randomly to positive and negative elements, so

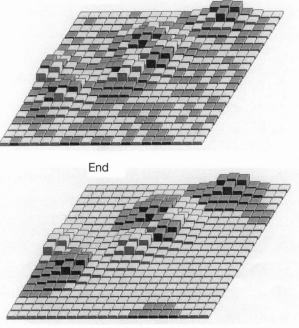

FIGURE 5.7. Self-organization in the self system.

the initial 60–40% distribution corresponds to weighted average values that vary around a mean of 0.2.

Figure 5.8 shows how dynamism, self-evaluation, and differentiation change over the course of simulation portrayed in Figure 5.7. At the beginning of the simulation, there are pronounced dynamics, with many elements changing their state. In the course of simulation, the number of changes decreases until an equilibrium state is finally reached. Since these changes occur in the absence of external influence, they reflect intrinsic dynamics. The most apparent change is the emergence of clusters, with randomly distributed positive and negative elements forming well-defined domains. The emergence of clusters reflects the local nature of influence among elements. If an element is surrounded primarily by elements of the same valence, its valence will not change. If, however, the element happens to be surrounded by elements with a different valence, it is likely to change its state to conform to these elements, although if it is highly important it may resist this influence.[2] As a result of this process, elements of similar valence tend to cluster and produce coherent areas of similar valence. Due to intrinsic dynamics alone, in other words, the self becomes organized in a fairly efficient manner.

In addition to the emergence of structure, the positivity bias in-

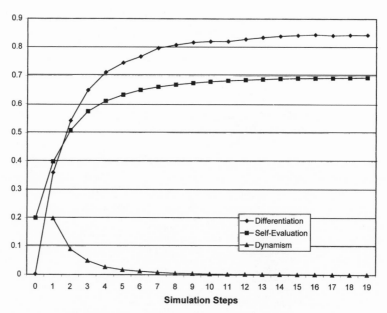

FIGURE 5.8. Change in properties of the self system.

creases, changing from the initial value of 0.2 to an asymptotic value of 0.64. In a disordered system, the proportion of both positive and negative elements in any given area corresponds roughly to the proportion of positive and negative elements in the system as a whole. This means that any given element is more likely to be surrounded by positive than by negative elements and thus likely to experience a pull in a positive direction. In a clustered situation, however, most elements are surrounded by elements of the same valence, so that only the elements on the borders of the clusters are subjected to conflicting influence. The emergence of differentiation thus stabilizes the self system. Although the proportion of positive elements increases, the negative elements that manage to survive tend to be important and hence resistant to further change. The mean weight of negative elements increases, in other words, as less important negative elements are eliminated. This result is consistent with research showing that although positive information is more prevalent than negative information in cognitive structures, negative information tends to be more important (Cacioppo, Gardner, & Berntson, 1997; Coovert & Reeder, 1990; Kanouse & Hanson, 1971; Peeters & Czapinski, 1990; Pratto & John, 1991; Skowronski & Carlston, 1989; Taylor, 1991). This conclusion regarding the average strength of minority elements has also been reached through analytical considerations (Lewenstein et al., 1993).

The intrinsic dynamics observed in these initial simulations are directly attributable to mutual influences among elements in the self system. Such influences presuppose a press for integration; in the absence of such a press, there would be no intrinsic dynamics and thus no self-organization. The strength of this press, though, can clearly vary in accord with contextual and personal variables. In some situations, for example, people are more accountable for their actions or are more likely to feel self-aware and concerned with issues of consistency (e.g., Carver & Scheier, 1981; Wicklund & Frey, 1980). Conditions that make the transmission of information more salient than the receipt of information also tend to heighten the concern with information integration (Zajonc, 1960). On the other hand, people may lack the cognitive resources necessary to achieve integration of diverse elements in these and other situations. This is likely to occur, for example, when people are under stress or experience cognitive overload (Bargh, 1997; Gilbert, 1993). Achieving integration presumably requires cognitive resources (Treisman & Schmidt, 1982), so anything that diverts such resources to other cognitive tasks can weaken integration tendencies. Even under conditions that promote self-awareness (e.g., the presence of an audience) or a concern with transmitting information, the particular demands in that context (e.g., performing a difficult or stressful task) may effectively exhaust the cognitive resources that might otherwise be used to achieve integration. Variation in press for integration, then, is clearly an important variable in the self system. We therefore manipulated this variable and examined its effects in the subsequent simulations.

Intrinsic Dynamics and Incoming Information

The self does not develop in a vacuum. To the contrary, self-understanding is an inherently social phenomenon that depends to a large degree on information mediated by interpersonal contexts. Were it not for such information, there would be no elements of the self to become organized. The sources of self-relevant information are diverse, reflecting such processes as social feedback, social comparison, self-perception of one's actions, perceptions of success versus failure, and so forth. The intrinsic dynamics of the integration processes that assemble the self are rarely left untouched by these sources of incoming information. To model the effects of these influences on the emergence of self, we started with an initially disorganized system, similar to the initial configurations employed in the simulations reported earlier, and varied the intensity and valence of incoming information.

In the first set of simulations, positively and negatively valenced information entered the system with equal probability. Note that this means that incoming information on average was less positive than the initial state of the self system (i.e., 60% positive elements). Operationally, we treated incoming information as a random variable with a mean of 0, signifying neutral evaluation, but with one of four different standard deviations around this mean to express different levels of intensity. In conditions with higher levels of intensity, the incoming information thus had stronger influence on the system, since the information had more highly positive and highly negative components. Information was introduced into the system by adding a random number, drawn from a normal distribution, to the weighted sum of internal influences on each element. This value changed randomly (within a given range of intensity), both across elements and simulation steps, so that the same element might experience a positive influence at one simulation step but a negative influence at the next step. Because of its random nature, information may be considered noise entering the system.

We also manipulated the degree of press for integration by systematically varying the strength of influence among elements. This was accomplished by multiplying the computed influence on each element by a value that was constant for a given round of simulations. The higher this value, the greater the weight attached to the summary evaluation associated with the other elements. A value of 1, representing high press for integration, means that each neighboring element has the same weight as the element itself. A value of 0.1, representing low press, means that the weight of each neighboring element is 10% of the element's weight.

The results of these simulations are displayed in Figures 5.9–5.11. Overall, the incoming information had much less effect when the press for integration was high rather than low. This is directly reflected in self-dynamism. Under high press for integration, only a very small proportion of elements (0.03) changed their state, even under conditions of high information intensity. Self-evaluation and self-differentiation also were largely unaffected by the intensity of incoming information when there was a high press for integration. Having sufficient cognitive resources available enables people to actively resist incoming information that might otherwise undermine their existing sense of self.

When there was a relatively weak press for integration, however, the intensity of incoming information had a marked effect on all three variables. In the absence of information, the influence from neighbor-

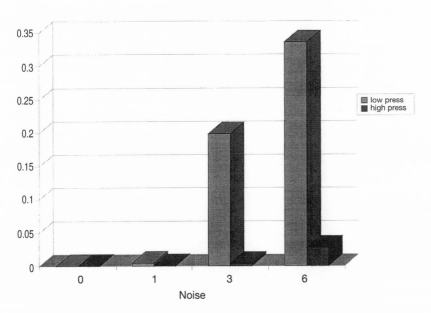

FIGURE 5.9. Dynamism by incoming information and press for integration.

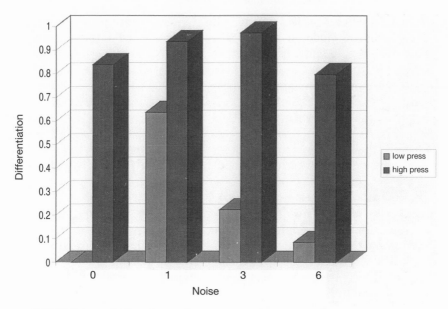

FIGURE 5.10. Self-evaluation by incoming information and press for integration.

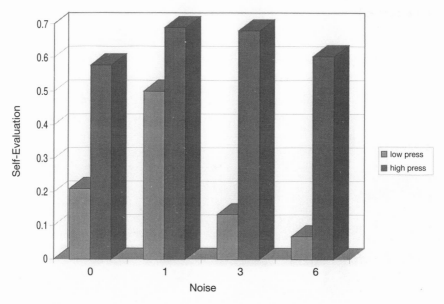

FIGURE 5.11. Self-differentiation by incoming information and press for integration.

ing elements is too weak to change an element, so intrinsic dynamics are at a minimum. In consequence, the system is highly reactive to any incoming information. In effect, the incoming information "shakes up" the system and thereby promotes intrinsic dynamics. Under low values of incoming information, relatively few elements changed their state in a single simulation step. The changes that did occur, however, were almost always in the direction of influence from other elements. Under these conditions, the system achieves the highest self-organization. There is relatively high differentiation and the positivity bias is strongly enhanced. Although the incoming information shakes up the elements, it is insufficient to independently dictate their value. This corresponds to a situation where external information is assimilated into a system only if it agrees with many of the system's elements and thus increases the coherence of the system. If the external influences are relatively weak, the shaking will result in an enhancement of the system's intrinsic dynamics and thus generate an increment in the system's differentiation and positivity.

Paradoxically, then, incoming information of a random structure increases the organization of the self, unless the system is overpowered by the amount of such information. This suggests that a person with a low internal press for integration benefits from social feedback and other sources of self-relevant information, provided the information is not too evaluatively intense. Such information has a way of facilitating the person's self-integration, even if its evaluative structure is essentially random and less positive than the person's existing sense of self. People may turn to others, not to learn specific things about themselves, but to facilitate their own internal process of achieving coherence in their self-concept.

This situation reverses dramatically with higher values of information intensity. In effect, the shaking becomes sufficiently strong that it dictates the dynamics of the system rather than facilitating the system's intrinsic dynamics. With a weak press for integration, the person's existing sense of self is insufficient to provide a basis for rejecting incoming information, making him or her highly vulnerable to social feedback and other sources of self-relevant ideas. Because the structure of incoming information is random, and because system elements change their state independently of their neighborhood context, higher order differentiated structures begin to decompose (or cannot be formed in the first place). The system loses intrinsic dynamics and simply follows outside influences. Because these influences are less positive than the initial state of the system, the positivity bias in self-evaluation diminishes. Lacking the cognitive resources to check for possible inconsistencies and conflicts among elements of the self, the system becomes vulnerable to new information from out-side sources. Without the capacity for rejecting incoming informa-tion, even patently absurd ideas may be initially incorporated into the self system without much resistance (Gilbert, 1993). This clearly cre-ates the potential for high vulnerability to external influence in self-evaluation.

Intrinsic Dynamics and Biased Incoming Information

In the simulations described thus far, incoming information was equal-ly balanced between positive and negative valence. Clearly, informa-tion relevant to the self is rarely balanced in this way in real-world set-tings. Feedback from other people commonly consists of flattering or unflattering judgments about oneself that tend to be self-reinforcing rather than self-negating. To capture evaluative bias of this kind, we ran further simulations in which a constant positive or negative value was added to incoming information, thus producing either a positive or a negative bias. To represent negative bias, the mean of incoming in-formation was changed from 0 to −2; to represent positive bias, the mean was changed to +2. The absence of information, meanwhile, was represented by a value of 0. We ran two sets of simulations to explore the effect of biased incoming information on the self system. In the first, we investigated the effects of valenced information on the devel-opment of the self system as a function of low versus high press for in-tegration. In the second, we investigated how a self system that has al-ready formed (i.e., a self that is positive, differentiated, and high in in-tegration press) reacts to valenced information.

Consider first the results for the effect of incoming information on the formation of the self system. In general, the results are consis-tent with the results of the simulations investigating the effects of ran-dom information, described earlier. Under conditions of high integra-tion press, the self system was able to resist incoming information, re-gardless of its valence. Under low press for integration, in contrast, the self system was strongly affected by incoming information. We found, for example, that negative incoming information was able to reverse the positivity bias and promote negative self-evaluation. Bi-ased information was also similar to random information in its effect on self-differentiation. Under high press for integration, information of either valence had little effect on the degree of clustering, although positive information tended to promote slightly greater clustering than did negative information. Under low press for integration, in-coming information of either valence tended to increase differentia-tion in the self system, a result that replicates the findings regarding the impact of noise. When the bias is positive, increased clustering is caused by the reversal of relatively isolated negative elements. When the bias is negative, increased clustering is caused by the reversal of positive elements that are surrounded by primarily negative elements.

Consider now the effect of biased information on a self system that has already formed. This set of simulations investigated how the self system reestablishes equilibrium after an exposure to positive versus negative incoming information. They differed in two basic ways from the previous simulations. First, the starting configuration reflected the typical final configuration of the earlier simulations—a strong positivity bias, a high degree of differentiation, and no dynamism because of its equilibrium state. Second, the valenced information was presented only at the outset instead of being supplied throughout the simulation steps. The information was introduced by reversing the valence of 15% of either the set of positive elements or the set of negative elements. The system was then allowed to run without the introduction of any further information. Each simulation was conducted under high press for integration. The results for self-evaluation and self-differentiation are presented in Figures 5.12 and 5.13, respectively. Each graph portrays the changes in these measures, with time 1 depicting the equilibrium of the system prior to the receipt of informa-

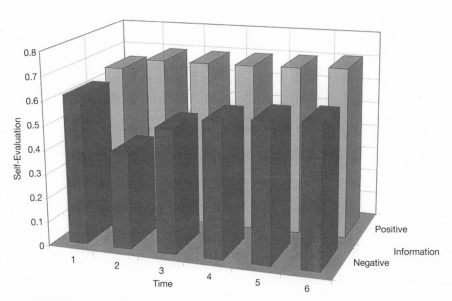

FIGURE 5.12. Self-evaluation by positive versus negative incoming information.

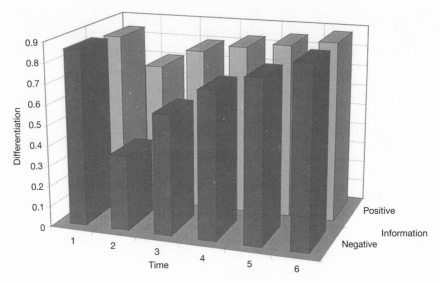

FIGURE 5.13. Self-differentiation by positive versus negative incoming information.

tion, time 2 depicting the state of the system immediately after the information was introduced, and the three succeeding times depicting successive simulation steps. Time 6 portrays the final equilibrium of the system.

For self-evaluation, negative information had a temporary effect, serving to decrease the proportion of positive elements at time 2. After three simulation steps, however, self-evaluation was restored to its original value (0.6). Positive information also produced an initial effect, serving to increase self-evaluation, although this effect was much less pronounced than the effect of negative information. Because of the positivity bias, fewer negative elements were available to be reversed. The increment in positivity in response to positively biased information diminished less than the corresponding decrement produced by negative information. The results for self-differentiation also revealed asymmetry between positively and negatively biased incoming information. Negative information served to disorganize an already organized system to a higher degree than did information biased toward positivity. In both conditions, however, the system's structure became fully reestablished after several simulation steps.

Taken together, these results show that the self system is quite immune to information that contradicts its current state when there is mutual influence among elements. Self systems with a positivity bias are especially immune to negative information. There is an immediate effect of such information, but because of the ongoing integration process the self fairly quickly regains its preexisting equilibrium. In view of the previous simulation results, however, it is clear that the effects of incoming information depend not only on self-evaluation, but also on the structural and dynamic properties that shape the process of integration and assimilation of information.

In other simulations, we have subjected the self system to repetitive instances of incoming negative information. As long as these instances were separated by a few simulation steps that allowed the intrinsic dynamics to promote reintegration, the effects were usually negligible. In essence, each new set of information entered a system that had already the eliminated the effects of earlier negative information. If all the negative information was amassed at the same time, however, the negative items provided mutual support and in effect established new areas of negative valence in the self system. This effect suggests why people with low self-esteem seem to be immune to positive feedback that is distributed over a long period of time (Swann, 1990). Such feedback could well promote change, however, if it was concentrated in time and effectively changed elements at a rate that exceeded the rate of self-integration processes. Indeed, low self-esteem people might be especially inclined to change in this manner, in view of the connection between low self-esteem and indices of uncertainty and poor differentiation (e.g., Kernis, 1993; Linville, 1985; Vallacher, 1978). In fact, poor differentiation may enable such people to accept any information that contradicts their negative self-image.

The cellular automata approach obviously oversimplifies the complex cognitive and affective machinery responsible for the emergence and maintenance of self-structure. This simplified model, however, is useful for revealing some generic properties of systems composed of many interconnected elements. It also exemplifies the basic rule that the stronger the dependence on other elements in a system, the less fragile and vulnerable each element is with respect to external influences. And from a strictly empirical point of view, the results observed in these simulations are compatible with well-established theory and research on the self and reinforce the findings on the intrinsic dynamics of self-reflection we described earlier in the chapter. Although the simulation approach is in a preliminary stage of development, it promises to provide a well-defined platform for integrating existing ideas and for developing and testing new predictions regarding the interplay between dynamics and structure in self-understanding. This approach thus serves as a model of qualitative understanding that holds potential for integrating principles of self with other complex systems in social life and the natural world.

SELF-CONTROL

Theoretical treatments of the self at some point invariably address the issue of self-control. Indeed, it is common to single out the capacity for self-control as one of the defining characteristics of human nature (e.g., Baumeister & Heatherton, 1996; Carver & Scheier, 1998; Duval & Wicklund, 1972; Vallacher, 1980). In general terms, the capacity for self-control simply means that people can inhibit the expression of their thoughts, feelings, and actions, and are capable of terminating these overt features of human experience once they are initiated. By the same token, self-control refers to the ability to initiate and maintain courses of action that run counter to one's impulses. People, in other words, are said to be uniquely capable of altering their ongoing processes of mind and behavior.

System Coherence and Self-Control

The exercise of such control implies the existence of another process beyond the ones being controlled. This executive or metacontrol process is commonly discussed in terms of self-awareness or self-directed attention (Wicklund & Frey, 1980). On this view, to be self-aware is to be aware of any discrepancies between a current action or action representation and some personal or social standard of appropriateness or desirability (Higgins, 1987; Vallacher & Solodky, 1979; Wicklund & Frey, 1980). These discrepancies are experienced as negative affect; the greater the deviation from whatever standard is salient, the greater the negative affect. The negative affect associated with such discrepancies is commonly discussed under the category of "self-conscious emotions" (Tangney & Fischer, 1995) and includes such states as embarrassment, guilt, and shame. People are motivated to reduce the perceived discrepancies so as to eliminate the negative affective state. In reducing discrepancies, or by avoiding them in the first place, people are said to exercise self-control over their impulses, egoistic desires, unacceptable feelings, and immoral thoughts. Self-awareness, in other words, is a vivid and unpleasant signal that one's state is not well coordinated with a relevant mental representation.

There is a clear parallel between this general depiction of self-control and the depiction of mind–action coordination presented in Chapter 4. The central idea is that when there is a breakdown in the coordination of mind and action, people experience negative emotion and heightened self-consciousness (Vallacher et al., 1998). This signal of ineffective coordination interrupts the behavioral sequence (Mandler, 1975; Simon, 1967) and induces people to recalibrate their mental representation of the act to match its performance difficulty. The self-focused attention induced by poor mind–action coordination is in marked contrast to the loss of self-awareness that is said to occur when one is in a state of flow (Csikszentmihalyi, 1990) or experiencing a dynamic orientation with respect to the environment (Wicklund, 1986). By this reasoning, when action is proceeding in an efficient, self-sustaining manner and produces feedback indicating that the mind is well-coordinated with the action's performance, there is no need for a control process to modify the action. In effect, the mind is called upon to inhibit current action and devise new action plans when mechanisms generating the action cannot cope with the demands and contingencies in the action context.

Self-control can thus be represented as a feedback loop in which the detection of low coherence in the self system triggers negative emotions and self-consciousness. Self-consciousness, in turn, triggers a change in the system's control variables that further disrupts the ongoing action and attempts to find a new mode for restoring coherence to the system. Viewing self-control in terms of system coherence rather than restricting this notion to features of the self-concept per se makes this phenomenon compatible with the notion of control in nonlinear dynamical systems and thus open to investigation with dynamical concepts and tools. Moreover, this perspective holds potential for integrating seemingly distinct forms of self-control operating at different levels of social reality. Thus, the dynamics at work in correcting simple behaviors or mastering new actions may be no different in principle than the processes of self-regulation associated with interpersonal relations or broad social norms.

Social Self-Control

Self-control extends beyond achieving coherence with respect to purely personal aims to incorporate feedback loops that are social in nature. The various structures of the self, after all, are dependent to a substantial degree on a number of interpersonal processes, including social feedback, social comparison, social influence, and self-verification. Ironically, it is by attending to the self-relevant information provided through these channels that the self achieves autonomy and some degree of independence from social support. As both empirical data (Vallacher et al., 1997) and the results of computer simulations (Nowak et al., 1997) indicate, the flow of even random external information relevant to the self may contribute to increased order in the self system, provided that the information does not overwhelm the system's ability to absorb it. As a result, self-control commonly involves maintaining coherence with respect to stable domains of social self-definition. Rather than acting only on the basis of personal pleasures and simple self-interest, people attempt to control their behavior so as to maintain coordination with internalized representations of the social environment.

It is noteworthy, but not all that surprising perhaps, that actions for which mind–action coordination is easiest and most natural to obtain are also those for which social norms are most likely to develop. Sex provides a case in point. This act represents what is arguably the most basic of all evolved psychological mechanisms. Its status as a powerful and fundamental impulse suggests that relatively little mind–action coordination is required for it to transpire with a fairly high degree of effectiveness. Yet virtually every culture surrounds sexual relations with a host of values, beliefs, and norms that function to restrain people from acting on their impulses. This makes good sense from the point of view of social coordination (Caporael & Brewer, 1995). Unrestrained sexual relations in a social system would pose serious risks to pair bonding and commitment to child rearing on the part of males, and it would promote considerable conflict within and between the sexes. Even in a culture such as ours that sets limits (albeit often ambiguous and inconsistent limits) on sexual behavior, suspected or feared infidelity produces considerable strain on a relationship and is the leading cause of spousal abuse and homicide by males (Wilson & Daly, 1992). Similar restrictions are placed on a host of other behaviors that do not pose much of a challenge for mind–action coordination and which represent basic sources of personal satisfaction or enjoyment. Societal restraint, by definition it seems, is at odds with personal gratification. Personal desires and impulses clearly have the potential for being in conflict with broader social and societal needs. From this perspective, the role of society is to disrupt certain natural tendencies toward mind–action coordination.

With this in mind, social norms are likely to conflict with an established self-structure that is resistant to change and well anchored by mutual support among elements. While individual elements of incongruent information are likely to be rejected by a coherent self-structure, elements of coherent social standards also support each other and therefore resist rejection. In this case, such elements may become the seed for a separate self system. Whereas the established self-structure attempts to achieve coherence with respect to other psychological structures and action, the normative self-structure attempts to achieve coherence with respect to the social environment. To the extent that these structures are independent of each other, people can function both as autonomous agents and as members of social groups and societies. This distinction corresponds to a well-documented distinction between private and public self (e.g., Baumeister, 1991; Fenigstein, Scheier, & Buss, 1975; Scheier & Carver, 1983). The private self is likely to supply standards of control in a situation where self-relevant feedback is provided in the process of self-reflection. The public self can override this process by supplying salient social standards by which one is expected to regulate one's thoughts and actions.

When the self-control mechanisms are part of a social feedback loop early in development, the private and public selves may be integrated and act as a single system. The social bases for self-control simply enhance internal bases for self-control. This confluence of self-control mechanisms is said to characterize so-called collectivist cultures (Markus & Kitayama, 1991), in which interdependence is emphasized at the expense of independence. This orientation toward self-control stands in marked contrast to that of Western societies—most notably, perhaps, the United States—in which independence is valued and reinforced more than interdependence. When a person from a Western society demonstrates a lapse in social self-control, pursuing his or her own interests and impulses to the detriment of the interests or needs of others, it is common for excuses and justifications to be offered. They are not always accepted, of course, but their success rate is sufficiently high that everyone seems attuned to their use. In Eastern societies, such as China and Japan, justifications and excuses are simply not relevant. People are expected to coordinate with others and with social norms, so any evidence that they have pursued their own personal concerns is a cause for social condemnation. In such societies, negative feedback is simply that—feedback produced by one's action that serves to regulate future action.

The integration between private and public selves is clearly possible in principle, but only in a very stable society is it likely to be complete. If social norms and standards change, a discrepancy between private and public self is likely to be recreated. In times of social transitions, then, one may expect a noticeable breakdown in the coordination between the individual and society. At the turn of the century, it is common for social commentators to bemoan the apparent breakdown in social coherence in certain Western democracies, as indexed by such disturbing phenomena as growing alienation and anomie, acts of violence and terrorism, loss of social concern, a decrease in the civility of public discourse, teen rebellion and suicide, and so forth. The different cultures and languages in modern society introduce healthy diversity into a culture and promote innovation and new forms, but such differences also produce enormous coordination problems when people from diverse backgrounds come into contact. The diversity of social norms, moreover, makes each of them seem somewhat relative or arbitrary and thus open to question. Rules are seen as agents of control rather than as unquestioned assumptions and guidelines for personal experience.

There are downsides of a more personal nature when there is a split between private and public self-control. In coordinating exclusively with interpersonal and societal norms, first of all, there is a potential for the disruption of action that might be enjoyable and rewarding at a personal level. No doubt, part of the mutual fascination among romantic partners is the promise of being able to coordinate personally and interpersonally at the same time. It is interesting that people who are most normatively controlled (i.e., authoritarians) and those who are most sensitive to direct interpersonal coordination (i.e., high in social desirability or need for approval) are typically the least spontaneous and happy, but the most guilt-ridden and anxious. It may be, too, that the pressures to suspend one's personal coordination in favor of interpersonal or normative coordination promotes the use of outlets that allow one to achieve something akin to flow. The use of drugs and alcohol, for example, is motivated in part by a desire to reduce self-awareness and to achieve a more harmonious mental and emotional state (Hull & Young, 1983). Baumeister (1991) made an argument along these lines with respect to "escaping the self." There is a certain burden associated with the public self; coordinating with the expectations of others and the larger society tends to be at the expense of impulse and personal desires. A person who feels excessively burdened in this way looks for outlets in which he or she can coordinate mind and action without the standards of society posing a disruptive threat.

Another danger follows from the perils associated with the suppression of thought and behavior. If thoughts and impulses are not discharged, they can become a preoccupation and a basis for obsession. Even simple thoughts and one-step behaviors are hard to suppress, particularly when one is depleted of cognitive resources (Wegner, 1994). Over a short time span, there may be a simple rebound or resurgence of suppressed thought or behavior. Over a longer time span, there is potential for a sudden and dramatic resurgence as increasingly long queues of undischarged components are accumulated. It may be that people whose private self is largely divorced from social norms, but who act in accordance with the latter nonetheless, are at enhanced risk for sudden and exaggerated acting out of impulses and fantasies. This possibility is clearly speculative at this point, although theory and research on the antecedents and consequences of thought suppression provide indirect support (see Wegner, 1989, 1994). In a study by Wegner et al. (1995), for example, participants who were instructed not to think about sex became as preoccupied with this topic over time as did those who were instructed to think about sex. More generally, this line of research has shown that the attempt to suppress a given thought or representation of behavior can lead to a resurgence of such states when cognitive resources are insufficient to maintain integration.

Clearly, not all social and personal problems can be attributed to a discrepancy between the private and public self. Nonetheless, to the extent that there is conflict between different self-control mechanisms, it is reasonable to expect a decrease in the overall effectiveness of control. When the private self calls for different actions than the public self, and if people act in accordance with the former rather than the latter, social control mechanisms are likely to be called into play to regulate individual behavior. Thus, many issues that would normally be controlled at the level of individual restraint in a stable social system become increasingly micromanaged by social and societal institutions (police, courts, politics). When personal means of self-control based on internalized values, norms, and principles fail, the diminution of self-control is compensated by an increase in social control over increasingly private aspects of behavior. Achieving a balance between private and social self-control is clearly a daunting task but one that cannot be sidestepped if we hope to enter the next millennium prepared to meet the challenges of increasing population, contact among diverse cultures, and dwindling resources.

THE SELF SYSTEM IN PERSPECTIVE

The self provides the means by which human experience is structured. It also imposes organization and control with respect to other psychological structures (e.g., social judgment) and provides a coherent basis for action. On the other hand, the self is itself subject to control and organization. Recognition of this dual nature of the self can be traced to the founding fathers of social psychology (e.g., Cooley, 1902; James, 1890; Mead, 1934) and has given shape to formulations of the self ever since. Despite large and significant differences among the wide variety of contemporary approaches to the self, they all share the assumption that the self is both the subject and the object of thought and judgment.

While it is relatively easy to see how self imposes control and organization on other structures, it is somewhat puzzling what imposes control and organization on the self. This puzzle brings to mind the philosophically untenable notion of the homunculus (see Ryle, 1949; Vallacher, 1980). The intuition here is that the idea of control implies directly the existence of a controlling agent, a superordinate higher level structure that imposes organization on the lower level structure. Acceptance of this idea immediately raises the question of what organizes *this* higher order structure, and so on, ad infinitum. Although the notion of a hierarchy of self is certainly reasonable (see Carver & Scheier, 1981), simply invoking yet higher levels hardly solves the basic problem, but rather leads only to an infinite regress. This paradox is partly solved by assuming that at some point, self-control is transferred to society, so that self becomes an element within a yet larger system. Nonetheless, both theoretical considerations and intuition point to the fact that the self can function autonomously to impose organization on itself and control its own processes. Although society may be critical for imposing norms and values that function as standards of self-control, it is ultimately the self that has the responsibility for checking inconsistencies with respect to such standards, imposing integration, and controlling courses of action aimed at meeting these standards. The question thus remains, how does one avoid the potential for infinite regress in self-control?

The phenomenon of self-organization, which has proven central to the dynamical systems approach, provides insight into this problem. Computer simulations as well as analytical considerations show that global order in a system may emerge from local interactions between system elements, without any higher order supervisory mechanism (Haken, 1982; Kelso, 1995; Progigine & Stengeors, 1984; Weisbuch, 1992). Self-organization in the self system reflects the ongoing process of integration, in which each element's value is verified with respect to other elements. As a result of this process of progressive integration, the self becomes differentiated, with clusters of interrelated elements sharing the same value. When the self becomes integrated in this fashion, the system loses degrees of freedom, and the unit of analysis may change from single elements to clusters of elements that correspond to various aspects of self, such as roles, domains, and self-schemata. In this case, support for a particular aspect of the self is not dependent on the fate of an individual element of that aspect, but rather derives from support from other elements and from higher order feedback relevant to the cluster as a whole.

Once a reasonable level of integration is achieved, the self is in a position to provide organization and control for other psychological structures and action. These functions operate in a feedback loop, in which the settings of control parameters depend on the coherence of self and, in turn, the coherence of self depends on the settings of control parameters. Poor coherence in this feedback loop can trigger negative emotions and self-consciousness, setting in motion processes to restore equilibrium. Even a smoothly flowing action may be disrupted in the process of coordinating with others. One may not have the means to coordinate with others, for example, or the demands for coordination may be in conflict with each other. In such cases, the self would be called upon to reset and redesign action. Incoherence may also arise from conflict with internalized social norms. In these cases, the normal flow of action is interrupted and the mechanism of self-control becomes the source of action generation. The potential sources of poor coherence exist at different levels, then, from the internal workings of the mind–action system, to the coordination of this system with the mind–action systems of others, and finally to the coordination of the mind–action system with the larger society in which it is embedded.

As noted at the outset, many theories of self are congruent with key assumptions of the dynamical perspective. Our aim in this chapter was not to point out flaws in other formulations, but rather to outline a dynamical approach to key issues concerning the self and to show how central concepts from the self literature can be captured by such notions as self-organization and self-control feedback loops. Viewed in this way, the self reveals the operation of mechanisms that are common to other domains of social psychological functioning, including social judgment, the mental control of action, close relationships, social influence, and the coordination of individuals and social groups.

NOTES

1. Note that self-evaluation and evaluative differentiation are largely independent of one another. Self-evaluation represents the (weighted) proportion of positive versus negative elements, whereas evaluative differentiation describes the grouping of these elements. A system may be both highly positive and highly differentiated, for example, if it contains very few negative elements that are confined to a compact region of the self system.

2. Note that elements on the borders of the simulation matrix are surrounded by five rather than eight elements and those in the corners are surrounded by only three elements. Clusters of negative elements in these positions thus have a slight survival advantage in that their relative isolation protects them against influence from conflicting elements.

6

↭

Interpersonal Dynamics

T O THIS POINT, THE FOCUS has been on individual level processes—
social judgment, action, and self-concept—that reflect dynamics
within the individual. Such dynamics are clearly rich and complex
enough in their own right. This complexity is magnified considerably
when two individuals become sufficiently attracted to one another to
establish a close relationship requiring the coordination of their personal patterns of thought, action, and self-reflection. Achieving such
coordination is not an easy matter, as is abundantly evident in the
enormous and sustained fascination throughout history and across all
cultures with romantic entanglements. Judging by the content of media that cater to popular interest (movies, music, literature, television
programming), no topic is guaranteed to attract greater interest than a
discussion of intimate relationships, even when those relationships involve people who are total strangers to the audience. This interest is
fueled in large part by the potential for both bliss and tragedy when
two individuals attempt to strike a balance between autonomy and
unity, between the dynamics each brings to the relationship and the
dynamics associated with the dyadic system they create. Not surprisingly, then, considerable theory and research in social psychology has
centered on the formation, maintenance, and dissolution of close relationships.

To this rich and extensive literature, we add concepts, considerations, and evidence reflecting a dynamical perspective. By depicting
close relationships as dynamical systems, many of the insights generated over the years are brought into even sharper relief. In providing
new concepts and research strategies, moreover, new insights and the
means by which these insights may be investigated are provided as

well. We focus in particular on two key features of dynamical systems: the coordination of individual elements to create a higher order system and the evolution of system equilibria. In discussing each feature, we present a formal model and preliminary results from computer simulations and experiments. In a concluding section, we reframe well-documented features of close relationships from a dynamical perspective.

THE COORDINATION OF DYNAMICS

It is common in social psychology to characterize relationships in terms of concepts such as attraction, power, and commitment. Such concepts play a prominent role in lay descriptions as well, but so do depictions that have a more dynamic feel to them. Thus, individuals in the throes of a romantic relationship are commonly said to "be on the same wavelength" or to "resonate with one another," whereas those in a less than fulfilling relationship are said to be "out of sync with each other." The intuitive wisdom here captures a primary aspect of a dynamical system: the coordination of individual elements to produce a higher order system. This is not to downplay the importance of aggregate characterizations such as affection, commitment, and the like. These characterizations, however, can be viewed as indicators of how well, and in what manner, the individuals in the relationship have managed to synchronize the patterns of thought, feeling, and action they bring to the relationship. By understanding the mode and depth of coordination in a relationship, then, one may be in a position to characterize the dyad in terms of the global parameters that are of focal concern in social psychological theory and research.

The Role of Coordination

For all their intensity, close relationships are also highly fragile phenomena. This is understandable when one considers the degree and depth of coordination required to couple the complex dynamics of two individuals. If such coordination is achieved, a higher order system is created that captures the essence of both individuals, while at the same time creating a new set of rich and pleasurable dynamics. But in view of the challenge posed by this coordination problem, it is not surprising that close relationships often contain the seeds of their own destruction, a fate that all too often transpires with minimal assistance from outside forces.

Coordination can take qualitatively different forms. Positive correlation is a very basic form, in which the behaviors or internal states of one person induce similar behaviors or states in the other person. Imitation and empathy capture this form of coordination. An equally simple form, but one with far different implications for the relationship, is negative correlation. In a relationship that has become antagonistic, for instance, the sadness of one person might induce satisfaction in the other and vice versa. Coordination can also take on more complex forms that reflect nonlinear relationships and higher order interactions between the partners' respective behaviors and internal states. Indeed, the synchronization characterizing some relationships may be sufficiently subtle and complex to confuse observers, or perhaps the partners themselves. In such instances, discerning the nature of the relationship may require plotting the behaviors or states of one person against the behaviors or states of the other person and looking for a well-defined pattern (see Chapter 2 for a discussion of relevant methods).

Beyond variation in its form, coordination can also vary with respect to the aspects of experience subject to synchronization attempts. The most basic unit of coordination is overt behavior. Thus, people can synchronize their interactions and relationships in terms of the rudimentary components of action, such as specific movements and gestures. Dancing and taking turns in a conversation represent this level of interpersonal coordination. Coordination, however, can also take place with respect to control parameters that set the stage for overt behavior. Thus, people in a relationship may attempt to synchronize their moods, perspectives, values, and internal rhythms, as well as their plans, goals, and other mental representations that serve to integrate basic aspects of overt behavior. Coordination with respect to such internal states would seem to have greater bearing on the quality of a relationship than would coordination with respect to relatively superficial and transient aspects of experience (e.g., rate of speech, movement characteristics). Both aspects of experience play an important role in the development and maintenance of close relationships, however. Issues of coordination with respect to each are discussed in turn.

The Coordination of Behavior

In its most basic form, coordination refers to the coupling of behavior patterns. This aspect of interpersonal coordination has been investigated from a dynamical perspective in the context of movement coordination (e.g., Beek & Hopkins, 1992; Schmidt et al., 1991; Turvey, 1990). In this line of research, pairs of individuals are simply asked to swing their legs. One person swings his or her legs in time to a metronome, and the other person tries to match those movements. This simple paradigm reveals several phenomena concerning synchronization of individuals' movements. First, synchronization may be in-phase, with people swinging their legs in unison, or in anti-phase, with people swinging their legs with the same frequency but in the opposite direction. Second, hysteresis is commonly observed. When participants are instructed to synchronize out-of-phase and the frequency of movement increases, at some tempo they are no longer able to synchronize anti-phase, and they switch their synchronization mode to in-phase. When the tempo decreases again, at some value they are able to coordinate out of phase again, but this tempo is significantly lower than the point at which they originally started to synchronize in-phase. The appearance of hysteresis shows that coordination in movement can be analyzed as a nonlinear dynamical system (see Kelso, 1995). The control parameter in this case is the tempo of movement. Yet more complex modes of coordination have been captured in this line of research (e.g., Baron et al., 1994; Kelso, 1995; Turvey, 1990).

These seemingly simple findings may be reflected in more complex social situations. When the tempo of behavior is increased, such as in a high-stress or panic situation, it may prove impossible for people to coordinate their respective behaviors in any other than an in-phase manner. In a crowded disco that suddenly bursts into flames, for example, it may be impossible for people to take turns leaving the room, although that is the only mode of coordination that would make evacuation possible. Instead, everyone tries to match the behavior of everyone else, thus preventing more complex modes of coordination from developing. In similar fashion, it may be difficult for members of a dyad to take turns in speaking in a stressful or otherwise emotion-inducing situation. Arguments have this quality, of course, but so do contexts defined in terms of excitement, anticipation, and other positive forms of affect.

In most life situations (aside from dancing, perhaps), interpersonal coordination involves more than simply swinging legs in unison. An interesting approach to capture more complex modes of coordination in motor behavior has been developed by Newtson (1994; Newtson et al., 1987). The basic idea in this approach is quantifying the intensity of behavior in an interval of time. Newtson assigns a single point for each body part that moves during the interval. Moving a leg or one's head would correspond to a single point, for example, whereas standing up would correspond to many points, because body parts change their configuration. In his research, human movements correspond to waves. Initial isolated movements (low scores) gradually combine and build to massive movements corresponding to high scores, which then dissolve back into isolated movements. When two people interact, the behavior of each of them may be represented as a wave. We can then describe the interaction as a temporal relation between the waves representing the behavior of each person.

Several interesting phenomena have been generated within this approach. For each individual, voice and nonverbal behavior tend to be highly intercorrelated, so that those who have a tendency to speak rather than listen also tend to gesture a great deal. When individuals are engaged in a conversation, they tend to alternate their speaking turns in a simple anti-phase pattern. More detailed analyses of the relation between verbal and nonverbal behaviors of the interactants has revealed that each person synchronizes his or her gestures (e.g., head nodding) to the other's voice. In research relevant to this point (Jaffe & Feldstein, 1970), cited by Newtson (1994), it was found that turn taking in conversation was rarely symmetrical. Each person in a small group had a brief pairwise conversation with everyone else. It turned out that each dyad had stable characteristic turn lengths for each speaker, with equal turn lengths being unusual. These turn lengths were replicated during a subsequent encounter two weeks later, and thus appeared to be reliable aspects of a dyad's pattern of coordination. These results suggest that each speaker's characteristic frequency was adjusted to the frequency of the partner.

Another phenomenon observed by Newtson (1994) is shadowing. Interactants often adopt the posture of their partners. If one person in a dyad crosses his or her legs, the other person will probably do so with 10 to 20 seconds. Coordination in this case can be characterized as synchronization with a time lag. Newtson points out that when interaction is somewhat difficult to follow or understand, the one having difficulty following the other is likely to assume a motionless posture, often by bracing the body, as with a chin on one hand. In a related vein, research on interaction synchrony (Tickle-Degnen & Rosenthal, 1987) and entrainment (McGrath & Kelly, 1986) suggests that positive interactions are associated with smooth coordination between participants. This essentially means that an individual synchronizes to the rhythms and movements of another person with whom he or she is interacting. Synchrony can arise both from mirroring of the other's movements and from an "out-of-phase" coordination of speech and movement during an interaction (Condon & Ogston, 1967). Such interpersonal coordination or synchrony can be observed at above chance levels by trained observers (Bernieri, Reznick, & Rosenthal, 1988). There is reason to believe that interaction synchrony helps to regulate smooth and efficient verbal exchange (Dittman & Llewellyn, 1969).

Behavior coordination takes place as well with regard to action at somewhat higher levels of action identification. Thus, the members of a dyad may engage in the same activities together (e.g., eating dinner, watching a movie), they may take turns in enacting certain behaviors (e.g., describing the day's events, taking a shower, providing one another back rubs), they may follow agreed-upon plans to achieve common goals (e.g., going shopping and preparing for a party), and they may agree upon a division of labor to achieve multiple goals (e.g., paying bills, doing laundry, deciding on a night's entertainment). These means of coordinating behavior are clearly not unique to close relationships; indeed, the very fabric of social life is defined in terms of coordination among people who may not even know each other (e.g., waiting in line at a movie theater, the scripted interaction between a store clerk and a customer). Coordination in a close relationship, though, is far more pervasive than it is in everyday encounters with strangers, colleagues, and acquaintances. Close individuals coordinate specific acts as well as behavior patterns across a wide variety of contexts, and the behaviors subject to coordination range from superficial transactions to deeply intimate encounters.

The Coordination of Internal States

The qualitative properties of a system's dynamics are determined by the setting of the system's control parameters. In a psychological system, control parameters refer to factors that are internal to the person. Some of these factors are variable, such as arousal, mood, mental set, and the availability of cognitive resources. Others, however, are more enduring properties of the person, such as temperament, personality traits, values, goals, and plans. In a close relationship, coordination commonly goes beyond the coupling of overt behavior to include the coupling of these internal states. To say that two people have achieved intimacy is tantamount to saying that they resonate with one another at a very deep level that transcends overt behavior. Such notions as empathy, perspective taking, and emotional compatibility capture this form of coordination.

Through the coordination of control parameters, people in close relationships essentially form a higher level system. Each person's idiosyncratic pattern of thoughts, moods, and other phenomenal states modifies and is modified in turn by the other person's pattern of intrapersonal processes. Because of the loss of independence this entails, the resultant system has fewer degrees of freedom than the sum of the component parts. To maintain the relationship necessarily entails relinquishing other avenues of behavior, such as dating other people or following impulses that do not involve the partner. At the same time, though, the higher level system may have more degrees of freedom than do each of the individuals comprising the system and thus may generate more complex dynamics than the individuals alone are capable of generating. In the context of the relationship, for example, two people can pool their talents, interests, and social contacts, thereby establishing new courses of activity.

Although the coordination of behavior and the coordination of control parameters seem to reflect very different psychological mechanisms, these modes of coordination are related. To begin with, the distinction between them is not as sharp as the extreme examples provided earlier would suggest. After all, an action can be identified at many different levels, not just in terms of physical movements on the one hand and abstract plans and goals on the other (Vallacher & Wegner, 1985). With increased levels of action identification, coordination becomes less tied to the precise nature of overt behavior and correspondingly more concerned with global behavioral properties (e.g., patterns, goals, values) that transcend physical movements. It is also the case that coordinating on the level of internal states can promote behavioral coordination. When the control parameters of two people are set at similar values, it is natural for their behavior to achieve coordination as well. Because they have a shared wellspring for action, people with synchronized mental and emotional states are in a position to coordinate their behavior without tracking one another's specific acts. Very subtle cues may be sufficient for sustained coordination of behavior, and these cues do not need to be provided on a frequent basis. Even when there is a cessation of behavioral cues (e.g., because of physical separation), people who have synchronized their mental states can continue to coordinate with respect to higher level representations of behavior (e.g., goals, plans, values). Thus, a close couple may be apart for a long time, yet remain synchronized in their decision making, reaction to events, and resistance to temptation. The persistence of high-level synchronization enables the partners to resynchronize very quickly at a more concrete level when they are reunited.

If, however, the settings of the control parameters of two people are very different, the maintenance of behavioral coordination is difficult, since the intrinsic dynamics of each system are very different. There is evidence, for example, that sibling differences in temperament can hinder effective emotional and behavioral coordination (Dunn & Plomin, 1990). In cases where individual's control parameters are highly divergent, coordination may be maintained only by being provided constant cues about one another's behavior. When someone is depressed at a party, for example, it is possible for him or her to match the behavior of others at the party, but this requires constant attention to what they are doing, and any lapse in attention is likely to lead to a breakdown in coordination, such that his or her actions suddenly decouple from the actions of others. Behavioral coordination in such situations is also relatively costly, since it requires sustained attention to the other person and the inhibition of one's own action tendencies.

The coordination of internal states is intuitively reasonable, but it is far from obvious how it is attained. Coordinating with someone at a concrete behavioral level is possible simply through imitation. However, one does not observe, say, a person's value in the same way that one observes his or her physical movements. To a certain degree, of course, internal states can be directly communicated through verbal and nonverbal channels. An important phase in the development of a close relationship, in fact, involves the explicit communication of one another's internal states, from momentary feelings to long-term hopes, dreams, and insecurities. Even without explicit communication, people can make inferences about one another's internal states from the observation of behavior (Jones & Davis, 1965). There is an extensive literature in social psychology concerning the means by which people gain insight into one another's motives, beliefs, values, and momentary bases for action (e.g., Fiske & Taylor, 1991; Gilbert, 1995; Hastorf et al., 1977; Higgins & Bargh, 1987; Nisbett & Ross, 1980; Wegner & Vallacher, 1977; Zebrowitz, 1990). These mechanisms can play a crucial role in gaining insight into someone's salient internal states for purposes of achieving coordination with him or her.

Internal synchronization with respect to mental and emotional states can also be achieved by sustained coordination on a behavioral level. The work associated with the facial feedback hypothesis, for instance, shows that when people are induced to mechanically adopt a specific facial configuration linked to a particular mood (e.g., disgust), they tend also to adopt the respective affective state (e.g., Strack, Martin, & Stepper, 1988). This matching of internal states to overt behavior is likely to be stronger when the behavior is interpersonal in nature. Even role playing, in which a person simply follows a behavioral script in social interaction, often produces pronounced changes in attitudes and values on the part of the role-player (e.g., Zimbardo, 1970). The tendency for overt behavior to resynchronize one's internal states provides an explanation for the effectiveness of behavioral coordination techniques associated with indoctrination. In the military and in certain religious organizations, for example, considerable emphasis is placed on the coordination of motor activities, often with a special role assigned to singing. The idea here is that the effect of co-ordinating to a common source on a behavior level goes far beyond behavior per se. Unless the person is explicitly concerned with resisting influence, he or she is likely to match to some degree his or her own control parameters so that he or she can spontaneously match the behavior of the others without much effort devoted to coordination of every single behavioral act. In effect, people internalize the rhythm and generate their own behavior from that source.[1]

The Quality of Coordination

Communication, inference, and behavioral coordination do not always produce coordination at the level of internal states. Communication can sometimes promote confusion rather than clarity, after all, and inferences regarding the internal states of another person are open to a host of distortions and biases (Nisbett & Ross, 1980). It is also possible for people to coordinate on a behavioral level without achieving coordination with respect to internal states. This is to be expected, for example, when the goal of coordination has primarily a self-serving purpose, as in social influence. In this case, the behavior is detached from one's internal state, true feelings, personal rhythms, and so forth. A Machiavellian personality, for instance, may display sadness when listening to someone's sorrowful tale or joy when listening to the person's recent successes. In neither case, however, is the listener's internal state commensurate with his or her overt behavior. In fact, the successful display of sadness may be associated with internal pleasure at the successful enactment of this behavior.

Faulty or incomplete coordination can also reflect differential willingness on the part of the relationship partners. One of them simply may not want to coordinate at a deep level. The tendency in this circumstance is for the other person to increase the amount of attention to coordination and to employ stronger signals. Because negative signals usually have greater impact than positive signals and are more difficult to ignore, they may be used when there is an especially heightened press for coordination. Negative signals are more likely to provide for momentary synchronization, not only because they are more salient, but also because the induction of a negative mood is likely to disrupt ongoing intrinsic dynamics of the interaction partner and thus set the stage for reorganization and renewed coupling. This idea is consistent with the role of coherence in psychological systems generally. Negative emotions signal poor coherence and interrupt ongoing dynamics. By doing so, they set the stage for new forms of dynamics that enable the system to reestablish coherence. Although all relationships no doubt experience this form of resynchronization from time to time, for some relationships, negative signals may provide the most common technique for resynchronizing partners. This is to be expected, for example, in mismatched or otherwise dysfunctional relationships. Thus, frequent arguments, guilt manipulations, and other means of inducing negative emotion provide the primary means of resynchronizing two people who cannot otherwise achieve coordination. One may ask, of course, whether coordination in such a relationship is worth maintaining.

Variability in the quality of coordination can also be traced to individual differences in relevant abilities. Such variables as emotional intelligence (Salovey & Mayer, 1990), social intelligence (Cantor & Kihlstrom, 1987), and self-monitoring (Snyder, 1974) capture this dimension of variation in interpersonal coordination. High self-monitors, for example, have the ability to coordinate with a wide variety of people, presumably because they match their internal states to those of their interaction partners. It is also the case that members of certain occupations, such as therapists, politicians, lawyers, and salespeople, require the ability both to follow the dynamics of others and to impose their own dynamics on others.

The Benefits and Costs of Coordinating Dynamics

Close partners do not need to observe and attempt to match one another's actions on a frequent basis. Such synchronization flows instead from tapping into a common wellspring for action. The partners to a close relationship, then, can traverse a whole spectrum of feelings together, and it is the shared nature of this experience that makes the feelings especially meaningful. By the same token, close partners can provide alternative perspectives to rescue one another from unpleasant mental and emotional states. Noting the sadness of a relationship partner, for example, a person might express optimism and enthusiasm so as to replace the partner's sadness with joy. The augmentation of complexity, moreover, may enable the two-person system to allocate responsibilities for complex tasks and thereby deal more effectively with various challenges and demands than each person could do individually. The notion of transactive memory (Wegner, 1986) captures this benefit of close relationships.

Coordination with respect to internal states has benefits that go beyond those generated for the two-person system. By synchronizing to one another in a relationship, each partner can synchronize his or

her own dynamics. As noted in Chapter 4, when the mind is not coupled to natural feedback coming from the environment, it can take off
on a self-perpetuating tangent. In the context of a close relationship,
though, each person can receive corrective feedback for internally driven thoughts and moods and thus dampen potential instabilities. In a
related vein, coupling to someone else's dynamics can provide coherence to the turbulent flow of thoughts and action plans experienced
during periods of introspection and self-scrutiny, and can help to bring
an emotional roller coaster under control. As demonstrated in Chapter 5, people differ in the structure and stability of their respective self
systems. Presumably, people who lack integration in this all-important
system can achieve stability and coherence by coordinating with the
perspectives of other people.[2] Although direct evidence has yet to be
obtained on this point, it is reasonable to suggest that a certain set of
psychological variables, including self-uncertainty, field dependence,
need for approval, and external locus of control make it likely that the
person will follow the dynamics of others, albeit with varying degrees
of success. These variables have in common the suggestion that the
person lacks stable intrinsic dynamics with which to coordinate on his
or her own terms with other people.

Although coordination of control parameters allows for smooth-
er and less effortful coordination of action, it does not occur without
cost. For one thing, there is reason to think that the achievement of
coordination of thoughts and feelings produces heightened excitement early on in a relationship, but that over time, the same level of
synchrony may promote boredom and disinterest in one another. It is
interesting in this light that the emotional quality of a close relationship may not be revealed until severe disruption of coordination occurs (see Berscheid, 1983). Ironically, the better synchronized two
people have become, the less intense the emotion they tend to experience in the context of the relationship. This lack of emotion may mo-
tivate one or both partners to terminate the relationship. Once the relationship is disrupted, though, negative emotion is experienced in
proportion to the concomitant coordination loss. In effect, negative
emotion signals coordination loss in a relationship in much the same
way that negative emotion signals poor coherence in other psychological systems (e.g., action, the self).

Coordination can be problematic in another sense. In readjust-
ing one's own internal states to those of the other person, one necessarily forfeits one's personal sources of intrinsic dynamics. In effect,
behavior is controlled with respect to the coherence of a higher order
system rather than with respect to the coherence associated with each
person's individual mind–action system. Sometimes, this can be a very

rewarding experience indeed. The feeling of togetherness and "oneness" promotes a transcendence of the self, a phenomenon that goes to the very heart of intimate relationships. This very experience, however, may be very threatening in other contexts. The loss of personal identity makes one vulnerable to the whims and unrecognized intents and plans of the other person. Intimacy, then, can be a very threatening prospect for most people and can promote actions intended to reestablish personal autonomy when the loss of individual identity becomes particularly salient.

The loss of personal autonomy may also promote actions that would be impossible if the person were acting on the basis of his or her personal action tendencies. The notion of deindividuation (e.g., Zimbardo, 1970; Diener, 1980) captures this loss of self-awareness and the concomitant transfer of control from one's own standards to the system of which one is just a part. When this happens, the coherence of the dyadic (or multiperson) system replaces the internal coherence of each person as the standard for action. As internal cohesiveness in the relationship becomes the standard for control, the respective individuals may engage in actions that might well be in conflict with the standards of each individual. [3]

MODELING THE COORDINATION
OF RELATIONSHIP DYNAMICS

Issues of coordination are critical in understanding biological and physical systems (e.g., Haken, 1978; Turvey, 1990). These issues can be investigated by modeling the "coupling" of separate dynamical systems. A particularly promising example of this approach involves coupled logistic equations, also referred to as coupled maps. The logistic map, described in Chapter 2, is the simplest system capable of displaying chaotic behavior. Depending on the value of its control parameter, each equation by itself may display qualitatively different types of behavior, from simple, fixed-point attractors to periodic regimes of differing periods to deterministic chaos. It has been shown that when the value of the dynamical variable (X) for one equation depends not only on its previous value but also to some degree on the value of X for the other equation, the two equations tend to synchronize (Kaneko, 1989, 1993; Shinbrot, 1994). This property has been used as a prototype for understanding synchronization underlying different collective processes in physics, chemistry, and biology (Shinbrot, 1994).

In this section, we use coupled logistic maps to model the synchronization of partners in close relationships (Nowak, Zochowski,

Borkowski, & Vallacher, 1997). The dynamics of each interaction partner are represented by a logistic equation. Each partner is characterized by two variables, a dynamical variable X and a control parameter r. The time evolution of X represents the dynamics of the person's behavior. In the absence of external influences (e.g., an interaction partner), the value of X depends on the value of X at the previous moment in time according to the equation. The type of intrinsic dynamics displayed by X depends on the value of r. Increases in the value of r (up to 4.0) generally result in increased complexity of the system's time evolution. For values of r between 0 and approximately 2.95, the system evolves toward a fixed-point attractor. For values between 2.95 and approximately 3.56, the system displays periodic behavior with periods increasing in a period-doubling manner. Above this value, the system behaves chaotically, with increasing complexity. In the present context, r describes an internal state (e.g., a mood, state of arousal, or mental set) that initiates and regulate behavior.

To capture the reciprocal influence between interaction partners, the state of each partner depends not only his or her preceding state but also on the preceding state of the other person. As noted, each person can influence the other either on the level of behavior (X) or at the level of internal states (r). By influencing one another on the level of behavior, the partners can achieve momentary coordination, whereas by matching the values of their respective control parameters, the partners achieve similarity with respect to prolonged patterns of behavior (e.g., periodic behavior of a given frequency, chaotic behavior with given complexity and irregularity). This model of coordination clearly has the character of a model of qualitative understanding. The simplifications are obvious. The dynamics of behavior cannot be directly represented by changes in the value of just one variable (X) and clearly many potential control variables may be relevant. Nonetheless, this model can highlight some emergent properties of relationships, in which individuals are viewed as separate systems striving for coordination.

Modeling the Coordination of Behavior

To say that the members of a relationship influence each other means that the behavior of one member impinges on the behavior of the other member. Formally, such influence is introduced by the assumption that the behavior of each partner at a given moment depends to a certain degree on the behavior of the other partner at the preceding moment. The coupling is done in a simple way, according to the following equations:

$$X_1(t + 1) = \frac{r_1 X_1(t)[1 - X_1(t)] + \alpha r_2 X_2(t)[1 - X_2(t)]}{1 + \alpha}$$

$$X_2(t + 1) = \frac{r_2 X_2(t)[1 - X_2(t)] + \alpha r_1 X_1(t)[1 - X_1(t)]}{1 + \alpha}$$

To the value of the dynamical variable representing one's own behavior (X_1), one adds a fraction, denoted by α, of the value of the dynamical variable representing the behavior of the partner (X_2). The size of this fraction (α) corresponds to the strength of coupling and reflects the closeness or mutual interdependency of the relationship. When the fraction is 0, there is no coupling on the behavior level. When the fraction is 1, in contrast, the person's behavior is determined equally by his or her preceding behavior and the preceding behavior of the partner. Intermediate values of this fraction correspond to intermediate values of coupling.

It has been shown that when the control parameters in a coupled system have the same value, the dependence between the respective dynamical variables causes the maps to coordinate fully, so that the values of X_1 and X_2 become identical (Kaneko, 1993). Obviously, the respective control parameters of two individuals are rarely, if ever, identical. Nor do relationships all have the same degree of interdependence. Our first simulation thus investigated the degree to which coordination depends on partners' similarity in their internal states (control parameters) and on their degree of interdependence (coupling). The value of r for one map (corresponding to one partner) was held constant at 3.67, which reflects the low end of the chaotic regime. We systematically varied the values of r for the other partner between 3.67 and 4.0, which reflects the highest value of the chaotic regime. These values are portrayed on the vertical axis in Figure 6.1. Because r for the first map is fixed, this axis corresponds to the difference between the control parameters of the two maps. We also systematically varied α, between values of 0 and .35. The horizontal axis in Figure 6.1 corresponds to this variable. Simulations were performed for each combination of the difference in r and the value of α. There were 900 divisions on the vertical axis and 1,024 divisions on the horizontal axis, so the crossing of these two dimensions resulted in 921,600 simulations. Each simulation, in turn, consisted of 800 steps.

For each simulation, we started from a random value of X for each person, drawn from a uniform distribution that varied from 0 to 1. We let the two coupled systems run for 300 steps, so that each system had a chance to come close to its attractor and both systems had a

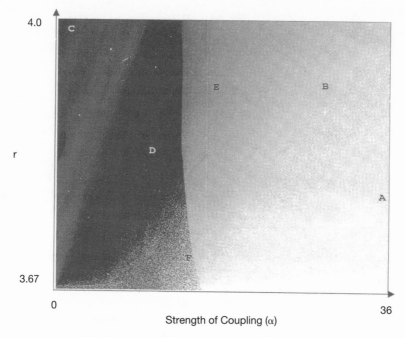

FIGURE 6.1. Coupled maps and relationship coordination.

chance to synchronize. For the next 500 simulation steps, we recorded the values of X for each system and computed the correlation between them. The brightness of each point on this graph corresponds to the value of the correlation, with white representing a correlation of +1.0, black representing a correlation of –1.0, and shades of gray representing intermediate correlation values.

The main result is straightforward and reflects the intuitions expressed in the previous section. In general, the correlation between partners' behavior increases both with α and similarity in r. Thus, there is an increase in brightness from the upper left to the lower right in Figure 6.1. This means that the larger the difference between the partners' control parameters, the stronger the coupling required to maintain a given level of coordination. For relatively strong mutual influence, as reflected in high values of α (> .35), full synchronization (i.e., positive correlation) occurs even for systems characterized by very different values of r. This suggests that when two people are highly dissimilar in their settings of internal parameters, they may nonetheless achieve a fair degree of coordination by directly influencing one another's behavior.

Against this general pattern, there are strong nonlinearities evident in Figure 6.1. For values of α close to 0, each system tends to evolve independently, as indicated by the generally gray area on the left side of the figure, regardless of their similarity in r. Within this region, though, there are also stripe-like structures of slight positive correlation (i.e., lighter gray) and slight negative correlation (i.e., darker gray). The direction of these stripes indicates that stronger values of α can compensate for increasing differences in r. With increasing α, the systems begin to coordinate in an anti-phase (i.e., negative correlation) manner, as indicated by the black structure in the figure. This form of coordination may correspond, for example, to turn-taking or compensatory behaviors. Note that the behavior of each partner tends to be more orderly (i.e., periodic) than it would be if it were evolving independently. This phenomenon is reminiscent of the control of chaos, in which each system stabilizes the other system's behavior (Ott, Grebogi, & York, 1990). For larger differences in r, α must be stronger for this form of coordination to occur. When the difference in r is very small, however, the two systems may coordinate in either phase or anti-phase manner, as indicated by the mixture of black and white points to the lower right of the black structure. With yet further increases in α, a phase transition from anti-phase to in-phase coordination occurs, as indicated by the sudden change from dark to light near the middle of the figure. After this transition, very complex forms of coordination occur, and the complexity of the coordinated system is greater than the complexity of each system. With further inceases in α and decreases in r, the systems begin to increase their degree of synchronization until they essentially mirror one another's behavior. As a result, the coordinated system loses its richness and complexity.

The letters A through F in Figure 6.1 correspond to specific combinations of r and α. Figure 6.2 shows the time evolution of coordination occurring for a single point within each of the lettered regions. Each picture is a scatterplot of the values of X from the two coupled maps, with the horizontal and vertical axes representing the values of X on a given simulation step for the respective partners. These values are plotted for 10,000 consecutive simulation steps. In general, these pictures capture the types of coordination described earlier. The straight line displayed in picture A indicates perfect correlation, reflecting complete synchronization in behavior. Picture B shows a high positive correlation, with one system limiting the values of the other system in a linear manner. The scatterplot in picture C indicates a lack of correlation in the behavior of the two systems. Picture D depicts periodic evolution (anti-phase coordination) of the two-map

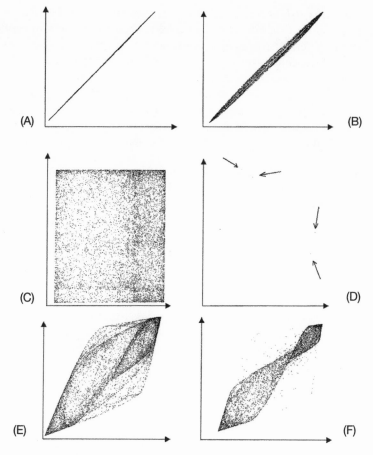

FIGURE 6.2. Types of relationship coordination.

system, with one map stabilizing the behavior of the other. The system evolves at period 4, so all the simulation steps cycle among four points. To enhance visibility, each point is indicated by an arrow. Finally, pictures E and F provide different examples of a nonlinear pattern emerging from some complex mode of coordination between the maps.

The results of these simulations provide three primary insights into the dynamics of close relationships. First, mutual control and strong interdependence can compensate for relatively weak similarity between partners. In this case, however, there is a strong potential for instability in the relationship. Thus, other simulations in this research program have shown that as soon as behavioral influence is broken, the dynamics of the two systems diverge rapidly if the systems have markedly different values of r. For small differences in r, the divergence is slower and because the overall forms of their respective dynamics are similar, the two systems can easily reestablish coordination when coupling is reintroduced. The second insight concerns the richness and nonlinearity of coordination phenomena in close relationships. Thus, there are strong exceptions to the general linear pattern described earlier. With increases in α, for example, two systems that are initially uncorrelated in their behavior may progress through a stage involving strong anti-phase coordination before achieving in-phase coordination. Even within this general nonlinear scenario, there are small regions where coordination takes on markedly different forms than that displayed in nearby regions.

The third insight is that the richest and most interesting dynamics are observed for relatively weak levels of coupling. Thus, when mutual influence is relatively weak, partners to a relationship may display a diverse repertoire of in-phase and anti-phase forms of coordination. Moreover, with very small changes in the strength of coupling, the two-person system may display rapid transitions from simple anti-phase coordination to very complex forms of in-phase coordination, and vice versa. This richness and complexity of interpersonal dynamics is very fragile, however, and tends to disappear when coupling is too strong. According to the simulation results, no enrichment of behavior in a relationship may be expected when the relationship is characterized by control over one another's behavior. Indeed, for partners with very high similarity in internal states, coordination is possible for extremely low values of mutual influence. This suggests that one can assess the similarity between people by noting how little influence is necessary for them to achieve coordination. In general, coordination can occur at very low levels of mutual influence, provided the partners are truly similar with respect to variables describing their internal states.

Modeling the Coordination of Internal States

Modeling the direct coordination of control parameters is relatively straightforward. All one needs to assume is that on each simulation step, the values of each person's control parameter drifts somewhat in the direction of the value of the partner's control parameter. The rate of this drift and the size of the initial discrepancy between the values of the respective control parameters determine how quickly the control parameters begin to match. This mechanism assumes that both interaction partners can directly estimate the settings of one another's control parameters. As discussed in the previous section, considerable effort in relationships may be focused on communicating or inferring these settings. Even with such effort, the exact values of the relevant control parameters may be difficult to determine.

Control parameters can also become coordinated through behavioral coordination. In this form of coupling, each person modifies the value of his or her own control parameter to match the other person's pattern of behavior. The exact value of the partner's control parameter is invisible to the person, but he or she remembers the partner's most recent set of behaviors (i.e., the most recent values of x) as well as his or her own most recent behaviors. By comparing his or her own behavior with that of the partner, the person adjusts his or her own control parameter until there is a match in their respective behavior patterns (Zochowski & Liebovitch, 1997). If the pattern of the partner's observed behavior is more complex than his or her own pattern of behavior, the person slightly increases the value of his or her own control parameter. If the partner's behavior is less complex than one's own behavior, on the other hand, the person decreases slightly the value of his or her own control parameter. In effect, each person can discover one another's internal state by monitoring the evolution of one another's behavior.

Figure 6.3 shows how the coordination between two maps develops over time as they progressively match one another's control parameters in the manner described earlier. This simulation was run for relatively weak coupling ($\alpha = .2$). The x-axis corresponds to time in simulation steps; the y-axis portrays the value of the difference between the two maps. The thin line corresponds to the difference in the dynamic variables, whereas the thick line corresponds to the difference in r. Over time, the difference in the respective control parameters of the two maps decreases, and the maps become perfectly synchronized in their behavior. This suggests that attempting behavioral synchronization with weak levels of influence and control over one another's behavior will facilitate matching of one another's internal states.

Figure 6.4 shows the results when the simulation was run with a stronger value of coupling ($\alpha = .7$). Coordination in behavior develops almost immediately, but the control parameters fail to synchronize, even after 1,000 simulation steps. This is because strong coupling causes full synchronization of behavior even for maps with quite different control parameters. Once the behavior is in full synchrony, the two maps do not have a clue that their control parameters are different. This would become apparent if the coupling were removed—the

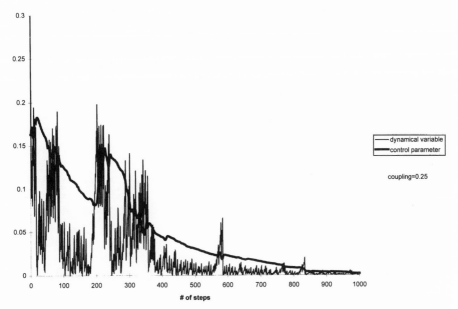

FIGURE 6.3. Development of relationship coordination under weak coupling.

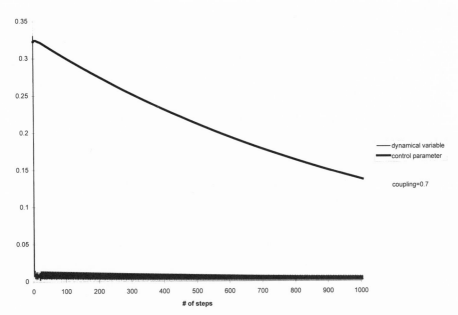

FIGURE 6.4. Development of relationship coordination under strong coupling.

dynamics of the two respective maps would immediately diverge. This suggests that using very strong influence to obtain coordination of behavior may effectively hinder coordination at a deeper level.

The aforementioned considerations and data suggest that there is an optimal level of influence and control over behavior in close relationships. Too weak an influence may lead to a lack of coordination, whereas too strong an influence may prevent the development of a relationship based on mutual understanding and empathy. The observation that high values of coupling restrict the range of possible modes of coordination suggests that intricate types of coordination are difficult when people strongly control one another's behavior. By the same token, relationships may have very rich dynamics and switch between different modes of coordination when the influence between the partners is not very strong. In a newly formed relationship, for example, the dynamics and coordination phenomena may be very surprising for both partners. On balance, the most desirable degree of coupling is one that allows for effective coordination, but keeps direct influence at a relatively low level.

We should stress that this work is in its beginning stages and thus one must exercise caution when generalizing the results to human relationships. Some parallels, however, are quite striking. The fact that strong influence can compensate for differences in intrinsic dynamics, for example, resonates well with intuitions regarding control in close relationships. Clearly, before fully accepting these results as applicable to human intimate relationships, one needs to perform empirical tests with actual relationships. Computer simulations, though, may help to generate the hypotheses to be tested, and they can highlight those phenomena (e.g., modes of coordination and transitions between them) that are worthy of special attention.

EQUILIBRIA IN CLOSE RELATIONSHIPS

Conventional wisdom suggests that people who are deeply in love experience no limits in their desire to be close to one another. It is not uncommon for love songs, romantic poetry, and bargain-basement paperback romance novels to convey fantasies of everlasting closeness, even the merging of identities. Romantic as this sentiment sounds, there is reason to question its validity. Consider, for example, the following story from the period of the Spanish Inquisition. It seems that a young man and a young woman in a Spanish village were very much in love and intended to marry. The Grand Inquisitor for this particular region of Spain, however, strongly opposed their relationship and decided to destroy it. His means of doing so was to have the young lovers tied together and remain bound for several days. This is about as close as two people can get. It turns out that after this experience, however, the lovers could no longer bear one another's company, or even cast their eyes on one another. At this point, the authority figure administered the ultimate punishment: He ordered the man and woman to marry.

The Formation of Relationship Equilibria

This story may well be apocryphal, but it conveys an important point about relationships. Simply put, there is a limit to how close two people really want to be. The partners to a relationship may harbor romantic visions of achieving unity, but the reality is that there are psychological limits to closeness, the violation of which can serve to destroy rather than enhance the relationship. Expressed in terms of systems concepts, the coupling of individual dynamics evolves toward an equilibrium expressing an optimal degree of coordination. When this equilibrium is disturbed, processes are set in motion to restore it. The notion of an equilibrium point for psychological closeness is well documented in research on proxemics and nonverbal behavior (e.g., Hall, 1966; Siegman & Feldstein, 1987). It has been demonstrated, for example, that when acquaintances are put in too close a spatial arrangement (e.g., a crowded elevator), they attempt to reestablish their preferred equilibrium for distance by engaging in compensatory behaviors, such as avoiding eye contact (e.g., Hall, 1966).

Physical distance and nonverbal behavior, of course, hardly exhaust the dimensions along which psychological closeness can be scaled. The choice of conversation topics, the degree of self-disclosure, the extent and form of self-presentation strategies, and perhaps most important, the level of commitment to the relationship, are all dictated by the preferred equilibrium point for intimacy and closeness on the part of relationship partners. Being further than desired from an equilibrium is associated with unpleasant feelings (e.g., dissatisfaction, longing, frustration) and a desire to be closer to the person. When contact is too close, however, the result might be boredom, discomfort, or in the extreme, even repulsion and aggression.

The classic depiction of conflict proposed over half a century ago by Miller (1944) provides a highly contemporary framework for understanding the formation of equilibria in relationships. Especially relevant here is the characterization of conflicts defined in terms of simultaneous approach and avoid tendencies, as described in Chapter 2. In this model, both the tendency to approach and the tendency to

avoid grow stronger with decreasing distance from a goal. The tendency to avoid, however, starts at smaller distances and grows faster than
the tendency to approach. As a result, the two gradients intersect at
some distance from the goal (see Figure 6.5). This point represents the
equilibrium around which a person is likely to oscillate. If the person
withdraws from the goal, the tendency to approach gets stronger and
draws the person closer. But if the person gets closer than the equilibrium, the avoidance tendency repels the person. This reasoning can
be readily extended to the establishment of equilibria in close relationships. No matter how simple a relationship may seem on the surface, there are certain to be factors pulling the partners apart, in addition to those that bring them together. The repelling factors may be
associated with the other person, or they may represent possible negative implications of being in a close relationship, such as loss of freedom and other social contacts.

When the repelling factors are constant, an increase in the attracting factors will promote a corresponding adjustment of the equilibrium, establishing it at a point closer to the person. By the same token, with a constant level of attracting forces, an increase in avoidance tendencies will result in a more distant equilibrium. It is interesting to consider what happens to equilibria when both approach and
avoid tendencies grow in strength. The resultant equilibrium may represent the same psychological distance, but because both the tendency to approach and the tendency to avoid are at higher levels, there

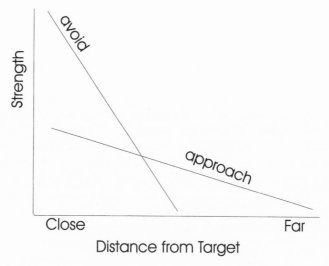

FIGURE 6.5. The approach–avoid conflict.

may be higher overall tension in the system. With this increase in tension, it becomes correspondingly likely that the relationship will be marked by dramatic shifts in sentiment and even behavior. This possibility is consistent with the notion of dynamic integration in social judgment generally (Chapter 3), and with the heightened volatility in feelings about relationship partners in particular (Guzik, 1996; Vallacher, 1995).

Hysteresis in Close Relationships

In any relationship, the degree of closeness depends not only on the mutual attraction between partners, but also to a large degree on the history of the relationship. After a relationship has formed, people are unlikely to end the relationship in response to some momentary setback or cost. Rather, a critical level of dissatisfaction must be reached, beyond which the relationship may suddenly collapse (e.g., Rusbult, 1980, 1983; Rusbult & Martz, 1995; Thibaut & Kelley, 1959). By the same token, people do not form a close relationship in response to their first positive experiences together. Indeed, it may take many rewarding experiences over an extended period of time before two people finally cross a threshold of mutual attraction and form a close relationship. This suggests that one may observe hysteresis in both the formation and dissolution of close relationships.

Hysteresis in close relationships was postulated by Tesser (1980; Tesser & Achee, 1994) within the context of catastrophe theory (Thom, 1975; Zeeman, 1976). The focal concern in Tesser's model is the conditions under which commitment to a romantic partner demonstrates sudden as opposed to gradual change as a function of social pressures against such involvement. Three factors are considered especially relevant to this phenomenon: two control factors corresponding to social pressure and emotional involvement, respectively, and a dependent variable corresponding to the strength of dating–mating behavior. According to Tesser's model, when there is relatively weak social pressure against dating, the relationship between emotional involvement and dating is linear: The greater the involvement, the more frequent and intense the dating behavior. When there is high social pressure against dating, however, essentially no dating behavior is observed until some level of relatively high emotional involvement is reached. Beyond this critical value, however, a strong dating relationship is suddenly established.

The opposite pattern is observed with decreases in emotional involvement: Once dating has occurred, gradual decreases in involvement decrease dating behavior only slightly. After some critical value is reached, however, the relationship is broken, and dating suddenly drops to a very low value. The degree of involvement at which the relationship dissolves is much lower than the degree of involvement necessary for dating to begin. Likewise, after the relationship is broken, small increases in involvement will not restore the dating behavior. Rather, involvement would have to increase to its original high value for the dating to become reestablished. The difference between the level of attractiveness at which the relationship is broken and reestablished defines the region of hysteresis. Tesser's model is portrayed in Figure 6.6.

The modern equivalent of catastrophe theory is the theory of bifurcations, which describes how attractors change as a result of change in control parameters (Ruelle, 1989). As noted in Chapter 2, the cusp catastrophe corresponds to a saddle-node or fold bifurcation. Consider the equilibrium of a system's behavior for high values of a control parameter for which hysteresis appears. The stability of the system is portrayed in Figure 6.7. The y-axis corresponds to different values of the other control parameter. The graph portrays an energy surface composed of hills and valleys; the left side of the graph shows the view from above, and the right side shows a series of cross-sections at places corresponding to the left side. In the energy metaphor, the natural tendency for this system is to minimize the energy. We can envision

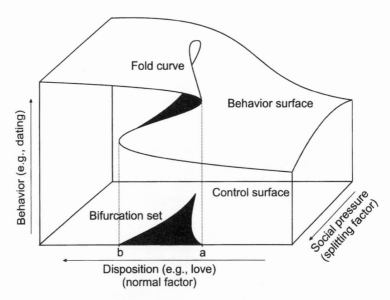

FIGURE 6.6. Love as a catastrophe.

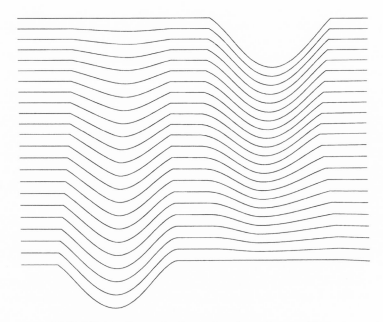

FIGURE 6.7. Energy landscape for relationship equilibria.

this as a ball rolling down hills and resting in valleys, which correspond to attractors.

For low levels of attractiveness, only one attractor exists, and any momentary increase in closeness will result in the restoration of equilibrium corresponding to a more distant relationship. For moderate levels of attractiveness, another attractor corresponding to a closer relationship appears. This attractor increases in strength with increasing levels of attractiveness. Despite the presence of this alternative attractor, it is not easy for the system to achieve it, because, in order to do so, the system has to cross an energy barrier (i.e., move uphill out of its present attractor). For high values of attractiveness, however, the first attractor gets progressively weaker and finally loses its stability, and the system jumps to the other attractor. This point corresponds to the sudden catastrophic change in Tesser's model. A reverse scenario can be constructed when starting from high values of attractiveness, where only the second attractor is present. Sudden catastrophic change in the relationship would again occur at the point where the second attractor loses its stability.

This description is analogous to the behavior of Tesser's model. Unlike Tesser's model, however, this model can specify what happens when the system travels outside its attractors. First of all, for weak per-turbations in the hysteresis region, and for all perturbations in regions where only one attractor is present, the perturbed system will tend to return to its original attractor with a force generally proportional to the strength of perturbation. For strong perturbations in the region of hysteresis, a very different phenomenon may happen. At some mo-ment, the system may cross the energy barrier separating the two at-tractors (climbing over the hill) and suddenly become pulled toward the other attractor. This model predicts that for relationship partners of intermediate desirability, the preferred and natural tendency would be to maintain distance in the relationship, with small and minor in-fluences promoting greater closeness being resisted. However, if con-ditions promote notably greater closeness (e.g., being on the same cruise ship for a few days) so that the cost threshold is crossed, the preference may reverse, and the person will seek an equilibrium of closeness.

This depiction of the dynamics of equilibria in close relation-ships is accurate as long as there are no random influences on the sys-tem. All biological and social systems, however, contain noise and random influences. Such influences act as a constant perturbation and can function to kick the system out of an attractor when the attractor becomes weak. When this happens, the system travels to the other at-tractor. At some moment, the noise may achieve sufficient strength to kick the system back into its original attractor. Near the transition points, then, the observed dynamics may consist of interlaced periods of closeness and distance. In this scenario, close relationships may progressively develop in a nonlinear way rather than through incre-mental changes in closeness. This model, then, converges to the cata-strophe model with respect to the change in equilibria in close rela-tionships. It goes beyond the catastrophe model, however, by describ-ing the system at nonequilibrium points and by proposing psychologi-cal mechanisms responsible for the appearance of equilibria and for change in equilibria.

Attractors of Love

This model was empirically tested by Kozlowska, Nowak, and Kus (1997). Their aim was to identify the attractors for relationships that varied with respect to relationship history, partner attractiveness, and social pressure. They asked unmarried male participants to indicate their likely behavior toward a female, portrayed in a photograph, in each of seven hypothetical situations. For each situation, participants were provided three behavior options: one that increased intimacy, one that did not change the degree of intimacy, and one that decreased intimacy. Extensive pilot testing was conducted to select photographs representing one of seven equally spaced levels of attractiveness and to select situations representing one of seven equally spaced levels of intimacy. Each participant indicated his behavioral choice for all 49 combinations generated by the crossing of attractiveness and intimacy.

Relationship history and social pressure were manipulated as between-subject variables. Participants in a past-history condition imagined that they had interacted with the female over a 3-week period on a cruise ship, whereas those in a no-history condition imagined that the female was a stranger prior to their interaction in the hypothetical situations. Social pressure was manipulated differently for the past-history and no-history conditions. In the past-history condition, pressure was created by involving the female's parents in the relationship. Under high pressure, the parents (who were rich and influential) liked the participant and presumably wanted the relationship to continue. In the low-pressure condition, the parents were not mentioned in the description. In the no-history condition, high pressure was created by asking participants to imagine that the female had an athletic and potentially aggressive boyfriend; in a low-pressure condition, there was not mention of a boyfriend. High pressure in the past-history condition thus acted to maintain the relationship, whereas high pressure in the no-history condition acted against relationship formation. The crossing of the history and pressure variables created four independent groups, each with between 15 and 17 participants.

Participants made their behavioral choices for situations of decreasing intimacy in the past-history conditions and for situations of increasing intimacy in the no-history conditions. The least intimate situations included seeing the female walking her dog or seeing her sitting in a coffee shop, whereas the most intimate situation involved the participant and the female waking up in bed together. The specific situations were constructed to be psychologically plausible (as determined by pilot research) and thus differed for the no-history and past-history conditions. In response to each combination of attractiveness and intimacy, participants were asked to indicate whether they would attempt to decrease the degree of intimacy with the female (scored as –1), maintain the degree of intimacy (0), or increase the degree of intimacy (+1).

The results are displayed in Figure 6.8. Each of the four panels corresponds to one of the four experimental conditions. The two upper panels correspond to the no-history conditions and the two lower panels correspond to the past-history conditions. The two left panels

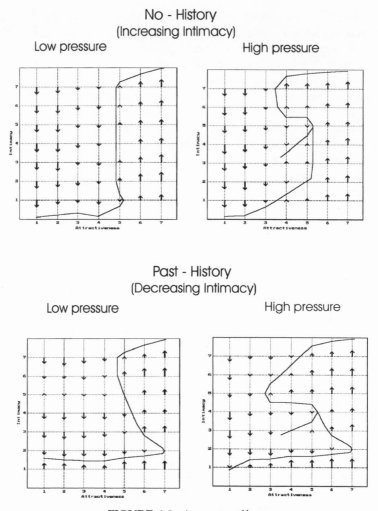

FIGURE 6.8. Attractors of love.

correspond to the low-pressure situations, the two right panels to the high-pressure situations. The horizontal axis in each panel corresponds to the seven levels of attractiveness, and the vertical axis corresponds to the seven levels of intimacy. The intersection of these axes define 49 situations for which participants were asked to indicate their intimacy preferences. The vector for each of these situations corresponds to the average preference across participants. The direction of the vector represents preference for increased intimacy (up arrow) versus decreased intimacy (down arrow), while the length of the vector represents the average strength of the preference. The solid line through each panel divides regions of the vector field containing vectors pointing in the same direction.

Inspection of each panel reveals a rather trivial effect: Participants preferred to be intimate with attractive females and to be non-intimate with unattractive females. The specific nature of this relationship is far from trivial, however, as it conforms to the bifurcation scenario postulated in the model. The attractors and repellors for each combination of history and pressure are indicated by the solid lines in each panel. A region of the line is an attractor if arrows on either side point to it, whereas a region of the line is a repellor if the arrows on either side point away from it. Note that the vector field as a whole is highly structured, with neighboring vectors pointing in the same direction, and that the attractors and repellors divide the vector space into coherent regions (i.e., vectors with the same direction). Note also that the attractors and repellors conform to a well-defined shape, indicative of highly structured patterns of changes in participants' preferences. These shapes differed for the low and high pressure conditions.

Consider first the low-pressure conditions. These participants preferred low intimacy with the female until a high level of attractiveness was reached (i.e., the fifth of the seven photos), at which point they switched to a preference for high intimacy. This pattern was observed whether the female was a stranger or an acquaintance. Contrary to expectation, the equilibrium did not vary in a linear manner with changes in attractiveness, but rather displayed a threshold function indicating the existence of two equilibria. This suggests that some form of implicit social pressure is always present when forming or dissolving a relationship. The lack of pronounced hysteresis, however, indicates that these equilibria did not exist at the same time.

Consider now the results for the high-pressure conditions. Hysteresis is apparent in both cases. Participants considering situations of increasing intimacy in the no-history condition preferred low intimacy until the female was highly attractive (the sixth photo), at which point their preferences switched to maximum intimacy. Those considering high-intimacy situations (the sixth and seventh photos), however, preferred to maintain or increase intimacy with females of intermediate as well as high attractiveness. This change of preferences with growing intimacy is analogous to crossing an energy barrier. The lower right panel shows a similar pattern for decreasing levels of intimacy in the past-history condition. Participants preferred high levels of intimacy until the female's attractiveness dropped to very low levels (the first or second photos), at which point they changed their preferences to low intimacy. When considering low-intimacy situations, however, participants preferred less intimacy even when the female was highly attractive (the sixth photo).[4]

These results suggest conditions under which changes in the level of intimacy are resisted versus accepted. Overall, there is a tendency to restore a preferred level of intimacy when this level is perturbed by new situations. If a partner's attractiveness is low, increases in intimacy are resisted, but if the partner's attractiveness is high, decreases in intimacy are resisted. In the hysteresis region, however, two intimacy attractors coexist and can become dominant. Small perturbations to a preferred level of intimacy are likely to produce a return to the current attractor. If one is already intimate with a partner of intermediate attractiveness, for example, slight decreases in intimacy will be followed by corrective increases. By the same token, if one has not achieved intimacy with this person, slight increases in intimacy are likely to be resisted. Beyond a certain point, however, changes in intimacy are likely to promote movement to the other attractor defining the hysteresis region. Thus, a person who has a nonintimate relationship with someone he or she considers moderately attractive may encounter this person in a psychologically close situation and subsequently desire to maintain this new equilibrium. On the other hand, an intimate relationship with a moderately attractive person may be dissolved if the partners find themselves in a situation that undermines the intimacy of the relationship.

This perspective suggests when external events are likely to be dampened versus amplified in a close relationship. For very low and very high attractiveness, the system will reestablish equilibrium, making even strong influences short-lived. But for moderate attractiveness, there is a threshold value for such factors, beyond which their effect will amplify rather than diminish over time, thereby promoting a qualitative change in the relationship. This perspective is also relevant to a seeming paradox involving cultural norms. In societies that place a high value on marriage, there tends to be considerable social pressure against casual contact between the sexes—the very thing that would seem to promote finding a marriage partner. This can be understood in terms of the threshold effects and hysteresis created by social pressure. It may be harder to form a relationship in the face of social pressure, but once a relationship is formed, it is more likely to be maintained, even if the attractiveness of the partners decreases. Ironically, then, obstacles to forming a relationship have a way of ensuring the stability of the relationship after it has become established. By the same token, relationships that are easy to form are also easy to break, once the initial attraction between partners begins to subside.

We should note that the results observed by Kozlowska et al. (1997) are consistent with Tesser's (1994) catastrophe model. In particular, the shape of the observed attractors and repellors closely resembles the shape of the cusp catastrophe he described. As noted earlier, however, bifurcation theory goes beyond a description of the changes in a system's equilibria to characterize the system's evolution as it restores equilibrium. The results obtained within this framework revealed an orderly structure to the vector field, indicating highly systematic behavior of the system even when it was far from equilibrium. This is noteworthy because biological (and presumably psychological) systems rarely act in isolation, but rather are constantly influenced by other systems and perturbed by the environment. Even if a static equilibrium exists, then, the system must continually attempt to maintain or restore this equilibrium.

INTERPERSONAL DYNAMICS IN PERSPECTIVE

A close relationship may be understood in terms of interpersonal coordination. People can coordinate on different levels, from the synchronization of simple movements to the matching of thought processes, emotional states, and values. This process may be modeled as the coupling of logistic equations, each capable of displaying complex dynamics by virtue of the setting of its control parameters. Coupling may occur with respect to dynamical variables, reflecting behavioral coordination, or with respect to control parameters, which corresponds to the matching of internal rhythms and moods. Different levels of coordination can to some degree compensate for one another, but their effects may be quite different.

When two individual systems establish coordination, a new, higher order system emerges. Each person loses some degrees of freedom due to the influence of the other person, but he or she also gains some degrees of freedom from being part of a larger system. From each person's perspective, there is an optimal level of coordination with the partner that establishes a desired equilibrium in the relationship. Too little coordination results in undesirable feelings such as loneliness and frustration, whereas too much coordination results in a loss of personal freedom, self-identity, and other aspects of personal dynamics. These forces toward restoration of equilibrium can be captured in terms of the approach–avoid conflict, with the relative strength of these tendencies dictating the desired degree of closeness in the relationship.

The dynamical perspective holds promise for integrating the seemingly unique properties of close relationships with other domains of personal and interpersonal functioning, including social judgment, action, the self, and social influence. In each of these domains, an emphasis is placed on coordination, although the elements to be coordinated are obviously different in each case. The disruption of coordination and the resultant breakdown in the system, moreover, is signaled by negative emotions and heightened self-consciousness, which in turn engage mechanisms aimed at reestablishing coordination. With respect to close relationships, if these mechanisms fail to reestablish coordination, the relationship may be severed, creating the potential for forming relationships within which coordination can be achieved.

We have concentrated on issues of coordination, but it is likely that other aspects of relationships can be incorporated into an explicitly dynamical framework. Indeed, a dynamical perspective on relationships is not entirely new to social psychology (e.g., Burgess & Huston, 1979; Gottman, 1979, 1993). Social exchange, for example, can be understood as the coordination between giving and taking, where both the utility of the resources and the timing of their exchange need to be considered. Kelley and Thibaut's (1978) model of interdependence is interesting in this regard, because it analyzes a relationship over time rather than characterizing it in terms of static qualities. Interpersonal behavior is investigated as ongoing repetitive interactions, in which the behavioral choices at one time create a different situation with a different payoff structure, which then generates new behavioral choices, and so on. The change in payoff structures, which is described by transformation matrices, comes very close to describing the principles governing a dynamical system. To date, however, the dynamical potential of social exchange theory has yet to be fully realized.

The dynamical perspective could be used to reframe a number of other key relationship concepts. Notions of equity and fairness, for instance, can be understood in terms of whether coordination results from mutual adjustment by both partners versus adjustment on the part of only one partner (e.g., Adams, 1965; Hatfield, Utne, & Traupmann, 1979; Homans, 1961; Lerner, Miller, & Holmes, 1976). In a related vein, power in a relationship is on the side of the person who sets the standards to which the other person must adjust his or her behavior or control parameters. Expectancies and differential roles, meanwhile, provide recipes for successful coordination (e.g., Wegner, 1986), enabling the individuals to maintain autonomy but yet fostering system-level coherence. Stability is another crucial feature of close relationships, and this notion occupies center stage in dynamical systems as well. Thus, two people may form a relationship based on the coordination of their behavior, and under many circumstances it may be indistinguishable from a relationship built on the deeper coordination of control parameters. However, when perturbed by external events—the availability of attractive alternatives to the present relationship, for example, or the temporary loss of coordinating behavioral signals—such relationships may become disrupted, revealing their inherent instability.

Considerable work remains to be done in order to establish the boundary conditions and range of application of the dynamical perspective. The key concepts explored in this chapter—coordination and equilibrium dynamics—clearly warrant further theoretical development as well as testing in both empirical and clinical contexts. At this stage in the development of the dynamical perspective, then, it is unreasonable to expect all the highly diverse factors relevant to close relationships to be fully integrated with respect to a small set of related principles. Dyadic relationships are of special interest from a dynamical perspective, however, because they provide the simplest example of a system in which the elements to be coordinated are individuals. Each element is itself an extremely complex system characterized by its own intrinsic dynamics. The basic question is how those individual dynamics coordinate in the formation of a higher order system. By gaining insight into this issue, we not only provide theoretical understanding of a central topic in social psychology, but also offer a new perspective for practical applications regarding the maintenance of close relationships.

NOTES

1. Even the anticipation of behavioral coordination with someone can promote a readjustment of one's control parameters so as to facilitate the impending interaction. Research on mental control, for instance, has found that people tend to match the expected mood of a future interaction partner, even if this means intentionally changing their current mood from happiness to sadness (Erber, Wegner, & Thierrault, 1996).

2. There is no guarantee, of course, that such attempts at coordination will take place in the intended manner. It is quite possible, in fact, that influence will work in the opposite direction, with the unstable person effectively putting an otherwise stable partner on a nonadaptive trajectory of thoughts and feelings.

3. We should note this phenomenon is not limited to close dyadic rela-

tionships. Even in ostensibly task-oriented groups, the members may become more concerned with synchronizing with one another than in dealing objectively with the task at hand (Janis, 1982). In such instances where mental coordination is the implicit goal, the group may engage in actions that to an outsider observer might appear misguided, and that might be seen as personally objectionable by the members themselves when personal identity is reinstated. Ironically, this discrepancy may be noticed only after the group action has failed or if the relationship should happen to dissolve. Tormented feelings of guilt may be the signal of self trying to regain control over action when the dyadic or group action fails or the respective social structure disintegrates.

4. Note the indication of a third attractor in the high-pressure conditions. Interestingly, the appearance of the third attractor is observed in biological systems for which hystersis is expected. It remains for future research to validate this finding and explore its meaning with respect to close relationships.

7

⤚

Dynamics of
Social Influence

PEOPLE DO NOT HAVE to be in love to influence one another. They do not even have to like each other that much. An abiding interest in changing one another's behavior and attitudes, in fact, is arguably the most pervasive feature of social life, a tendency that finds expression any time two or more people encounter each other. Although influence attempts are often resented, even actively resisted, such attempts clearly serve important functions. It is only because of the potential for influence that a group can be considered more than simply a collection of individuals. The various mechanisms of influence are largely responsible for the coordination of individuals' thoughts, beliefs, and actions necessary for collective action, and by providing for interpersonal accommodation, such mechanisms put a check on the impulses and penchant for self-interest that would otherwise characterize personal behavior. And in attending to the demands, expectations, and suggestions of other people, the individual is provided external cues for resynchronizing his or her intrinsic dynamics, in much the same way that a person's circadian rhythm is continually synchronized by clocks and other environmental cues.

This chapter explores the dynamical underpinnings of social influence at two levels of analysis. We consider first the means by which people attempt to control or shape one another's thoughts, feelings, and actions. Depending on how such attempts resonate with the influence target's intrinsic dynamics, they can meet with outright success, impassivity, or resistance. We then consider influence in social groups. We focus on the interpersonal forces that operate simultaneously on group members and with the macrolevel processes that emerge from the aggregate aspects of influence. We present a model designed to capture the dynamics of social influence in a group context. This model is tested through computer simulations, the results of which are consistent with formal analytical considerations. In a concluding section, we illustrate how this dynamical model of influence leads to the coupling of otherwise independent attitudes and thus provides an avenue for the emergence of ideology in groups and societies.

THE DYNAMICS OF INDIVIDUAL INFLUENCE

From a dynamical perspective, influence can occur in one of two general ways. The first mode of influence involves tracking the target's overt acts and verbal expressions, employing various strategies to promote desired behaviors and suppress undesired behaviors. In focusing on overt behavior, this mode of influence may succeed only in producing public compliance, with the target of influence simply doing what is expected or demanded of him or her. The second mode of influence involves resetting the person's control parameters and in this way changing the basis for the target's subsequent thoughts, feelings, and actions. If successful, this general approach goes beyond eliciting public compliance to generate private acceptance and internalization of the influence agent's agenda.

Influencing Behavior

Perhaps the most basic way to influence someone's behavior is make rewards and punishments contingent on the enactment of the behavior. For decades, experimental psychology was essentially defined in terms of this perspective, and during this era, a wide variety of reinforcement principles was generated and validated. The extension of these principles to social psychology was always complicated by the undeniable cognitive capacities of humans and the role of such capacities in regulating behavior (e.g., Bandura, 1986; Zajonc, 1980). Nonetheless, several lines of research trading on behaviorist assumptions are represented in social psychology (e.g., Byrne, 1971; Staats, 1975, 1991). With respect to social influence, this perspective suggests simply that people are motivated to do things that are associated with the receipt of pleasant consequences or the avoidance of unpleasant consequences. Thus, people adopt attitudes, become attracted to one another, change the frequency of certain behaviors, or take on new activities because in effect they have been trained to do so.

As noted early on, this perspective never really achieved mainstream status in social psychology. One might think that social influence would be an exception, however. Reinforcement, after all, is defined in terms of the control of behavior, and in view of the self-interest premise in virtually all theoretical traditions in social psychology, it is hard to imagine how the promise of reward or threat of punishment could fail to influence people's thoughts, feelings, and actions. Yet there is abundance evidence that this is precisely the case. Over the last several decades, in fact, reinforcement assumptions have come to serve as a convenient strawman for more enlightened accounts of motivation and influence that give star billing to people's higher level cognitive capacities and proclivities. Two aspects of human thought and judgment have been emphasized in such accounts.

The first is people's seemingly unrestrained capacity for interpretation. In broad form, this simply means that the objective properties of a stimulus—or of a behavior, for that matter—do not have a direct mapping onto people's representation. Stimuli that might seem to be unequivocally desirable, such as food or money, may be viewed primarily in terms of their negative consequences or disadvantages. Thus, food might represent the potential for weight gain, and money might be tainted because it is viewed as a means to get people to do things they normally would not do (Deci & Ryan, 1985). The importance of interpretation is arguably more pronounced with respect to behavior (e.g., Trope, 1986; Vallacher & Wegner, 1985). No matter how intrinsically pleasurable a behavior might seem, people can find a way to reframe it in negative terms. Thus, relaxing in the sun can represent wasting time, playing sports may signify risking injury or the possibility of failure, and sexual relations for some may be synonymous with immorality, a lapse in self-control, or the risk of life-threatening illness.

Of course, the role of interpretation could itself be interpreted in terms of reinforcement principles. If food, for example, is negatively valued because it represents weight gain, perhaps this is because food has been associated with weight gain through personal experience or excessive exposure to mass media. The second aspect of phenomenal functioning, however, is not so easily reconciled with the reinforcement perspective. This aspect centers on people's capacity for self-reflection and the self-concept that results from this process. As discussed in Chapter 5, people employ integrated subsets of their self systems for purposes of self-control. The true test of self-control comes when people are enticed by an opportunity for immediate self-gain that would produce a discrepancy with an internalized frame for self-evaluation. Such dilemmas are common in everyday life. A student may have an opportunity to cheat on an exam and improve his or her grade, a man or woman may experience seduction by someone other than his or her spouse, and a wallet without an apparent owner may suddenly appear in one's path. As potentially rewarding as these opportunities might be in terms of a purely hedonic calculus, they may well go unembraced because of the signal of poor coherence they would produce with respect to relevant domains of one's self system.

At the least, interpretation and self-reflection complicate the application of reinforcement principles to social influence. A more likely conclusion is that these features of human experience can serve to invert the predictions offered by this perspective. Since the late 1950s, several lines of research have converged on the idea that rewards, commonly operationalized as monetary incentives, not only fail to change attitudes and behavior, but also they may actually produce precisely the opposite effect. In one common paradigm, participants are offered a material reward for engaging in an activity (e.g., Bem, 1967; Deci, 1975; Festinger, 1957; Harackiewicz, Abrams, & Wageman, 1987; Lepper, Greene, & Nisbett, 1973). Although a wide variety of moderators have been identified, a consistent finding here is that participants' motivation to perform the activity at a later time is undercut rather than enhanced by the prospect of reward (Lepper & Greene, 1978). This effect occurs both for unappealing activities (e.g., boring and repetitive tasks) and for activities that would seem to be intrinsically enjoyable (e.g., painting, solving puzzles). Across a wide variety of actions, then, if participants are influenced at all by the promise of reward, it is in a direction opposite to what was intended.

Various theories are offered for this "reverse incentive" effect; most trade on the capacity for interpretation (e.g., Bem, 1967; Lepper et al., 1973), although accounts emphasizing something akin to self-concept distress are still serious explanatory contenders (e.g., Aronson, 1992). A separate line of research in support of self-concept mechanisms centers on the concept of reactance (Brehm & Brehm, 1981). According to this notion, the mere fact that influence is being exerted to change one's opinions or behavior provides a reason for embracing the target opinion or behavior all the more strongly. Presumably, heavy-handed influence constitutes a threat to one's general sense of self as an autonomous agent. A similar theoretical account for the failure of rewards to influence people in a straightforward manner emphasizes people's concern with self-determination (e.g., Deci & Ryan, 1985). These accounts are consistent with the perspective on self-control provided in Chapter 5. By acting in opposition to influ-

ence, one reasserts one's self and thereby enhances coherence with respect to the self system as a whole.

More generally, external reinforcement contingencies are not effective in producing long-term change in people's behavior. A variety
of social influence principles have been developed over the years that
specify processes that do not rely on reward–punishment considerations (see Cialdini, 1988). As social animals, people have a natural
tendency to embrace the thoughts and behaviors of others, whether
through compliance (Milgram, 1974), modeling (Bandura, 1986),
conformity to group standards (Asch, 1956), or empathy (Hoffman,
1981). As long as this tendency is not contaminated by explicit concerns with obtaining rewards or avoiding punishment, influence attempts based on it are likely to go beyond simple behavioral compliance to reset control parameters that initiate and maintain action. In
the foot-in-the-door paradigm (Freedman & Fraser, 1966), for example, obtaining a person's cooperation to perform a small behavior
without a promise of reward tends to have a powerful effect on the
person's attitude, which in turn ensures maintenance of the new behavioral tendency.

Resetting Control Parameters

Attempts to influence a person's attitudes and actions directly meet
with equivocal success at best, and often promote stronger commitment to the person's preexisting state (e.g., Kiesler, 1971). The problem is that change must take place with respect to a person's control
parameters, not simply with respect to the momentary output of the
psychological system in question. Patterns of thought and behavior
are generated in accordance with a person's internal state, so if an influence agent is to have any hope of engendering meaningful change
in such patterns, he or she must find a way to reset the values of the
relevant internal state. From a dynamical perspective, the resetting of
control parameters is difficult when the system is well integrated and
stable. To promote change in behavior, then, it is necessary first to
destabilize the system. Once destabilized, the system is primed for resynchronization by incoming information.

On this view, influence may meet with success if the target of influence does not have an integrated cognitive structure with which to
resist influence. Someone with a poorly defined self-image with respect to morality, for example, may be unable to resist the temptation
to cheat on an exams, may take advantage of opportunities for extra-
marital sexual escapades, and may pocket the contents of lost wallets.
And when offered rewards for engaging in a task, someone who is un-

able to provide a coherent interpretation of his or her own for the task may come to see it simply as an opportunity to make money. Rather than engaging the task with their own interpretation in mind, in other words, people in a disassembled mental state accept the depiction offered by the influencing agent. In effect, the erratic dynamics of thought associated with a disorganized mental structure are dampened and form a stable pattern when provided organizing information from an external source.

This perspective is useful for understanding why the settings of some internal factors (control parameters) allow for successful external influence. Under most circumstances, when a person has a well-integrated and stable cognitive structure, it is pointless and counterproductive to challenge his or her attitudes head on. A more effective strategy is to undermine the person's cognitive structure in some fashion and then provide cues to resynchronization. The various manipulations of cognitive load (e.g., Gilbert, 1993) may have this effect since, as demonstrated in Chapter 5, cognitive resources are necessary to achieve and maintain integration in psychological systems. In similar fashion, a variety of other transient mental states are likely to render people open to all manner of suggestion. Thus, distraction, preoccupation, fatigue, and stress tend to make people susceptible to incoming information in support of a conclusion regarding a social attitude or a person's attributes, even if the information is logically irrelevant to the conclusion (e.g., Chaiken, 1980; Gilbert, 1993; Petty & Cacioppo, 1984).

A general strategy for resynchronizing people's attitudes and goals follows from the emergence process of action identification theory, discussed in Chapter 4. Research on this process has established that when people do not have an integrated representation of what they are doing, they become highly susceptible to coherent perspectives on the action provided by others (Vallacher, 1993; Vallacher & Wegner, 1987). This tendency has also been observed with respect to the identification and evaluation of other people's actions (Vallacher & Selz, 1991). Extrapolating this idea to social influence is a straightforward matter. In this scenario, the influencing agent first induces the person to consider the topic in question (e.g., a course of action, an attitude, a person) in concrete, low-level terms. Thus, an action can be described in terms of its mechanistic details, an attitude topic could be disassembled into a set of separate points, and a stimulus person might be described in terms of specific behaviors rather than traits.

From this state of disorganization, the person is likely to experience a strong press for integration. Left to his or her own devices, the person might emerge with a higher level frame for the topic that reflects past positions or perhaps one that reflects a new integration altogether (Vallacher et al., 1998). However, if the influence agent offers a message that provides the missing integration before the person has demonstrated emergence on his or her own, there is a strong likelihood that this message will be embraced as an avenue of emergent understanding, even if it is at odds with the person's prior conceptions (e.g., Wegner et al., 1984). Even new conceptions about the self may be embraced when the target is provided social feedback during a period of induced low-level identification of his or her social behavior (Wegner et al., 1986). Although the emergence process has been demonstrated primarily with respect to people's identification of their own action, the underlying assumptions and mechanisms reflect basic principles of self-organization in nonlinear dynamical systems, and as discussed in preceding chapters, there is reason to think that it is manifest in psychological and social systems generally.

Certain dimensions of individual difference are also associated with openness to influence, and these too can be considered from a dynamical perspective. These include self-uncertainty (e.g., Swann & Ely, 1984), level of personal agency (Vallacher & Wegner, 1989), field dependence (Witkin et al., 1962), external locus of control (Rotter, 1966), and low cognitive differentiation (Bieri et al., 1966). Although these constructs are based on different assumptions, each can be seen as a manifestation of weak structure in a relevant psychological system (i.e., action, other people, society, the self). Lacking internal integration, the person utilizes incoming information as a frame around which he or she can achieve a sense of coherence.

It may not be necessary to destabilize people's internal state directly in order to reset their control parameters in service of social influence. Because control parameters are linked directly to intrinsic dynamics, any factor that changes people's temporal pattern of thought or behavior may promote a corresponding change in the underlying mental state. Experimental research demonstrating a causal link between rapid speech and persuasion is consistent with this idea (MacLachlan & Siegel, 1980; Miller, Maruyama, Beaber, & Valone, 1976). Although inferences regarding the speaker's attributes are clearly relevant, this effect may reflect an increase in the rate of thinking on the part of the target audience to match the rate of incoming information. Intrinsic dynamics of thought characterized by relatively high speed are a sign of instability and openness to different perspectives (Vallacher & Nowak, 1994c).

Music is an especially effective means of resynchronizing the rhythms of thought and behavior (Jones, 1976), and it has been used throughout history to engender various states of consciousness. The film industry and television advertising, of course, play on this link to the tune of billions of dollars in revenue. Qualitatively different rhythms in music are employed to create such states as sympathy, excitement, fear, and relaxation, over and above the informational content of the episode or message presented. To promote sadness and empathy regarding a victim's plight, for example, one would be well advised to associate the visual images and factual information with slow tempo as opposed to uptempo music. In effect, people change their internal settings to match the rhythm associated with incoming sensory information.

CELLULAR AUTOMATA MODELS OF SOCIAL INFLUENCE

Social influence represents more than an attempt to control someone's thought and behavior. Although influence strategies certainly are employed for purposes of manipulation, social influence processes also serve far loftier functions in social life. Indeed, social influence is what enables individuals to coordinate their opinions, moods, evaluations, and behaviors at all levels of social reality, from dyads to social groups to societies. This process of coordination may take different forms, and, as discussed earlier, can happen at different levels of social reality. The particular focus here is influence in social groups. At this level, many details and subtleties of the form that influence takes may be disregarded. What is most important is the reciprocal nature of the influence process, in which each individual is influenced by his or her social contacts and in turn influences these contacts. The concern, in other words, is not with how a particular individual is influenced, but rather with how patterns of individual-level influence combine to form group-level phenomena, such as public opinion.

We assume influence processes on the group level consist of multiple feedback loops, where each individual affects and is in turn affected by opinions, beliefs, and attitudes of other group members. Although these processes are probably very complex in nature, they can be understood in terms of dyadic interactions, in which individuals attempt to coordinate with respect to both behavior and underlying control parameters. In this section, we consider cellular automata as models for such processes. These models portray simpler dynamics than do other models, such as coupled logistic maps, but they enable one to capture important aspects of the way individual-level dynamics are combined to produce group-level processes.

A Dynamical Model of Social Influence

In a social group, each individual both influences and is influenced by the social context. Considerable research has shown that influence can be described in terms of two universal functions. The first describes the combined effect of different people on a single person; the second describes how a single individual's influence is divided across different people. Three critical variables are common to both functions: the number of people influencing or being influenced, the respective strength of these people, and their immediacy to one another (Latané, 1981). Whether the group influence on an individual concerns conformity in an Asch paradigm or in a in a naturalistic setting (e.g., agreeing to sign a petition), stage fright, or interest in news media events, the influence of a group grows as a power function of the number of people involved, usually with an exponent of approximately 0.5. This means that the joint effects of a group exerting influence grow as a square root of the number of people in the group. Influence also grows in proportion to the strength of the individuals exerting the influence. Strength represents the potential for influence, and refers both to relatively stable individual characteristics (e.g. social status or persuasion skills) and topic-relevant variables (e.g., motivation to persuade others). Finally, influence depends on proximity and appears to decrease as a square of the distance. Latané, Liu, Nowak, Bonavento, and Zheng (1995), for example, showed that the probability that two people will discuss matters of mutual importance decreases as a square of the distance between their physical locations.

The joint effect of these three factors can be described as a multiplicative function of strength, immediacy, and number. The reciprocal of this function, meanwhile, describes how social influence is divided among the individuals in a group. The diffusion of responsibility in a group captures this idea, in that the influence each group member experiences is inversely related to the number of other group members. Research on bystander intervention, for example, has shown that a victim is more likely to receive help when there is a single witness than when there are multiple witnesses to his or her plight (e.g., Latané & Darley, 1968). Research on social loafing, meanwhile, has found that individuals commonly exert less effort on a task when performing as a member of a team than when performing alone (e.g., Latané, Williams, & Harkins, 1979), although there are important exceptions to this phenomenon (e.g., Kerr, 1983).

This depiction of social impact provided the basis for the cellular automata model of social influence developed by Nowak et al. (1990). In this model, each individual is characterized by his or her opinion on a topic, persuasive strength, and position in a social space. The distance between two individuals in social space is inversely related to their immediacy vis-à-vis one another. In the original model, individuals were assumed to have one of two opinions on an issue (e.g., either for or against a particular referendum), but in later versions this restriction was relaxed, so that many positions were possible on an issue (Nowak et al., 1993). The social group is modeled as a cellular automata consisting of n individuals located on a two-dimensional grid (see Figure 7.1). Each box in Figure 7.1 corresponds to an individual. The color of the box denotes the individual's opinion, and the height of the box corresponds to the individual's strength.

The model assumes that each individual discusses the issue with other group members. In so doing, he or she assesses the degree of support for each position. The opinions of those who are closest and have the greatest strength are given most consideration (i.e., are weighted most heavily). An individual's own opinion is also taken into consideration and is weighted most heavily by virtue of immediacy. The basic decision rule is simple. Each individual adopts the opinion that was most prevalent in the process of social interaction. The strength of influence of each opinion is expressed by the following formula:

$$I_i = \left[\sum_1^N \left(\frac{s_j}{d_{ij}^2} \right)^2 \right]^{1/2},$$

where I_i denotes total influence, s_j corresponds to the strength of each

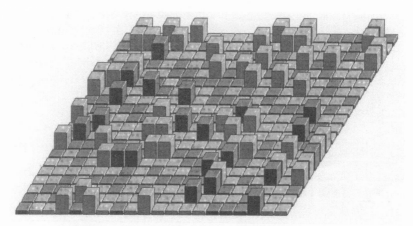

FIGURE 7.1. Cellular automata model of social influence.

individual, and d_{ij} corresponds to the distance between individuals i and j.

In the simulations, one individual is chosen (usually at random), and influence is calculated for each opinion in the group. If the resultant strength for any opinion is greater than the strength of the individual's current opinion, his or her opinion changes to match the prevailing opinion. This process is performed for each person in the group. This procedure is repeated until there are no further changes. This typically requires several rounds of simulation, since a person who previously changed his or her position to match his or her neighbors may revert to the original opinion if the neighbors change their opinions. A typical simulation outcome is shown in Figure 7.2. In the first picture, there is a majority of 60% and a minority of 40%. The second picture shows the equilibrium reached after six rounds of discussion. Now the majority is 90% and the minority is 10%. Note that the minority opinion survives by the formation of clusters of like-minded people and that these clusters are usually formed around strong individuals.

Social Order Parameters

These two outcomes—polarization and clustering—are reminiscent of well-documented social processes. There is evidence, for example, that as a result of group discussion, the average attitude in a group becomes more extreme in the direction of the prevailing attitude in the group (e.g., Moscovici & Zavalloni, 1969; Myers & Lamm, 1976).

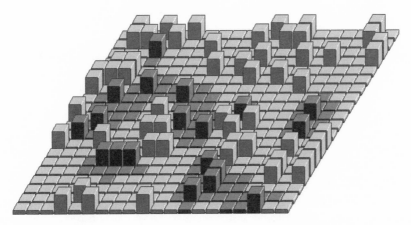

FIGURE 7.2. Typical outcome of social influence processes.

The same underlying phenomenon was discussed in political science by Noelle-Neumann (1984), who noted that a slight difference in opinion before an election can be transformed into a landslide by individuals who want to be on the winning side. In the simulation model, polarization is due to the greater (on average) influence of the majority opinion. In the random initial configuration, the average proportion of neighbors holding a given opinion corresponds to the proportion of this opinion in the total group. The average group member is thus surrounded by more majority than minority members, and this difference results in more minority members converted to the majority opinion than vice versa. Nevertheless, some majority members are converted to the minority opinion because they happen to be located in the vicinity of an especially influential minority member, or because by pure accident, more minority members happen to be at this particular location.

Clustering is also highly pervasive in social life. In fact, it is hard to conceive of a social phenomenon that does not demonstrate clustering. Attitudes, for example, have been shown to cluster in residential neighborhoods (Festinger, et al., 1950). Farming techniques, political beliefs, social movements, religions, fashions, and so forth also display pronounced clustering. Clustering reflects the relatively strong influence exerted by neighboring individuals. Social interaction can be seen as a means of sampling the distribution of opinions in a social group. If opinions are mixed randomly, such a sampling process gives a reasonably accurate portrait of the distribution of opinions in the larger society. If opinions are clustered, however, such an estimation process will yield a highly biased result. The opinions of those in the nearest vicinity will be weighted the most, and the prevalence of one's own opinion is likely to be highly overestimated. The maintenance of minority opinions is thus enhanced in a highly clustered society. Because of this effect, opinions that are in the minority in global terms form a local majority. Only individuals on the borders of clusters are exposed to contrary opinions to a significant degree. Even here, some minority members may be relatively strong or located next to someone who is. Higher strength can counteract the prevalence of the majority opinion and thus protect the border of the cluster.[1]

Polarization and clustering are order parameters of social influence processes. This was demonstrated by Lewenstein et al. (1993), who used the tools of statistical mechanics to analyze the dynamical model of social influence. In this approach, changes in the distribution of opinions are expressed in the form of differential equations. In effect, a high-dimensional system composed of many interacting individuals can be described as a low-dimensional system composed of several differential equations. In such a description, one does not describe individual changes in opinion, but rather the evolution of proportions of each opinion in the group. This work revealed polarization and clustering to be order parameters of the process of opinion change at the group level. It can be noted as well that measures of polarization and clustering have been developed that can characterize these variables both with respect to computer simulations and to real social groups (Latané et al., 1994).

Conditions Necessary for Polarization and Clustering

Both computer simulations (Latané & Nowak, 1997) and analytical considerations (Lewenstein et al., 1993; Nowak, Lewenstein, & Frejlak, 1996) have identified variables that are responsible for the dynamics observed in this model. Three features in particular are especially important for the emergence of polarization and clustering: the existence of individual differences in strength, nonlinearity in attitude change, and the local nature of influence dictated by the geometry of social space. Individual differences, first of all, are often indispensable to the survival of minority clusters. This conclusion resonates well with evidence regarding the importance of leaders for the survival of minority positions. The literature on brainwashing (e.g., Schein, 1956), for example, suggests that the importance of individual differences for preventing unification was clearly recognized by those who employed such techniques. For this reason, natural leaders were commonly removed from the group before attempts were made to brainwash prisoners of war. By counteracting the sheer number of majority opinions, the strength of leaders stops minority clusters from decaying. It can be noted that as a result of social influence, individual differences in strength are likely to become correlated with opinions. This is because the weakest minority members will most likely adopt the majority position, so that over time, the average strength of remaining minority members will grow at the expense of the majority. This scenario provides insight into the observation that individuals advocating minority positions are often more influential than those advocating majority positions.

There are three basic configurations by which minority clusters containing leaders can survive (Nowak et al., 1996; Nowak et al., 1993). These configurations are displayed in Figure 7.3. In the leader and followers configuration (A), a single leader is encircled by a ring of followers. The followers can sustain their opinion because of the strong support provided by the leader. The relationship is symbiotic, since the followers make it easier for the leader to sustain his or her

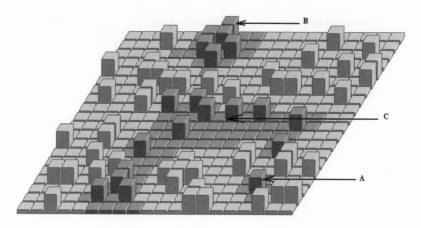

FIGURE 7.3. Configurations of social space.

opinion. Thus, the followers provide additional support to the leader and, more important, they isolate the leader from the direct influence of the majority. In the stronghold configuration (B), several strong individuals are grouped together, and this cluster is surrounded by weaker group members. This configuration is extremely stable, more so than the leader–follower configuration. Even if one of the strong members switches to the majority opinion, the opinions of the other strong members can often bring him or her back to the minority position. In the wall configuration (C), the leaders are located near the borders of the cluster, forming a wall that protects weaker group members from the influence of the majority. In this configuration, even a relatively small number of leaders can protect a relatively large group of followers. The wall does not need to be contiguous; just a few leaders can serve as guards at widely separated points and effectively protect the interior of the cluster.

The second important feature is nonlinearity in attitude change. Abelson (1979) has shown that when individuals move incrementally toward the opinions of their interaction partners as a result of social influence, the outcome of simulations is invariably uniformity, with no minority clusters. In the present model, however, a strong form of nonlinearity is assumed, namely, a threshold function. Opinions are presumed to be categorical in nature, with individuals holding their opinion and switching dramatically from one category to another rather than incrementally on a dimension of judgment. Computer simulations (Szamrej, Nowak, & Latané, 1992) have demonstrated the critical importance of nonlinearity in the attitude change rule, of which the threshold function is simply the extreme case. Whereas a linear change rule implies a normal distribution of attitudes, a nonlinear change rule implies that attitudes in a group should have a bimodal distribution. Latané and Nowak (1994) have shown that both types of distributions can be observed. As discussed in Chapter 3, the critical variable here is attitude importance. For unimportant (e.g., uninvolving) attitudes, a normal distribution tends to be observed, with intermediate values of the attitude emerging as the most common in the group. For important issues, however, attitudes display a bimodal distribution, with almost no individuals occupying the intermediate points on the attitude scale. This suggests that one way to achieve consensus in a group is to decrease the subjective importance of the topic in question.

The third crucial feature of the model concerns the geometry of the space in which individuals interact (Nowak, Latané, & Lewenstein, 1994). People obviously do not communicate equally with all members of a group, nor are their interactions often random. We can approximate different communication patterns with different geometries of social space. This approach has two advantages. First, it allows for visualization of patterns of opinions emerging from interactions. Second, it allows one to make links between the geometry of interaction space and dynamics of influence. In most of the simulations, social space is portrayed as a two-dimensional matrix of n rows and n columns. This is consistent with interactions that are governed by physical proximity, such as those in neighborhood structures, town squares, and the like.

By constraining the spatial structure of interactions, the geometry of social space dictates the nature of cluster formation, the shapes of the resultant clusters, and the probability of their survival versus decay. Consider first a group in which there is virtually no geometry, in the sense that everyone is equally spaced from everyone else, so that each individual interacts equally with all members of the group. Under these conditions, minority opinion may survive for a relatively long time if high value is placed on one's own opinion and individual differences are strongly pronounced (Lewenstein et al., 1993). However, because the social space lacks structure, minority opinions cannot cluster. Geometry may be said to be lacking as well when the interaction patterns in a group are random. In this case, minority opinion rapidly decays, and the group converges on the majority position (Lewenstein et al., 1993).

Other geometries may be used to capture different types of communication structures (Nowak et al., 1996). It is possible, for example, to envision one-dimensional geometry, in which people interact mainly with neighbors to their left and right. This corresponds, for example, to a row of houses along a river or a village stretching along a road. In this case, strong clustering occurs because of well-pronounced local interactions between nearest neighbors. There is no polarization, however, because individuals on the borders of clusters interact equally often with minority and majority members. The members of the majority do not have a persuasive advantage, because in one dimension they cannot encircle members of the minority.

In a hierarchical geometry, people are divided into groups, subgroups, and so forth (Lewenstein et al., 1993; Nowak et al., 1996). The distance between any two individuals in a hierarchical structure depends on the level at which they both belong to a common unit; the higher this level, the greater the distance. Thus, there is very little distance between two individuals in the same subgroup, greater distance between two individuals who share the next highest level but not the same subgroup, greater distance yet between two individuals who share the next higher level but not the two prior levels, and so on. In a university structure, for example, two individuals in the same research group are close, two individuals from different research groups but the same department are less close, two individuals from two departments within the same college are yet less close, and two individuals from different colleges are farthest apart. In hierarchical geometry, the formation of clusters follows this progression in distance. Borders of clusters will almost invariably coincide with subgroups at some level. The structure of opinions therefore follows the structure of social interaction. Once formed, clusters will be very stable, because most of the interactions happen among individuals belonging to the same group, with correspondingly less interaction as distance increases in the hierarchy.

Yet more elaborate geometries for social space can be envisioned (Nowak et al., 1994). In real social interactions, many different geometries are likely to co-occur and thus determine the dynamics of social influence. Consider the multiple means of communication in a community, for example. The availability of telephones, E-mail, and common areas for shopping and recreation clearly add many dimensions to the effective geometry in which interactions occur. The properties of all these geometries and their combined effects play a significant role in determining the shape of social processes.

Control Parameters of Social Influence

Many variables in the cellular model produce only small quantitative effects, but a few variables strongly affect the course of dynamics observed. Three variables in particular play a critical role and thus qualify as control parameters of group-level social influence processes. One of these, referred to as bias, reflects unequal *a priori* attractiveness of the various attitude positions. For present purposes, we assume that the attitude positions in a group do not differ substantially in their relative desirability. When this condition is met, two variables dictate the nature of the dynamics observed: the level of noise and the magnitude of self-influence.

Without influences external to the group, and in the absence of randomness, minority clusters would exist forever once they reached an equilibrium. Of course, in the real world, everyone is subject to a variety of influences beyond social influence within a group. These influences include such things as personal experiences, communication from people outside the group, and selective exposure to media. These factors may be modeled as random influences and referred to collectively as noise. The value of noise may be added to the social influence experienced by each person. Noise may sometimes cause a person to adopt a different opinion than the one suggested by social influence. If the noise is relatively small, such changes in opinion happen rarely and the basic scenario of the model is not significantly affected.

When noise is present, there are no absolute equilibria indicating stabilization of attitudes for the simple reason that a randomly induced change is always possible. Nonetheless, well-defined clusters are formed, and these may exist for a very long time. A small value of noise does not change this picture in a radical way, even if, from time to time, some of the weaker minority members change their opinion. Usually, their own group can bring them back into the fold. Even noise that is relatively weak on the average, however, may take on a high value from time to time. In the presence of strong random influences, clusters may lose their stability. Somewhat larger random influences may cause one of the leaders to change his or her opinion, and if the leader is part of a wall protecting a minority cluster, the cluster will start to decay. This decay will terminate if another strong person happens to be on the border and thus in a position to protect the minority members. The cluster in this case will reach a new equilibrium. In the presence of noise, this scenario may occur several times before a cluster vanishes. The dynamics here may reflect long periods of relative stability intermixed with rapid decay. For obvious reasons, this scenario is referred to as *staircase dynamics* (Lewenstein et al., 1993).

Analytical considerations have shown staircase dynamics to be a general scenario of decay in a variety of complex systems, including those in which there are no individual differences. A decline in health, for example, is usually characterized by periods in which the decline is negligible followed by periods of rapid deterioration, during which several biological systems worsen in a short period of time. The staircase scenario may have implications as well for a variety of social systems. With respect to societal collapse, historical accounts suggest that many institutions experience sudden deterioration and collapse, while another group of institutions may be left relatively intact. A new equilibrium is then reached that may persist for some time, followed by a new burst of institutional collapse, and so forth. More generally, systems are composed of subsystems of interdependent elements, so that when one element of a subsystem fails, it places an extra burden on the elements to which it is interconnected, producing a ripple effect throughout the subsystem.

Self-influence represents the weight an individual attaches to his or her own opinion as compared to the opinions of others. This variable reflects such psychological states as self-confidence, belief certainty, and strength of conviction. Self-influence is assumed to be perfectly correlated with strength, although its absolute value is determined by dividing strength by a constant to represent self-distance. Self-distance reflects the relative importance of one's own opinions relative to others and varies as a function of the topic or social setting. For example, when an issue is new and confusing, self-distance is relatively high for all group members, reflecting the fact that no strong opinion has been formed, and members are thus open to external influence. When an issue is familiar and personally important, however, self-distance is set at a low value, reflecting the general openness to self-influence on the part of all group members. Because self-distance is constant across all members, however, it represents a variable property that is perfectly correlated with strength.

The dynamics of social influence are determined by the value of self-influence relative to the total influence of other group members. When self-influence is very low, individuals may switch their opinions several times during the course of a simulation. Decreasing values of self-influence also tend to destabilize clusters. For topics characterized by relatively high self-distance, then, one can observe heightened dynamics leading to unification based on the majority opinion. If self-influence is greater than the combined influence of others, however, there are no dynamics in the absence of noise. The introduction of noise may destabilize opinions, even when there is strong self-influence. Because noise works jointly with social influence, the changes caused by noise will most often be in the direction of majority influence. Hence, the introduction of a random factor that by itself would not favor any opinion can neutralize the effect of self-influence and enhance the effect of majority opinion. Very high values of noise, however, may dilute the effects of social contacts as well, producing random changes in opinion.

Cellular Automata Models in Perspective

Cellular automata are clearly quite useful in modeling the dynamics of social influence. Indeed, they are useful in modeling any social process in which each individual's state is dependent on the states of other individuals in his or her local neighborhood. Because they are quite flexible with respect to the nature of updating rules, they are able to capture qualitatively distinct influence processes. It should be noted, though, that the rules of cellular automata are commonly relaxed in social science applications, as compared to their applications in the physical sciences. Thus, in order to capture variables believed to be important in understanding social processes, it is common to include characteristics of elements beyond their state and location. In the model we have described, for example, considerable emphasis was placed on individual differences in strength. In models concerned with social interdependence (Chapter 8), meanwhile, consideration is given to individual differences in resources, preferences, and strategies—characteristics that have little meaning in the modeling of physical phenomena.

Although cellular automata models are flexible with regard to individual differences and updating rules, they are rigid with respect to social structure. In the two-dimensional lattices employed in the model of social influence, for example, each individual interacts with either four neighbors (in von Neumann structures) or eight neighbors (in Moore structures). Such constraints may prove useful in models of qualitative understanding, where it is important to define some local neighborhood. The two-dimensional grid, for example, is well suited to represent the likely contacts among individuals in a town or village. The inflexibility of such structures, however, is unreasonable in light of research demonstrating the potential for complex and changeable social structures (e.g., Friedkin & Johnson, 1990). People who are widely separated in social space can nonetheless strongly influence one another, for example, and it is also the case that individuals differ a great deal in the number of social contacts they have.

The inflexibility of cellular automata also makes them inadequate for modeling the development of social structure from individual interactions. As discussed in Chapter 6, for example, there is often bidirectional causality between the states of individuals and the connections between them. Closeness can lead to convergence in opinions, as in the model we have presented, but it is also the case that interpersonal ties are more likely to be formed between people who hold similar views (e.g., Byrne, Clore, & Smeaton, 1986; Newcomb, 1961). Although the latter case may be captured in cellular automata by allowing for movement to a new location (e.g., Hegselman, 1994; Shelling, 1969), it is not possible to form only a single relationship in the new neighborhood. Rather, the individual necessarily adopts the entire structure of social ties in the new location, despite being enticed there by similarity with only one of the neighbors. In other words, the structure of social relations is dictated by the geometry of social space used in cellular automata rather than reflecting individual choices.

Cellular automata may be limited in their generalizability to social reality for another reason. In everyday interactions, it is clear that social influence does not always have its intended effect. Indeed, quite the opposite commonly occurs. An individual who adopts a particular position may influence some people to adopt the same position, but he or she may make others less likely to do so. The occurrence of such reactance effects (Brehm & Brehm, 1981) may in fact be diagnostic of the relationship between the individuals involved. Balance theory (Heider, 1958), for instance, holds that people are inclined to adopt the attitudes of some people (e.g., those they like) but to reject the attitudes of other people (those they do not like). A member of a political party thus may be predisposed to accept the positions of the leaders within his or her party, but to shift away from the positions espoused by the leaders in opposition parties. Cellular automata are not equipped to accommodate the potential for negative social influence, however, because social ties are not a flexible property of individuals, but rather are dictated by the geometry of social space.

In summary, cellular automata models are ideal for investigating individual differences and a wide variety of rules expressing mechanisms of individual change in the context of social groups. This approach is also attractive because it enables visualization of the emergence of group structure. At the same time, though, cellular automata are inflexible in their depiction of social ties, a feature that makes them less than ideal for investigating individual choice in social contacts and the potential for negative as well as positive influence between individuals.

ATTRACTOR NEURAL NETWORK MODELS OF SOCIAL INFLUENCE

As noted earlier, social connections are sometimes negative and can thus promote reactance in response to influence attempts. There is also reason to believe that social structures are constrained in their evolution, with certain patterns of connections more likely to emerge and stabilize than others. According to balance theory (Heider, 1958), for instance, it is unlikely that two people who dislike each other will form a common sentiment relation with a third person. Extending this simple principle to large groups suggests that social structures will evolve toward some equilibria rather than others, with many possible structures never realized because of their psychological instability. Both of these features—the possibility of negative social relations and the impossibility of certain social structures—can be modeled with attractor neural networks. These models have in fact achieved widespread popularity, particularly in cognitive neuroscience, because of their ability to handle different types of connections (i.e., excitatory and inhibitory), and because they capture the tendency to evolve toward well-defined equilibrium (attractor) states (see Hopfield, 1982).

Individuals and Their Connections

Although attractor neural networks were originally designed to model brain function, it is possible to recast their architecture as representations of social groups and even societies. In this interpretation, each neuron corresponds to a single individual, and the connections between neurons correspond to the relations among the individuals comprising the group. This general description is actually quite similar to the characterization of social networks (Wasserman & Faust, 1994). Attractor neural networks have two advantages over social network models, however. First, in attractor neural networks, one can map the relationship between structure and dynamic properties. Second, these models provide formal operators for dealing with negative as well as positive connections, and with graded connections of either valence.

There are two types of dynamics in attractor neural networks. The first type corresponds to learning and involves changes in the connections between neurons, with the neurons themselves remaining stable. The changes in connections are defined in terms of a learning algorithm, which guarantees that the desired configuration of neurons, corresponding to a memorized pattern, functions as an attractor. In social terms, such changes reflect the formation and dissolution of social relations based on the opinions, moods, and attitudes of group members. Because such changes converge on attractors, only certain configurations of opinions, moods, and so forth are likely to be observed in a social group. This feature makes attractor neural networks relevant to issues in close relationships (Chapter 6) and social inter-dependence (Chapter 8).

In the second type of dynamics, corresponding to recognition, the states of neurons change, but the connections among neurons remain stable. The idea is that each neuron tries to adjust its state to the total input it receives from other neurons, from the environment, and from noise (i.e., random influences). The neuron adopts an excited state if the sum of all these inputs exceeds a certain threshold. If the summed input fails to exceed this threshold, meanwhile, the neuron adopts a low value corresponding to a nonexcited state. Viewed in terms of social networks, each node (i.e., neuron) corresponds to an individual, and the dynamics correspond to changes in the opinions, moods, or attitudes of individuals as a result of influence exerted through existing social ties with other individuals.

It is common in this approach to treat nodes as binary, with each adopting either a +1 or a −1 value, corresponding to high and low states, respectively (see, e.g., Hopfield, 1982). As it happens, the qualitative properties of the dynamics in such networks are very similar to the dynamics observed in networks in which elements can adopt continuous values (see Hopfield, 1984). Because attractor neural networks based on binary nodes are easier to understand, however, we describe them and develop their implications for the dynamics of opinion change. The Hopfield (1982) model in particular provides a nice illustration of how attractor neural networks can be utilized to represent the dynamics of social influence.

In a Hopfield-type network, each node is connected to every other node, with each connection being symmetrical. The strength of the connections between nodes i and j represents the degree to which the state of j influences the state of i, and vice versa. Connections are represented by positive numbers, corresponding to excitatory influence, or by negative numbers, corresponding to inhibitory influence. The influence of j on i is expressed as the product of j's state (+ 1 or −1) and the strength of the connection between i and j. If there is an excitatory connection between i and j, in other words, j will influence i to be in the same state, whereas if there is an inhibitory connection between i and j, j will influence i to be in the opposite state. Each node tries to adjust its state in the next moment of time ($t + 1$) to the total input it receives from the other nodes, which may be expressed as a sum of all the inputs at time t:

$$h_i(t) = \sum_{j=1} J_{ij} s_j(t).$$ (1)

In this equation, $h_i(t)$ represents the total input that i receives from other nodes at time t, J_{ij} describes the connection (i.e., its sign and strength) from j to i, and $s_j(t)$ describes the state of j at time t. If the sum is greater than some threshold (often set at 0), the node will adopt a high state at the next time moment; if lower than this threshold, the node will adopt a low state. For a threshold value equal to 0, the updating rule may be written as

$$s_i(t + 1) = \text{sgn}[h_i(t)]. \qquad (2)$$

The function "sgn" has a value +1 whenever $h_i(t)$ is positive and a value of –1 whenever $h_i(t)$ is negative. The dynamics may be realized in either a synchronous updating, in which the state of each node at one time is based on the states of all its connected nodes at the previous time (i.e., all the nodes are updated simultaneously), or in a Monte Carlo updating, in which one node at a time is randomly chosen and its state is updated based on the states of all other nodes (i.e., the nodes are updated sequentially). These two updating rules typically produce highly similar outcomes.

In a social interpretation, positive connections represent relationships in which the two individuals influence one another to have similar moods, attitudes, and so forth, whereas negative connections represent a reactance-like influence between the two individuals. Although positive and negative connections typically correspond to positively valenced relations (i.e., friendship, attraction, etc.) and negatively valenced relations (i.e., dislike, resentment, etc.), respectively, the sign of a connection can also represent strategic decisions concerning coalition formation rather than the affective quality of the relationship. Thus, a person may have a neutral feeling at best toward someone else, but still adopt that person's position on a given topic because he or she wishes to have the backing of the person on another issue.

Attractor Social Networks

It is common for a person to be influenced by two or more other people. This feature of social relations can be considered in light of Heiderian principles of relationship structure (Heider, 1958). In balanced triads, for example, the distribution of opinions is stable, since all the pairwise relations support the distribution. If all the relationships are positive, everyone tends to have the same opinion. If one relationship is positive and two are negative, meanwhile, the persons connected by a positive relationship will share an opinion, while the third person will have a contrasting opinion. In unbalanced triads, on the other hand, no single configuration of opinions will satisfy existing relationships. If all three relationships are negative, for example, or if two are positive and one is negative, the opinion structure is necessarily strained and hence unstable. This requirement can be relaxed somewhat in attractor networks, however, because the actual configuration of opinions will depend on the relative strength of pairwise connections. Thus, even an unbalanced triad may tend toward stability if one of the connections is weaker than the others and can be effectively ignored.

Social relationships typically extend far beyond a triad. In large social systems, individuals can reasonably be expected to have multiple relationships. Even if the majority of these relationships are characterized by weak ties, they can nonetheless have a significant impact on a given individual when their effects are summed (Flache & Macy, 1996). If the connections within a group are primarily positive, the dynamics are relatively simple: after some time, everyone will converge on the same opinion. However, if there is a significant proportion of negative (inhibitory) connections (e.g., greater than 30%), the dynamics become much more complex. In fact, there may be several equilibria of opinions for a given set of connections. In the Hopfield model, for example, when connections are symmetrical, the number of potential uncorrelated equilibria is approximately $0.14\,n$, where n is the number of individuals. For asymmetrical networks (e.g., Gardner, 1988), the number of equilibria can approach $2n$.

Some equilibria, however, are more stable than others. To understand the dynamics of social networks in the presence of several equilibria, it is helpful to employ an energy metaphor. Given a set of connections, every configuration of states of nodes can be assigned a specific value of a so-called energy function. The energy of a given state corresponds to

$$E = -\tfrac{1}{2} \sum_{j \neq i} J_{ij} s_i s_j. \tag{3}$$

J and s are used in the same way they were used in equation (1). The energy is computed by summing these terms over all the connected nodes. In the fully connected model, this corresponds to the summation of all possible pairs of nodes, with the exception of the node with itself. Metaphorically, one can imagine a landscape in which hills correspond to high energy and valleys correspond to low energy. Figure 7.4 presents a simplified depiction of such a landscape.

In this figure, the x-axis corresponds to configurations of states of

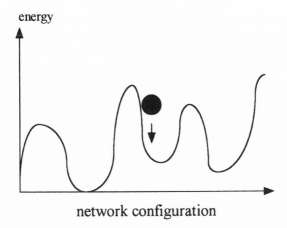

energy

network configuration

FIGURE 7.4. Energy landscape for attractor social network.

nodes, such that neighboring points differ by the state of one node, and the y-axis corresponds to the energy of each configuration. Each valley corresponds to a local minimum in the energy function (i.e., an equilibrium state), with the depth of the valley depicting the strength of the equilibrium. Dynamics of the network consist of the descent from any state to the closest equilibrium. Metaphorically, picture a ball rolling down a hill until it reaches a valley, at which point it comes to rest. The dynamics of attractor networks, in which each node adjusts its state to the total signal coming from other nodes, corresponds to the descent on the energy landscape.

This definition of an energy function may be seen as a formalization and generalization of the Heiderian principle of balance (Heider, 1958). Although Heider's concept of balance refers to the amount of incoherence and conflict that people experience in a given social network, the formalization of this concept is limited to triads. His depiction, moreover, does not take into account the fact that some relationships are clearly stronger and more important than others. The energy function allows for precise characterization of the degree of conflict in a social network of any size and takes into consideration not only the direction (i.e., positive or negative), but also the strength of the relationship between any pair of individuals.

If influence among nodes were the only source of dynamics, once a system achieved an equilibrium state—even the most shallow of valleys—the dynamics would cease. In social reality, of course, direct influence from other people is not the sole source of opinion change. A person's opinion depends on such things as the recall of idiosyncratic memories, communication from outside the group, and mass media exposure. The joint effect of all such factors may be represented as a random influence on each individual. In attractor neural networks (as in cellular automata models), random influences are commonly referred to as noise. Noise is typically added as a random number to the summed input of all the connections for each individual.

The introduction of noise can qualitatively change the dynamics of social influence in groups. Under certain conditions, in fact, noise can make a given individual change his or her opinion in a way that is contrary to social influence. The larger the magnitude of the noise relative to the value of social influence, the more likely that this will occur. If the value of noise relative to the value of social influence is very small, its influence is correspondingly subtle. Larger relative values of noise, on the other hand, tend to destabilize weak equilibria. This occurs because the introduction of randomness can cause the system to evolve in such a way that the energy function increases rather than decreases. By extension, with increases in noise, correspondingly stronger equilibria become unstable. Finally, for some value of noise, no equilibria will be stable, so that the system evolves randomly.

The extrapolation of these ideas to social influence is straightforward. The greater the proportion of outside and random influences on individuals' opinions, the weaker the role of equilibria produced by the structure of social relations within the group. In terms of the energy landscape metaphor, noise in effect shakes the landscape, causing the ball to leave relatively shallow valleys and settle in the deepest valleys. For yet higher values of outside and random influences, opinions begin to evolve independently of the internal group pressure. All the equilibria hence become unstable, and the change of opinions resembles a random process.

The Emergence of Ideology

Social relations are often stable regardless of the opinion in question. In this case, the same network structure applies when group members hold positions on multiple issues. We can examine how the relationship among different opinions evolve by portraying the initial distribution of each opinion as a corresponding configuration of states of nodes and observing how these configurations change as a result of social influence. In a sense, we model the group as it discusses each issue in turn and note the resultant equilibrium for each issue. The number of possible equilibria is limited and scales linearly with the size of the group. As noted earlier, the maximum number of equilibria cannot be greater than $0.14n$ in networks with symmetrical connections (Hopfield, 1982) or greater than $2n$ in networks with asymmetrical connections (Gardner, 1988). In reality, the maximum number of equilibria is considerably smaller, especially when some issues are especially important for the group, resulting in some equilibria being very strong. If the number of issues is small, each starting configuration may end up in a separate equilibrium. Opinions on these issues may be uncorrelated. But if the group members hold positions on a number of issues that exceeds the number of equilibria, several opinions will have to share a common equilibrium and thus become correlated among the group members.

In the absence of significant values of noise, even subtle equilibria should be visible, so that relatively many starting configurations end up in separate equilibria. With increases in noise and the concomitant destabilization of weak equilibria, a smaller number of strong equilibria can be achieved. With even stronger noise, all the opinions may evolve to the strongest equilibrium of the system in a process reminiscent of simulated annealing (Kilpatrick, Gelatt, & Vecchi, 1983). At this point, all the issues have become correlated. This process is reminiscent of the emergence of ideology in a society (Converse, 1964). As Converse noted, issues that were previously uncorrelated develop correlations over periods of time. In similar fashion, the process of emergent correlation among attitudes and opinions may provide the basis for forming ingroup identity (e.g., Brewer & Kramer, 1985; Tajfel & Turner, 1986). Obviously, this line of reasoning does not take into account the logical implications of the content associated with particular issues. A hard line on fighting crime, for example, implies being in favor of more money for the police force, mandatory sentencing for people convicted of crime, and more prisons. What the model suggests, however, is that correlations may also emerge among issues that do not have any logical implications for one another. Hairstyle preference, for example, does not seem to have any logical bearing on the abortion issue, but according to the model, opinions regarding these topics could become correlated within subgroups.

For yet higher values of outside and random influences, each opinion begins to evolve independently of the internal group pressure. All the equilibria hence become unstable, and the correlations among issues begin to dissipate. At extremely high values of noise, the correlations vanish altogether. In terms of the energy landscape metaphor, as the landscape is shaken in a subtle manner, those balls that are resting in very shallow valleys roll into deeper ones. With progressively stronger shaking of the energy landscape, the balls gather in increasing deeper valleys. At some point, however, even the deepest valleys cannot contain the balls jumping in response to energy. Hence, the balls begin to jump randomly and independently of one another. In the social interpretation, this is tantamount to the decoupling of attitudes and opinions, with each attitude and opinion becoming susceptible to different outside and random forces.

Due to social influence, even unrelated issues are likely to become correlated as the issues achieve their respective local equilibria. Since the number of equilibria changes as a function of group size, it is possible for societies to hold uncorrelated positions on many issues, as long as interpersonal relationships (as opposed to, say, media influence) are the primary means of opinion change. In relatively small groups, however, it will be unlikely for even a small number of opinions to remain uncorrelated. It follows, then, that it is much easier for small groups to become cohesive than it is for larger groups, a conclusion that is consistent with work on group dynamics (Cartwright & Zander, 1968).

These considerations assume that social influence is the only force affecting opinions. Obviously, opinions are affected by other factors, such as vested interests and self-influence. Also the structure of relations may change as a function of the issue in question. These factors complicate predictions about the exact number of possible equilibria in a group. The general line of reasoning regarding the relationship between variables, however, remains valid.

Attractor Neural Networks in Perspective

Neural networks models are appealing models of social relations, but it is also the case that neurons are not people and that brains are not groups or societies. There are, in fact, some potentially crucial differences between neural and social networks. Some of these differences can be handled by modifying the assumptions and rules of neural network models to accommodate well-established principles of social psychology. But there are other differences that pose serious challenges for future work in this area. In this section, we consider the features of human psychology that are open to realization in neural networks, as well as those that may prove highly difficult to capture in neural network models.

The primary goal of neural networks is to code a large number of complex memories and then retrieve them on the basis of minimal cues. The primary goal of social networks, on the other hand, is to provide for the often-difficult coordination of individuals' thoughts, emotions, and interpersonal actions. Social relations, after all, are a mix of cooperative and competitive tendencies. Some goals are best served through cooperation, but the fact that resources are often scarce, or at least zero-sum, means that competition is to be expected in many circumstances. Social relations thus should form in such a way that they can accommodate both cooperation among those with shared goals and competition among those with conflicting goals. So whereas the architecture of neural networks should be optimized for complexity, the architecture of social networks should be optimized for social coordination. To accommodate the necessary social rules, standard learning algorithms of neural networks may need to be modified.

The equilibria of a neural network may have a very complex structure. Accordingly, learning algorithms are formulated to accommodate a maximal number of memories. If the evolution of social ties simply mimicked such algorithms, the resultant social configuration could prove incomprehensible for group members, making the coordination necessary for social action virtually impossible to attain. Indeed, there is reason to believe that in contrast to neural networks, social networks evolve toward simplicity in both structure and dynamics. So although unbalanced triads in neural networks allow for multiple equilibria and hence a rich set of memories, Heiderian principles (Heider, 1958) state that unbalanced triads tend to evolve toward balance. Thus, a friend of our friend tends to become our friend, an enemy of our friend tends to become our enemy, and an enemy of our enemy tends to be become our friend. Such processes aimed at minimizing frustration in a social network eventually lead to the emergence of two groups characterized by positive ties internally and negative ties (i.e., conflict) with one another.

It is possible to provide for yet further simplification of this type of social structure by representing each group with a single node, with the members of each group having a positive connection to the group's node. The relation between conflicting groups, then, can be represented by a single, very strong negative connection between the respective group nodes. To a certain extent, this characterization of social structure captures important features of the emergence of ingroup identity (e.g., Brewer & Kramer, 1985). In this formulation, the number of connections is effectively reduced from N^2, representing the case where each individual is connected to every other individual, to $2N$, representing the case where each individual is simply connected to his or her own group node. This simplified structure obviously provides a much more efficient mechanism for ingroup coordination of thoughts, feelings, and actions.

Attractor neural networks are characterized by symmetry between positive and negative connections, as well as between similarity and dissimilarity. In social life, however, there is a pronounced tendency to avoid negative relations and displays of dissimilarity. Negative evaluations of people, for example, are displayed less frequently but are given greater weight in social relations (e.g., Cacioppo & Berntson, 1994). It is possible to represent this type of asymmetry in attractor networks by simply assigning a higher number to negative states (e.g., –2) than to positive states (e.g., +1). The greater the asymmetry in the frequency of positive versus negative states, the greater the compensatory weighting of these states. In a related vein, it is typically the case that negative social relationships tend to be broken rather than maintained in the same way that positive relationships are. This means that the resultant social structure tends to be heavily biased in favor of positive relationships. By virtue of their very infrequency, however, the few remaining negative relations are likely to be especially salient, thereby increasing their effective strength. In principle, this manifestation of positive–negative asymmetry could be coded into attractor networks, although this task has yet to be undertaken.

In most attractor neural networks, it is assumed that each neuron reacts to the influence from other neurons, but does not influence itself in an explicit fashion.[2] This stands in contrast to the potential for self-influence associated with people's capacity for self-reflection. Research has shown that when people adopt a position on an issue and are made privately or publicly self-aware, there is a tendency for them to embrace the position even more strongly and become correspondingly resistant to influence attempts (e.g., Wicklund & Frey, 1980). It may prove possible, though, to implement this feature of self-awareness in attractor network models. Quite simply, self-influence can be represented as a connection from a node to itself, with the strength of this connection corresponding to the magnitude of self-influence. This form of influence would have the effect of stabilizing the dynamics of the network. In terms of the energy landscape metaphor, it effectively serves as friction to slow down the movement of the ball, thus enabling the cessation of movement in areas that are not completely flat (Nowak, Lewenstein, & Tarkowski, 1994). If self-influence were to become very strong, meanwhile, the dynamics of opinion change would slow considerably and perhaps even cease altogether.

UNCHARTED TERRITORY IN SOCIAL INFLUENCE

Cellular automata and attractor network models are formal tools developed in mathematics and physics to understand the dynamics of complex systems composed of many mutually interacting elements.

As such, they allow for precise description of structural and dynamical properties that are not easily captured with traditional tools. At one level of description, for example, the Hopfield learning rule is simply a restatement of the similarity–attraction relationship. However, it goes beyond the verbal description of this relationship by enabling one to state precisely the evolution of the connections between two individuals holding particular positions on an issue. It also allows one to couch the dynamics of any given dyad in the context of other dyads in a larger social structure defined in terms of this relationship. Moreover, given the set of all connections in the social structure, the Hopfield rule allows for precise description of all possible equilibria and their respective strengths. In addition, one can follow the change in each configuration of opinions in the social network and describe the resulting equilibrium.

In the physical sciences, an enormous amount of work has been devoted to formulating general laws concerning the dynamics of cellular automata and neural networks. The results of this work may be applied to social reality, once it is clear how these models can be instantiated in terms of social processes. It can be noted in this regard that many of the central theoretical issues concerning cellular automata and neural networks have already been resolved. Currently, we are witnessing a fascinating set of applications of these models to issues that spill well beyond the borders of the physical sciences to capture the essence of key social psychological processes (see, e.g., Kunda & Thagard, 1996; Read & Miller, 1998; Smith, 1996). If we successfully map these models onto social networks, a rich set of practical applications is likely to be developed. It may be possible, for example, to predict the course of social processes well into the future and with greater precision than is currently possible. Perhaps more fascinating, it may be possible to influence the course of social processes and thereby solve social problems, such as social polarization and fragmentation.

It should be kept in mind, though, that people are not cells on a grid or neurons in a brain, and that social relations are not the same as neighborhood structures or synaptic connections. To be sure, there are important formal similarities between network models of brain and society, and many of the differences that exist are of little substantial consequence. Some differences, however, may prove to be crucial for understanding how people change their opinions, moods, and attitudes in a social context. First of all, people may use much more complex decision rules that are the result of factors other than whether social influence exceeds a certain threshold. Although such rules are difficult, if not impossible in principle, to implement in attractor social network models, some relatively complex decision rules have been incorporated into cellular automata models (e.g., Hegselman, 1998). A second fundamental difference concerns the goal-oriented nature of human cognition and action (e.g., Carver & Scheier, 1998; Gollwitzer, 1996; Miller et al., 1960; Powers, 1973; Vallacher & Wegner, 1987). Individuals are not simply reactive, as implied in both cellular automata and neural network models, but rather are active and instrumental in their behavior. The structure of goals may guide thought and behavior in ways that are not easily represented in such models.[3]

Perhaps the most important characteristic of human psychology is the capacity for consciousness. Individuals are not only subject to influences, but they are also conscious of the influence being exerted and can make an effort to resist it. For this reason, social relations do not always evolve in accordance with similarity of opinions and other formal rules. Instead, the rules of social relations may be reflected in consciousness and modified at will to match self-defined values and other prepotent conscious concerns. In this sense, consciousness and reflection create a barrier between individual decisions and factors influencing these decisions. Consciousness can therefore complicate to a high degree the rules of individual behavior and thereby undermine the rules of social dynamics. It may prove possible, of course, to incorporate simple effects of consciousness into both cellular automata and network models. But pending ambitious attempts in this regard, it is an open question whether the full panoply of effects attributable to human consciousness can be captured by formal descriptions, even in principle.

One should not look upon models of cellular automata and neural networks as replacements for social psychological theory and insight. Clearly, a great deal of work remains to be done before cellular automata and attractor network models achieve the status reserved for mature models of social reality. In view of its impressive track record in other areas of science, though, we suspect that this approach—which can be referred to as computational social psychology (Nowak & Vallacher, 1998; Nowak et al., 1998)—will emerge as one of the dominant paradigms for understanding group and societal dynamics. In this role, it is likely to provide both integration to a vast number of seemingly independent phenomena and to generate new lines of theory and research in the years to come.

NOTES

1. Clustering can result from two other mechanisms. In one, individuals relocate near others who have similar opinions. In simulations incorporat-

ing this mechanism (Szamrej, 1989), polarization is diminished but clustering is enhanced. The third mechanism reflects common reactions to local conditions. No social influence concerning fashion, for example, is needed to explain why people in Arctic regions wear warm clothing.

2. In some models, self-influence has an implicit form. This occurs when the new activation value of a neuron is determined by increasing or decreasing the current activation value of the neuron by a value proportional to the input from other neurons. This stands in contrast to a situation where the new value of a neuron is not governed by its previous value. This mechanism functions to smooth the dynamics of a neuron and bring it through a succession of closely related values rather than rapid jumps that might otherwise occur. Clearly, in humans, self-influence has a different form and meaning.

3. It may be possible, however, to describe each individual as a neural network rather than a single node. In such a description, very complex cognitive processes, perhaps even those pertaining to goals, may be captured. To date, this possibility has not been explicitly investigated.

8

⟨⟩

The Individual
and Society

SOCIAL PSYCHOLOGY IS A VERY ambitious discipline. Most fields of inquiry are careful to delineate the issues they feel prepared to tackle. In social psychology, however, everything is fair game. Virtually every nuance of interpersonal function has been explored at one time or another, from the exchange of glances in everyday interactions to the unfolding of passionate relationships. Social psychology also differs from other sciences in its willingness to cross different levels of analysis in pursuit of theoretical understanding. Thus, attention is given to the nature of individual thought processes and to the relations between groups in a society. All this diversity has had the unintended and lamentable effect of creating a highly fragmented field, with little, if any, theoretical synthesis available for the inexhaustible supply of principles and empirical generalizations (Vallacher & Nowak, 1994b). There is little coherence within a given level of analysis (e.g., group-level processes) and unclear linkages between phenomena at different levels of analysis (e.g., social judgment, group decision making).

Our aim in this concluding chapter is to suggest what a dynamical perspective has to offer with respect to these concerns. We first discuss the utility of dynamical principles and methods for identifying invariant properties that cut across different levels of social reality, and the rules by which one can specify linkages among different levels. We then discuss different variations on the persistent dilemma between individual self-interest and the concerns of the social groups to which individuals belong. Different models have been proposed to

250

deal with this issue, but they all have in common the assumption that coordination at the group level is an inevitable result of interactions among egoistic individuals. The link between the individual and society is then discussed with respect to issues of social change and transition. The tension between forces toward stability versus change is examined in the context of a formal model that has proven successful in capturing the trajectory of societal transitions. The present and future identity of dynamical social psychology provides the focus for the concluding section. We summarize the benefits of viewing human social experience from the perspective of nonlinear dynamical systems, but we also stress the importance of remaining cognizant of the uniqueness of human experience when viewing the subject matter of social psychology from this perspective.

LEVELS OF SOCIAL REALITY

One of the most challenging problems in social psychology concerns the relation between micro- and macrolevels of description. For the most part, social psychological theories tend to be couched in terms of a particular level of description, with little if any explicit coordination with theories at different levels. Thus, the set of laws and mechanisms pertaining to group-level processes tend to be independent of the laws and mechanisms pertaining to processes at the level of the individual actor. It is clear, however, that no level of structure and function operates in isolation. So although an individual's behavior is strongly influenced by the social context in which he or she functions, it is equally true that each individual creates the social context for other individuals through his or her interactions with them. The exact nature of this mutual dependency is not easy to describe in traditional approaches to social psychology.

Levels of Description and Invariant Principles

Research on the behavior of nonlinear dynamical systems has established that vastly different topics can be understood in terms of a common set of principles (e.g., Cohen & Stewart, 1994; Haken, 1982; Prigogine & Stengers, 1984). Thus, the same general principles apply to such otherwise diverse phenomena as laser pulsation, autocatalysis in chemical reactions, predator–prey relations in population biology, and weather patterns. Although each of these phenomena consists of fundamentally different kinds of components (e.g., atoms vs. foxes and rabbits), it is the nature of the influences among the components, rather than the nature of the components themselves, that determines the behavior of interest. Both autocatalysis and predator–prey ratios, for example, show periodic evolution under certain values of each system's control parameters. Viewed dynamically, in other words, highly diverse phenomena in science, representing different levels of analysis, conform to remarkably similar principles. In fact, the invariant nature of dynamical systems across phenomena and levels of analysis has fueled optimism that this perspective may represent an integrative framework for science as a whole.

With this in mind, it may prove possible to describe social psychological phenomena at different levels of description with recourse to a set of invariant principles. Regardless of the topic, the task is essentially one of identifying the relevant components and the nature of their mutual influence. Connectionist models, for example, employ the same concepts—nodes and connections—to describe phenomena as distinct as brains, minds, and societies. General properties exhibited by connectionist models are therefore invariant across these levels of description. Thus, the brain can be investigated in terms of individual neurons that influence each other through synaptic connections, the mind can be understood in terms of cognitive and affective elements that become configured to create thoughts and feelings, and a social group can be explored as a set of individuals in which mutual influence is governed by social relations. Extending this analysis yet further, one can view society as a system composed of diverse social groups that interact in positive or negative fashion, and one can explore international relations in terms of nation-states that influence each other in a variety of ways.

This is not to deny that different levels of description are associated with unique principles and psychological laws. Individuals are clearly different than groups, for example, and each of these levels of description requires a specific theoretical language and set of research tools. For this reason, considerable precision is required when discussing phenomena at different levels and when considering how phenomena at different levels are related to one another (see Vallacher & Nowak, 1997). Still, it is hard to ignore the integrative power of the dynamical systems approach. Phenomena at different levels of description may well differ in fundamental respects, but characterizing these phenomena as dynamical systems allows one to employ many of the same formal tools to characterize the relations among elements and the resultant dynamics at the system level. As noted in Chapter 7, for instance, neural network models can be used to describe the structure of connections among neurons in the brain and the structure of relations among individuals and groups in a society. This in no way means that the same processes carry influences between neurons and between people. It does mean, though, that on an abstract mathematical level, important aspects of how neurons influence each other and how people influence each other can be expressed in similar terms.

Emergent Properties and Levels of Social Reality

Social psychology has a long-standing concern with the relationship between different levels of description. It is fair to say, in fact, that the debate regarding reduction versus emergence has done more than has any other issue to create opposing schools of thought in psychology in general (see, e.g., Dennett, 1991; Hofstadter, 1979) and in social psychology in particular (e.g., Gergen, 1994; Harré & Secord, 1973; Rosnow, 1981). There are many who feel that each level of description can be reduced to more basic levels, with fundamental principles couched in terms of individual function. On this view, cognitive, emotional, and behavioral processes are sufficient to generate group-level and even societal-level phenomena. Others argue, instead, that each level of description must be understood on its own terms, with principles that bear little or no relation to the principles characterizing higher or lower levels. This point of view is often expressed in terms of emergence (e.g., Durkheim, 1938). When individuals form groups, for example, new modes of thought and behavior seem to arise that bear little similarity to the modes of thought and behavior characteristic of individuals.

The dynamical perspective suggests that both sides of the debate contain elements of truth. The phenomena at a given level of social reality are often unique and not easily reduced to principles describing phenomena at lower levels. At the same time, though, emergence has a well-defined meaning in dynamical systems theory, and this meaning is useful in understanding how the phenomena at one level of description give rise to distinct phenomena at higher levels of description. The elements at different levels of analysis may be related to each other in two ways. First of all, each element on the higher level may represent a collection of elements on the lower level. Thus, neural assemblies each represent a set of individual neurons, a social group represents a collection of individuals, and so forth. In this type of hierarchy, the elements at different levels may be described with respect to the same variables. One can therefore talk about the political attitudes of an individual and the political attitudes of a social group. Such a characterization, of course, presupposes at least some minimal degree of coordination among the group members in their attitudes. When levels of social reality are defined in terms of increasing aggregation, the hierarchy reflects increasing levels of generality. The same variable, in other words, is simply applied to an increasingly broader domain.

In a fundamentally different mechanism for building hierarchies, introduced in Chapter 2, the elements at a given level correspond to order parameters for the elements at a lower level. Haken (1978), for example, suggested that thoughts may be order parameters for brain states. Note that thoughts and brain states are of a very different nature and that the meaningful characterization of each requires different variables. Extending Haken's example, evaluation may be an order parameter for thoughts, and dynamic versus static integration, introduced in Chapter 3, may be an order parameter for evaluation (Vallacher & Nowak, 1997). Yet higher level order parameters can be defined in this example if one broadens the scope to consider the coordination of evaluation among interacting individuals. In particular, the degree of clustering of attitudes in a social group may be considered an order parameter for group-level evaluations (Nowak et al., 1990; Latané et al., 1994), as discussed in Chapter 7. When levels of social reality are defined in this way, the hierarchy reflects qualitatively different variables that typically differ in their level of abstraction. The derivation of order parameters at each level eliminates many variables from the description; in effect, a large number of variables are replaced with a single, qualitatively different variable reflecting an emergent property.

Although we have emphasized the influence of lower level interactions on the development of higher level variables, it is also widely recognized in social psychology that higher level variables influence the operation of lower level elements. Once a group-level norm has developed, for example, it serves to regulate the behavior of individual members of the group. In like manner, cultural values and beliefs affect the behavior of both groups and individuals in a society. The individual, in other words, both influences and is influenced by his or her social context. This bidirectional causality between different levels of social reality can be readily captured in terms of dynamical systems.

Synergetics provides one of the most formally elegant tools for characterizing the linkage between levels of social reality (see Weidlich, 1991; Weidlich & Haag, 1983). In this approach, the behavior of each individual is described by a set of differential equations, referred to as "slave equations." Dynamical properties at the systems level are described by a different set of differential equations, referred to as "master equations." The dynamics of each individual depend on the state of the system. This is achieved by making control variables in the slave equations dependent on the values of dynamical variables in the master equations. A change of state in the global system thus changes the patterns of individuals' dynamics. The global state of the system, meanwhile, is a function of the aggregated states of all the individuals in the system. In particular, the collective output of individual states and actions influences variables in the master equations. Specific methods of synergetics allow for the progressive elimination of variables on the individual level, resulting in a set of equations describing dynamics of the system as a whole. With respect to the individual and society, this means that social reality may be understood both as a set of individuals and as a single, higher order unit (i.e., the group). Separate rules can be specified to capture the dynamics of a single individual versus the dynamics of the group as a whole. One can also specify how the state of the group affects each individual, and how distributions of states of individuals influence the group.

DILEMMAS OF INTERDEPENDENCE

One of the great puzzles of social psychology is how cooperative and altruistic behavior can emerge against the backdrop of self-interest (Kelley & Thibaut, 1978). Interdependence is a basic feature of human experience, but quite often the consequences of ignoring one's shared fate and operating in accordance with egoistic concerns are not recognized or experienced directly. In the tragedy of the commons (Hardin, 1968), for instance, a farmer may be motivated to overgraze an area of land shared with other farmers. In the short run, doing so provides the farmer an advantage over his neighbors. In the long run, however, ignoring the interdependence in this situation will result in suffering not only for the neighbors but also for the farmer.

Mixed Motives in Social Relationships

The dilemmas of interdependence have most often been examined empirically in the context of the Prisoner's Dilemma Game (PDG). The PDG, which is defined in the formal context of mathematical game theory (Luce & Raiffa, 1957), represents a particularly interesting example of a "mixed-motive" situation. A mixed-motive situation is a situation in which a behavioral option with the most favorable outcome also carries the greatest risk. In the context of social interaction, each participant experiences mixed motives when he or she must choose between maximizing his or her immediate gain and minimizing long-term losses. The PDG essentially pits a motive for competition and self-enhancement against a motive for cooperation and mutual gain with someone else.

The PDG is couched in terms of the following scenario. Suppose that two people are taken into custody on suspicion of having committed an armed robbery. Conviction for robbery is impossible without a confession from at least one of the suspects. Each suspect has two alternatives: Cooperate with the other suspect by refusing to confess, or defect by confessing to the crime. The interrogation of each suspect takes place in a separate room, so that they are unaware of each other's decision to cooperate versus defect. They are told that if both of them confess, they both will be convicted, and the prosecution will recommend moderately harsh sentences for both. If neither confesses to the armed robbery, they both will be prosecuted for a lesser charge, the illegal possession of firearms. If one confesses but the other does not, the one who confesses will be free as a result of a plea bargain, while the one who does not confess will receive the maximum punishment for the armed robbery. In this case, each suspect is better off confessing, regardless of the other suspect's decision. For both of the suspects, it is much better if they both cooperate by not confessing. If each suspect follows individual concerns, however, they both end up confessing and thus receive a poorer outcome. The situation thus captures the essence of conflict between self-interest and the interest of the group. What is good for an individual introduces the worst outcome on the group level.

This formal model has been widely used in economics, political science, and sociology to model different types of conflict situations. It has been used in political science, for example, to analyze the arms race between the superpowers. Thibaut and Kelley (1959) used this paradigm to model a variety of mixed-motive situations in social interaction. In this approach, participants interact as members of a dyad. Each participant is confronted with a choice to cooperate or compete with the other participant and makes this choice without knowing the choice of the other participant. The payoff matrix for their choices is scaled in terms of subjective utility, with each entry in the matrix representing the subjective value of expected outcomes. A positive value means that the outcome is expected to be rewarding, whereas a negative value means that the outcome is expected to be costly or punishing relative to a reference point defining the break-even value. Figure 8.1 depicts a commonly employed payoff matrix.

The Emergence of Cooperation

A general perspective on the dilemma of self-interest versus cooperation, employing the PDG approach, is provided by genetic algorithms (e.g., Holland, 1975, 1989). Genetic algorithms apply principles of bi-

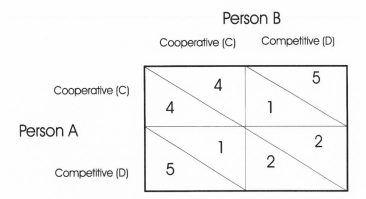

FIGURE 8.1. Payoff matrix in the Prisoner's Dilemma Game (PDG).

ological evolution to model changes in populations of individuals. Each individual is represented as a sequence of bits of information, corresponding to a sequence of genes. These genes undergo mutation with a small probability that they will change when transmitted to offspring. Mutation brings diversity into the population. The process of selection decreases diversity by eliminating the least fit individuals (i.e., gene sequences). The fitness of individuals is specified by a so-called fitness function designed to characterize how well each individual can cope with the task the simulation is intended to solve. Individuals who are relatively fit are allowed to replicate (i.e., produce offspring) to compensate the loss of individuals in the selection process. A process called crossover mimics sexual reproduction by allowing individuals to exchange whole sequences of genes. In the course of simulation, the fitness of an average individual increases. The genetic algorithm approach is very popular in the modeling of complex adaptive systems, with applications to problems in mathematics, physics, engineering, and other disciplines where analytical solutions cannot be derived.

In the social sciences, Axelrod (1984) has used computer simulations to illustrate how cooperation can emerge among individuals who are oriented toward maximizing their own self-interest. In these simulations, individuals play repetitive PDGs with other individuals. The choice whether to cooperate versus defect on a given round is regulated by individual strategies. Genetic algorithms are used to generate evolution of these strategies. Each individual begins with a random sequence of genes that generates choices reflecting different strategies. Those individuals who acquire the least profits in their interactions with many others are eliminated from the population, whereas the rest are allowed to multiply and produce offspring. New combinations of genes are produced through mutations.

At the beginning of the simulation, there is usually a strong increase in the frequency of defection, since defection produces higher payoffs regardless of the choice made by an interaction partner. After some time, however, the frequency of cooperative choices begins to grow, reflecting the higher adaptive value of strategies capable of cooperation. Although cooperative choices produce lower outcomes in any single interaction, in the long run, this strategy has a chance of inducing cooperation in one's partner, yielding higher profits for both. Cooperative strategies prevail by generating profits while playing with other cooperative strategies. In the long run, defection strategies are maladaptive because they turn other strategies into defection. Their initial prevalence is due to encounters with highly cooperative strategies incapable of retaliation. Such strategies are eliminated as the proportion of strategies capable of both cooperation and retaliation when faced with defection grows in the population.

In a recent development, Macy, Skvoretz, and Bainbridge (1995) showed how meaningless characterizations achieve meaning in the course of social interaction. In their simulations, individuals play the PDG along the general lines employed in Axelrod's simulations. These individuals, however, are randomly equipped with some characteristics that are visible to other individuals. By chance, certain of these characteristics may be more common among those who cooperate than among those who defect. After some time, those characteristics are perceived as predictive of whether a given individual will cooperate or defect. This recognition, in turn, shapes the behaviors of others toward him or her. Thus, others start to exhibit more collaborative behavior toward such individuals, which in turn produces even more collaboration on their part. The reverse scenario is observed for those characteristics that initially happened to be slightly correlated with defection. As the result of social interactions, then, initially meaningless characteristics become meaningful and reliable predictors of social behavior.

Hegselman (1994, 1998) has taken a somewhat different tack in addressing the issue of social interdependence. His specific concern is the emergence of social support networks in a society. In his simulations, individuals live on a two-dimensional grid containing some unoccupied sites. The individuals play a two-person "support game" with all of their immediate neighbors. Each individual is characterized by some probability of needing help. A needy individual is clearly better off if he or she receives help from a neighbor. Providing help to a neighbor, however, is costly. The most preferred neighborhood for each individual is thus one in which he or she can obtain the degree of help needed while minimizing the help provided. From time to time, individuals are provided a migration option that enables them to move to a more desirable location within a certain radius. Results demonstrate that support networks can evolve among rational egoists who are differentially endowed, and who are motivated to choose partners in an opportunistic fashion. The emergent networks, however, tend to be highly segregated. Individuals who have a moderate probability of becoming needy tend to form relationships with one another, and also with individuals from somewhat higher and lower risk classes. Interestingly, the individuals belonging to extreme risk classes—those with very high or very low probabilities of needing help—have the most difficulty in establishing support relations. If they do manage to form relationships, their partners tend to be from the same risk class.

Competition among Strategies

Messick and Liebrand (1995) modeled the consequences of different strategies in the PDG. Each interactant, located at a fixed position in a two-dimensional lattice, plays a PDG with one of his or her nearest neighbors. On each trial, the interactant chooses whether to cooperate or defect according to an updating rule, which is defined by the strategy assigned to all interactants in a given simulation. In the "tit-for-tat" strategy, each interactant makes a choice that imitates the choice made on the preceding trial by his or her neighbor. In the "win–cooperate, lose–defect" strategy, the interactant with the greater outcome cooperates, whereas the interactant with the smaller outcome defects. In the "win–stay, lose–shift" strategy, interactants who perceive their situation as winning continue to behave in the same fashion on the next trial, whereas interactants who perceive their situation as losing change their behavior on the next trial. Note that these strategies are not defined on the basis of rational choice rules, but rather represent psychological considerations based on locally available information. The results of these simulations show that in relatively small groups, equilibrium tends to be reached fairly quickly, as all the interactants converge on a particular choice. In relatively large groups, however, each strategy leads to continuous dynamics characterized by the coexistence of different behavioral choices. Over a long period of time, though, each strategy does lead to specific proportions of cooperating individuals. These general proportions tend to be maintained at the group level, despite the fact that the interactants may continue to change their choices.

Nowak and Borkowski (1995) have extended this paradigm to model competition between socially defined strategies. They introduced a set of strategies in addition to those described by Messick and Liebrand (1995). These included "modeling," in which the individual imitates the choice made by his or her most successful recent partners, "cooperation with in-group," in which the individual always cooperates with others in his or her own ingroup, and "fixed strategy," in which the individual cooperates at a given level of probability, regardless of the partner's choice. In the simulations, all the strategies were randomly assigned to individuals who are situated on a two-dimensional matrix. Initially, each individual is equipped with certain resources. Those resources can grow or diminish as a result of the interactions with others, according to the PDG payoff matrix. If an individual runs out of resources, he or she is eliminated from the game, creating an empty place on the matrix. If an individual's resources exceed a certain threshold, he or she may produce an offspring, provided there is an empty place in the local neighborhood. Resources are then divided with the offspring, and the offspring inherits the strategy of the parent. There are no mutations to the strategies in this game. In a variation on this game, individuals can migrate if they are close to a more profitable neighborhood.

Each interaction is most likely to take place with a different individual. However, an individual's choice is influenced by his or her previous interactions. This feature was introduced to capture the tendency for people to react not just to their specific interaction partners, but also to their experience with a "generalized other" (Mead, 1934). Thus, for example, an individual who has experienced exploitation in his or her previous interactions may be biased in his or her choice in subsequent interactions with different individuals. This models the fact that many social interactions are not repeated and thus do not provide a person an opportunity to reciprocate, reward, or punish the specific individuals with whom he or she has interacted.

The simulations usually develop according to one of two scenarios. In the first, an increasing number of individuals defect and in a relatively short period of time, all individuals run out of resources and everyone dies. In the other scenario, there is also an increase in the number of defectors at the outset, and a significant portion of the individuals eventually die as a result. However, islands of cooperators are formed. In a process of mutual cooperation, high resources are produced and these islands expand. The islands usually consist of one strategy or two coexisting strategies. A high level of cooperation is typically restored to the whole group, offspring fill up the empty spaces, and several clustered strategies coexist for a long time in the society. One of the strategies eventually wins the game by increasing to 100%. This strategy tends to be either "tit-for-tat" or "win–stay, lose–shift."

It is interesting to consider the situations that distinguish these two very different scenarios. Stated differently, what conditions are necessary for survival of a society in a social dilemma situation? The strongest predictor of survival in the simulations was the distance between individuals. If interactions were limited to the closest neighbors, defectors suffered by ruining the local neighborhood, and they were quickly eliminated from the society. If interactions were allowed to take place over relatively large distances, however, a defecting individual was able to find victims for a long time. The effect of ruining others and turning them to defection did not come back to haunt the defector. Thus, a large area was affected before the defector could feel any impact of his or her behavior. In the meantime, the large resources accumulated through defection with cooperators allowed the defector to produce several offspring. Cooperators were eliminated first, but eventually, the defectors could not survive, because there were only fellow defectors left with whom to interact. In some simulations, individuals were allowed to move away from unprofitable neighborhoods. This factor was also very detrimental to the well-being of society. Immediately after ruining one neighborhood, defecting individuals moved to another cooperating neighborhood that they would then proceed to ruin by turning these individuals into defectors. Whenever cooperating individuals were able to form an island and engage in mutually beneficial cooperation, a defecting individual would move into the neighborhood and destroy the cooperation among the individuals there.

The severity of the PDG was also manipulated in these simulations. This was achieved by adding or subtracting a constant from all cells of the payoff matrix, providing for asymmetry between gains and losses in either direction. The effects of this manipulation were almost paradoxical in nature. The more severe games (those in which it was easier to lose than to gain resources) led to much higher probability of survival at the societal level. This was because turning one's neighborhood toward massive defection was much more costly and thus quickly eliminated the individual who started the chain of defection. When the games were generous (i.e., when it was easier to gain than lose resources), the destructive effects of defection on the neighborhood were less pronounced. Defectors did not sink together with their neighborhood for a relatively long time, and because of their short-term advantage over others, this strategy had ample opportunity to become more frequent. Ultimately, the society with a high percentage of strategies likely to defect could not find cooperative solutions and became extinct. This finding suggests that it might be easier to achieve cooperation in a society living under harsh conditions (e.g., scarce resources, external threats, etc.) than in a society spoiled by well-being.

Taken together, the observed effects of these three factors suggests that the likelihood of achieving cooperation in a society is enhanced by strong and immediate links between individual choices and their consequences for the individual. If such links are weak and delayed in time, the social system may lack the necessary corrective feedback to assure long-term survival. The crime rate is clearly felt by people, for example, so correction through the justice system to prevent crime is quite likely. The degradation of the rain forest, on the other hand, may be more dangerous than a high crime rate in the long run, but because people do not feel feedback between their own actions and their well-being as a function of such destruction, moves to stop the destruction are relatively weak. If everyone began experiencing difficulty breathing immediately after the loss of an acre of rain forest, the destruction would no doubt cease in short order.

Although cooperation is essential for societal coordination, a society characterized only by this tendency may be highly vulnerable to exploitation—and even extinction. This point was driven home in simulations by Lomborg (1992). His simulations followed the general lines of Axelrod's (1984) approach but introduced some noise (randomness) into the interactions. He also assumed that individuals who exhaust their resources and end up with net losses are eliminated from the population. While running a long-term simulation in which practically everyone adopted highly cooperative strategies, Lomborg observed a curious effect: After some time, such populations would suddenly turn to massive defection, which resulted in extinction. This resulted from the creation through mutation of especially vicious strategies characterized by frequent defections, which would win against virtually every other (cooperative) strategy. But when this strategy succeeded in eliminating the other strategies, it could not cooperate with like-minded individuals and thus could not exist among its own.

In societies characterized by a diversity of strategies, a different scenario was observed. Most of the time, these societies did not do as well as the fully cooperative societies because of the existence of defecting individuals, interactions with whom lowered everyone's profits. Whenever a vicious strategy developed, however, only a temporary decline in the well-being of the society was observed. Mildly vicious individuals in the society would turn to full defection when playing with the vicious intruders and thus prevented them from spreading throughout the population. When the intruders were eliminated, however, the mildly vicious individuals were able to find cooperative solutions among themselves and thereby create the groundwork for the reemergence of more cooperative strategies. This finding suggests that societies benefit from diversity. Societies composed of different types of people are more flexible, adaptive, and able to contain dangerous processes. It is important, then, that the variety of ideas and lifestyles in a society do not converge to uniformity. This is a very real danger when some of these characteristics are in a clear minority. As discussed in Chapter 7, the prevailing views and characteristics in a society have a tendency to eradicate minority characteristics.

We also noted in Chapter 7, though, that minority opinions are protected by the creation of clusters. Preservation of an infrequent language in a multilingual society, for example, depends not only on the global proportion of the two languages, but also on the ability of the minority language to cluster by forming a local community. If the process of migration in a society is high, such that individuals relocate apart from similar others, such clusters are disrupted. So although it is critical that interaction takes place among diverse types of people in order to promote mixing, it is also important to create conditions in which people with minority opinions and other characteristics can survive by clustering with similar others. Those within clusters have the opportunity to interact with and receive the support of like-minded individuals and thus are protected from exposure to the potential devastating influence of dissimilar others. Diversity, which is made possible by the existence of local cultures, may not be optimal for the productivity of the society as a whole at any given point in time, but it may be essential in promoting the adaptive potential for the society and its long-term survival.

SOCIAL CHANGE

Society as a whole can be viewed as a dynamical system. As such, it should be possible to characterize basic properties of societal dynamics in the same way that one characterizes dynamical phenomena at lower levels of social psychological reality. Thus, one may ask whether large-scale social systems display the sorts of dynamic patterns observed with respect to social judgment, action, the self, close relationships, social influence, and intergroup relations. In a general sense, this is almost certainly true. Societies clearly demonstrate the potential for both change and stability, and it is not unreasonable to suggest that these tendencies can be traced to the interactions among elements comprising the society and the manifestation of such dynamics in the context of external (i.e., international) events.

The Nature of Social Transitions

With this agenda in mind, the social and political transitions that have taken place in Europe near the end of the 20th century provide especially relevant and fascinating subject matter for investigation. The importance of these transitions has prompted concerted efforts at understanding how social transitions in general occur. Fortunately, during these transitions, a rich and diverse set of relevant material was gathered in the form of survey research, interviews, documents, and statistical data. This material has made it possible to test existing theories of social change and to construct new theories if need be. On the basis of preliminary analyses, it appears that theories developed on the basis of data from stable societies do not provide an adequate model for understanding the dynamic nature of social transitions. How can we explain that in almost all of the countries in the former socialist bloc, the communist parties experienced strong defeat in the first free elections, climbed back to victory in many countries in the second election, and then lost again in subsequent elections? Why is it that changes introduced to improve the economy by reducing political control over economic decisions resulted initially in strong economic decline? Why did the victory of a movement based on solidarity principles result in the growth of social conflicts?

The social transitions in Europe comprise very complex processes, with many factors specific to each country shaping the exact course of the country's transition. At a certain level of abstraction, however, social changes can be said to occur in two qualitatively distinct ways. One type of change is slow and incremental. Certain opinions, esthetic preferences, and lifestyles, for example, gradually become embraced by larger segments of the society. This pattern of change generally occurs when everyone incrementally changes his or her own evaluations, opinions, or preferences. The other type of social change is fast, abrupt, and nonlinear, occurring in a manner that is remarkably similar to phase transitions, as described in physics. It is this type of change that more commonly characterizes social and political transitions. Thus, "islands of new" form in the "sea of old," in a manner similar to the formation of gas bubbles in a liquid that is nearing the boiling point. As the transition progresses, those islands or clusters grow and become connected, and begin to encircle the remaining islands of old. During social transitions, then, two distinct realities coexist—the reality of the old and the reality of the new.

Social transitions consist of changes that occur both at the level of social institutions and at the level of individuals' attitudes and behaviors. Our focus here is on changes at the level of social groups. For social transitions to occur, it is usually necessary for some global factors to change. In the case of the recent transitions in central and eastern Europe, the critical global factor that changed was the status of the Soviet Union. Nonetheless, the influence of global factors on society is usually mediated by social interactions. In Chapter 7, we described how minority opinion can survive if it can create coherent clusters. Clustering fosters the preservation of diversity in a society, which promotes plasticity and adaptive potential. This is especially true when environmental conditions change. Clusters of minority opinion under the right circumstances may turn into seeds of transition because of their greater adaptive value. In other words, for the transition to occur, an initial minority has to become the majority.

In the models of social influence described in Chapter 7, the minority could prevent its own decay, but it could not grow. These models assumed, however, that all opinions and attitudes are equally attractive. This rarely is the case in the real world. Some attitudes are more functional, more compatible with the society's value system, or are simply more salient because of external factors such as mass media influence. During social transitions, such externally based preferences usually change. We can incorporate the global effects of external factors in our model by introducing "bias" into the rule describing changes in opinions. Bias is introduced by adding a constant to favor one of the positions, which acts in addition to the effects of social interaction. In effect, individuals' opinions not only reflect social influence, but are also based on preferences that are independent of social interactions. In principle, very strong preferences can overwhelm the effects of social influence, although this is unlikely to occur in practice.

These ideas were tested in simulations based on cellular automata models of social influence, similar to those described in Chapter Seven (Nowak et al., 1993). Figure 8.2 shows the typical course of social influence processes when there is a bias favoring the minority position. We start from a configuration of 10% minority, randomly distributed in the population (panel A). If not for the presence of bias, the minority opinion would not be able to survive, because it is insufficiently frequent to form coherent clusters. In the presence of bias, the minority opinion begins to grow (panel B). The growth by itself is not surprising, since we have added bias to facilitate such growth. Note, however, that the new opinion forms clusters around the origi-

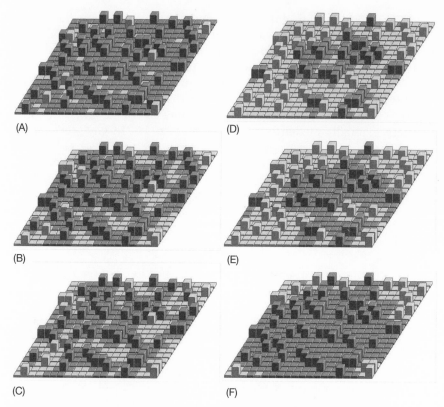

(A)

(B)

(C)

(D)

(E)

(F)

FIGURE 8.2. The growth of minority opinion in society.

nal seeds of the new opinion. As the transition progresses (panel C), the clusters of new continue to grow and begin to connect. This connection between clusters is critical to the process of transforming the minority into a new majority. When the clusters of initial minority become fully connected, the initial majority is reduced to islands. Finally, a new equilibrium is reached, in which, despite the bias toward the new opinion, clusters of the old opinion still exist, well-entrenched in the sea of new (panel D).

Inspection of panel D might suggest that the transition is irreversible. The initial majority is reduced to 20%, so that any voting or referendum would be overwhelmingly won by the new opinion. This is reminiscent of developments in post-Communist countries, where all the referendums and elections were won decisively by anti-Communist parties. In Poland, for example, not a single communist candidate was elected to Parliament in its first free elections. Close in-spection of panel D, however, reveals that the initial majority was re-duced to its strongest members, who now survive in strongholds. Pan-el E shows the new equilibrium when the bias favoring the new opin-ion is withdrawn. The attractiveness of the new opinion dissipates when people begin to experience the costs of the transformation that has occurred. The proponents of the old opinion grow to 50% (panel E). Panel F shows a reversal of bias, corresponding to sentiments fa-voring the old opinions, causing the new opinion to be reduced to 20%. We should note that it took about 40 simulation steps with the bias favoring the new opinion for the new opinion to prevail, but it took just five simulation steps for the old opinion to rebound. The sit-uation, however, has not returned to its original configuration. Now the *new* forms strongholds that can survive the pressure of the majori-ty. When social sentiments change again, it will be easy for the *new* to launch an offensive from these strongholds.

This scenario may explain why, in almost all European countries of the old socialist camp, post-Communist parties suffered a humiliat-ing defection but were able to win the next election. People who were prominent (i.e., strongest) during the Communist era tended to form networks in which they supported one another, in line with our depic-tion of strongholds. In the course of economic transformation, these individuals tended to join the new economy while preserving their old political alliances and social connections. This suggests that pure-ly political forces may be insufficient for a complete social transition. Our analysis suggests, however, that social transition may become irre-versible when preferences for the new are positively correlated with strength. This may happen through economic mechanisms. Joining the new economy is associated with improvement of one's own per-sonal economic situation. In the case where social context inhibits rather than facilitates social changes, the strength allows one to break through this inhibition and join the new economy.

Facilitating Social Change

This model suggests that different actions can be undertaken to facili-tate social change depending on the type of change characterizing a society. If the mode of change is incremental, factors such as tax pref-erences and information campaigns that affect all members of a soci-ety should be most effective. If the society is undergoing a social tran-sition, however, highly targeted actions are likely to be more effective. Individuals inside clusters have already made their changes, and they are likely to remain with the new because of the support they receive through social contacts with others in the cluster. Individuals far from a cluster, however, are unlikely to sustain a change even if they make one, because they lack appropriate social contact and support. The most effective strategy is to allocate effort to the borders of clusters in the form of an information campaign, legal support, and tax breaks. The strongest members (i.e., the leaders) on the borders should be especially targeted. It is also important to facilitate connections between different clusters.

Strategies based on this model may prove useful in combating various social problems, such as the spread of drug use, teen pregnancy, and criminal behavior. In this approach, one would start by identifying natural leaders of a social network. The initial intervention would be targeted to a subgroup of interconnected high-status group members who are relatively open to the new position (e.g., sports instead of crime). All the initial resources would be targeted to converting this select group to the new position. When this is achieved, resources would be switched to people from their vicinity (e.g., family members, friends) in an effort to create an interconnected network in which people support one another in their new attitudes and behavior. Such a growing group would be connected with other groups that have received similar interventions, perhaps through sport competitions or discussion groups. If the groups reach some critical mass and the movement is able to sustain itself, resources can be gradually withdrawn and reallocated to other social networks in line with the model. Computer simulations allow one to test the effectiveness of different specific interventions within this general scenario. Such simulations were in fact used with high effectiveness to design a large-scale social program for unemployed young people in Poland (Nowak et al., 1993).

In summary, although it may be desirable to attempt the facilitation of social change on a global level, the process of change in a transitional society occurs in an uneven manner, with local environments most susceptible to intervention strategies. Agents of change should thus concentrate their effects on pockets of society containing preferences for the new agenda. This in effect creates seeds that may grow to form clusters. If these clusters develop connections with each other, there is a chance that the new agenda will overcome the old. This perspective suggests that the future may often coexist with the present. Some elements of the diversity that surrounds us may in fact be harbingers of future global states of the system. It may be very difficult, however, to say at present which local clusters provide a window on the future, and which are simply aberrations that will pass without leaving any traces.

THE IDENTITY OF DYNAMICAL
SOCIAL PSYCHOLOGY

There is a danger that the dynamical systems perspective may prove *too* appealing for those looking for a new paradigm for social psychology. Many of the key concepts and principles, such as attractor, bifurcation, self-organization, and chaos, have an intuitive resemblance to a host of personal and interpersonal phenomena. Thus, it is tempting to suggest that constructs such as attitudes and goals are attractors, to note an analogy between decision making and bifurcation, to suggest that the mind is fractal, or to say that life is chaotic and unpredictable. Many of these intuitions may ultimately prove to be correct, of course, and it is natural that the early stages in the development of a new paradigm should emphasize insights and ideas regarding potential applications of the paradigm. It is important to keep in mind, though, the distinction between ideas and intuitions, on the one hand, and hypotheses and theories, on the other hand. In science, there is a context of discovery and a context of proof. Enthusiasm must therefore be tempered with caution, and there must be a concerted effort to maintain rigor when attempting to apply the dynamical perspective to the subject matter of social psychology.

Caution is especially relevant when considering certain of the tools and methods that have been generated within this perspective. Many of these have been adapted from the work on nonlinear dynamical systems in mathematics and the physical sciences. In view of the uniqueness of human experience, one should look carefully at the nature of dynamical models, critically examining their assumptions and the relevance of these assumptions for investigating social psychological dynamics. In this section, we attempt to provide such perspective. We first compare and contrast the assumptions of the dynamical models depicted throughout the book, with an eye toward identifying their respective resonance with basic assumptions about personal and interpersonal processes. We then discuss those features of human experience that are unique, qualitatively distinct from other classes of phenomena in nature, and how well these features can be modeled and understood with a dynamical systems approach. In the final section, we summarize what we feel to be the primary advantages of framing the subject matter of social psychology in explicitly dynamical terms.

Dynamical Models in Perspective

Throughout this book, we have described formal models that capture different facets of dynamism in social experience. Particular emphasis has been placed on models of cellular automata, attractor neural networks, and coupled maps. Each approach represents a distinct formalism of nonlinear dynamical systems, in that it portrays a set of elements that interact with and influence one another over time. Through these mutual influences, the elements become coordinated in some fashion, so that the system as a whole can be characterized in terms of emergent properties. As a result, individual elements lose some degrees of freedom reflecting their own characteristics but gain degrees of freedom associated with the characteristics of other elements and with the larger system within which they are coordinated. As we have illustrated, this general scenario characterizes different levels of social reality, from the coordination of thoughts to the coordination of social groups. Each formalism, however, captures different aspects of the coordination process. The points of contact and difference among the approaches are easiest to appreciate with respect to social coordination in groups, simply because each approach has been considered in the context of this general topic. Cellular automata, attractor neural networks, and coupled maps are based on somewhat different assumptions, and these assumptions constrain the manner in which each approach characterizes the nature of individuals and interpersonal relations. Each approach is associated with its own blend of benefits and drawbacks, making it difficult to declare one of them clearly superior to the others.

The models of cellular automata illustrate how people with different characteristics coordinate their opinions, beliefs, and attitudes through social influence processes. The regularity of spatial structure in cellular automata makes it easy to identify the emergence of group-level patterns (e.g., clustering of like-minded individuals), and the straightforward interpretation of elements makes this class of models relatively easy to relate to empirical phenomena, whether experimental findings or descriptions of societal conditions. By characterizing social relations in terms of the geometry of social space, meanwhile, this approach can make use of computer simulations and analytical tools to relate the structure of social relations to the dynamics of social processes. And because cellular automata are used to model different types of social processes, this class of models provides the best hope of integrating social influence processes with other types of processes operating within groups, such as those associated with the dilemmas of interdependence. The regularity of spatial structure in cellular automata, however, limits the generalizability of these models to real-world social processes. These models also assume that neighbors all influence one another in a similar manner, a feature that has questionable psychological reality.

Attractor neural networks provide a more realistic description of the structure of social relations. Any type of social network, in fact, can be portrayed as an attractor neural network. Unlike cellular automata, attractor neural networks can model qualitatively different forms of influence (i.e., negative and inhibitory as well as positive and excitatory) as well as variation in the importance of different social connections. Attractor neural networks are also advantageous in that they can portray the bidirectional relationship between social influence processes and the development of social relations. Thus, this class of models is ideally suited to investigate how the states (e.g., opinions) of individuals change as a result of social influence, and how the structure of social connections changes to accommodate different distributions of such states.

In both cellular automata and attractor neural networks, individuals are assumed to be basically passive, ready to respond to external influences but with no intrinsic dynamics available to mediate such influences. As we have stressed throughout the preceding chapters, however, the potential for internally generated dynamics is one of the most fundamental and fascinating properties of human beings. In the absence of external forces of any kind, people display patterns of thought, feelings, and behaviors that can be meaningfully characterized and measured. This potential clearly complicates the coordination problem. Coupled logistic maps provide a formal tool that allows one to incorporate the intrinsic dynamics of individuals into an interpersonal context. In this approach, each individual in a group is modeled as a logistic equation that can display qualitatively different types of intrinsic dynamics, depending on the value of his or her control parameter. Thus, each individual's internally generated thought or behavior can conform to a constant equilibrium, display different values of periodicity, or undergo chaotic evolution. This is clearly preferable to simply characterizing individuals in terms of their position with respect to an attitude topic. Coordination in this class of models may be achieved either by coupling the values of variables, which corresponds to the synchronization of behavior, or by matching control parameters, which corresponds to the coordination of the mental and emotional underpinnings of behavior.

One could argue that coupled maps provide the richest platform for modeling social coordination. We should note, however, that it is difficult to find exact correspondence between the states of dynamical variables and control parameters in such maps, on the one hand, and measurable psychological properties, on the other hand. It is also the case that coupled maps are new to social psychology—to our knowledge, in fact, this approach has never been implemented before—so their ability to capture social psychological phenomena remains to be demonstrated. At this stage in the development of this formalism, coupled maps have the status of models of qualitative understanding and thus are difficult to map directly onto experimental procedures for purposes of empirical verification.

In summary, different formalisms are optimal for capturing different aspects of social psychological dynamics. At this point, it is an open question whether one of these models will ultimately prevail, or whether some synthesis of the features in each will someday provide comprehensive characterization of the diverse features of interpersonal (and intrapersonal) dynamics. It should be stressed as well that these formal models, regardless of their individual fascination, need to be related to empirical findings and observations. One cannot claim to have achieved true understanding of interpersonal dynamics until the phenomena captured in empirical research are modeled with these formalisms, and these formalisms in turn have generated predictions that are verified in empirical research. Formal models, in other words, cannot substitute for social psychological theory and research. To the contrary, they must be constructed and refined in accordance with the content of social psychology.

The Uniqueness of Human Experience

Dynamical systems theory clearly does not exhaust the ways in which the dynamism of interpersonal processes can be framed and investigated. We feel this perspective is quite likely to do what it is designed to do: to describe the basic properties of dynamics and the associated structures that generate dynamics, in human thought, emotion, and behavior. But no matter how well this perspective succeeds in providing such description, it is irrelevant in principle to the description of other crucial aspects of human experience. In a sense, this is true for the application of dynamical systems to any field of inquiry. Every area of science ultimately must be understood in its own terms. Laser physics, meteorology, and predator–prey relations are all dynamical processes that can be modeled in much the same way at a very general level, but clearly each application involves different elements and mechanisms of coordination. This ultimate limitation seems especially true for psychological and social processes. Dynamical systems theory can tell us how specific mechanisms combine to jointly produce a system's dynamics, but it cannot provide complete information about the nature of those mechanisms. Nor can this perspective hope to capture the content of personal and experience. People's thoughts, for example, may well conform to a trajectory that can be characterized formally in terms of attractors and order parameters, but the rich and idiosyncratic features of the thoughts themselves are beyond the purview of dynamical tools and methods.

Dynamical systems theory thus can never substitute for a science of social psychology per se. Social psychology is uniquely equipped to provide deep insight into such uniquely human phenomena as consciousness, personal meaning, self-awareness, and romantic love. Notions such as self-organization and dynamics only make sense, after all, with respect to the content of specific values and concerns. The dynamical perspective can provide the boundary conditions and constraints for the development of social psychological theory, but it is the social psychologist, not the physicist, who must flesh out this outline. Physics allows for many possible worlds, but we happen to live in only one of them (Gell-Mann, 1994). It is up to social psychology to describe the uniqueness of our personal and interpersonal worlds.

In this regard, it is noteworthy that social psychology never lost sight of the unique nature of thoughts, feelings, and actions in an interpersonal context. Even in the heyday of behaviorism, most social psychologists talked freely of people's attempt to structure their experience, find meaning, maintain personal consistency, and behave independently of formal and informal social pressures. Such features of experience are testament to the potential for internally generated dynamics in the subject matter of social psychology. The maintenance of this worldview is remarkable in light of the way social psychology was viewed by many in the so-called hard sciences. It was not uncommon for researchers in physics, chemistry, and biology to trivialize the efforts of social psychologists, claiming that not only was the field soft and unscientific, but also that it could not even measure its own variables with any degree of precision, much less develop formal mathematical models.

It is an intriguing irony that as the physical sciences evolved in the 1980s, so did their respect for the agenda of social psychology. With their discoveries concerning complexity, internally generated dynamics, nonlinear relations, and unpredictability, scientists came to appreciate the deep insights concerning these matters that were developed close to a century earlier at the very beginning of social psychology. This appreciation has even translated into new areas of application that overlap with concerns traditionally confined to those in the social and brain sciences. The complexity of the brain, for instance, is a focal point for understanding complexity in general by many in physics. Societal processes, meanwhile, have become the subject of investigation by mathematicians, physicists, and biologists, because of the similarity of these processes to complex systems in their respective disciplines. Emergence, internal causation, and nonlinearity are concepts that have begun to unite rather than separate social psychology and other fields of science.

The application of dynamical concepts and methods thus serves to enhance rather than diminish the uniqueness of social psychology. Unlike the traditional application of natural science assumptions, the dynamical approach provides full expression to the complexity and malleability of human experience. When viewed in this way, there is no reason to ignore the potential relevance of dynamical systems to social psychology. Nothing fundamental about the field need change, nor should it change. To the contrary, the dynamical perspective enables us to be more explicit than ever about the issues that defined social psychology in its infancy. Since that time, the physical sciences have matured to the point that they can appreciate what social psychologists have known all along. In their attempt to capture the complexity and dynamism of processes in the physical sciences, scientists have developed a wide variety of algorithms, formal tools, and new empirical approaches. By adapting these methods to the special nature of human experience, social psychology is poised to undergo a profound transformation that may change the theoretical and topical landscape of the field.

For the first time, then, social psychology can make contact with the physical sciences without forfeiting its identity as a distinct discipline concerned with all that is fascinating in human experience. Unlike earlier attempts to establish contact with the approach of physics, chemistry, and biology, social psychology this time is doing it on its own terms. Because concepts such as internal causation and complexity have a long history in social psychology, it is likely that this contact will benefit the physical sciences with deep insights, while gaining from the these fields a useful set of tools with which to penetrate the mystery responsible for these insights—all in all, a remarkably fair trade between social psychology and the physical sciences.

Toward Coherence in Social Psychological Theory

Perhaps the most important role for dynamical systems in social psychology lies in its potential for integrating scattered theories and empirical findings. Social psychology usually describes only one direction of what is really a reciprocal feedback, only one step of what is really a repeated, iterative process, and only a single mechanism removed from the system in which it operates. Nonlinear dynamical systems theory provides tools by which the scattered pieces of the puzzle can be put together. This role is exactly the same as that played in other areas of science and is largely responsible for the enthusiasm with which this perspective was greeted in the 1980s. In fulfilling this role, it can discover similarities and identify invariant principles among diverse and seemingly unrelated phenomena. What makes this approach particularly attractive for social psychology is that although it provides for precise description for various phenomena, it does so without sacrificing an appreciation for the intrinsic underpinnings and complexity of human experience. To the contrary, it is ideally suited to provide relatively simple explanations for some highly complex social psychological phenomena.

Dynamical systems theory also provides for integration of social psychology with other disciplines of science. It offers common formalisms, analytical techniques, research methods, and, most important, suggestions concerning the most fruitful directions for scientific investigation. The ability to observe the same mechanisms operating in different systems produces deeper understanding of the phenomena under investigation and promotes the integration of science as a whole. In view of the central role of complexity and intrinsic dynamics in all facets of human experience, it is conceivable that the theory of dynamical systems may find more applications in the investigation of social and psychological processes than in the investigation of processes within the domain of the physical sciences.

Nonetheless, the dynamical perspective is only beginning to make its presence felt in social psychology. Although a number of promising dynamical models have been developed, it remains to be seen whether they can capture in a comprehensive fashion the defining features of personal and interpersonal experience comprising the subject matter of social psychology. Many specific topics remain to be investigated with specific models or empirical techniques reflecting an explicit dynamical perspective. At this point, then, many plausible claims are necessarily speculative in nature. We hope, however, that throughout this book, we have been able to highlight the potential of the dynamical approach, and that for some phenomena we have succeeded in demonstrating the manifestation of this potential.

FURTHER ITERATIONS

We clearly believe the dynamical systems perspective has much to offer the field of social psychology. The knowledge gathered within this approach has been readily adapted to other branches of science, both physical and social (e.g., economics, political science, sociology). This has occurred not only because the concepts map well onto the concepts and primary concerns of these sciences, but also because describing phenomena in dynamical systems terms usually brings with it deep insights concerning likely mechanisms to be operating, new phenomena likely to be observed, an ability to distinguish the possible from the impossible, and ideas about new ways to study the phenomena and analyze the results. Because laws formulated in the theory of dynamical systems concern all systems that have similar relations among elements, each branch of science may apply these general laws to their phenomena of interest.

The successful application of the dynamical systems approach to social psychology, however, ultimately will depend on the ability and willingness of researchers to go beyond metaphors, intuitive similarity, and general statements. Dynamical systems theory is a precise scientific formulation that generates testable formulations and provides tools for verifying such formulations. The interpretation of social psychological phenomena in terms of this formulation must therefore fulfill strong requirements of science. It is compelling to think of goals as attractors, for instance, but this suggestion is ultimately empty unless one specifies the properties of a dynamical system that produce such attractors and provide means of empirically demonstrating that the system in fact converges on them over time. In like manner, noteworthy changes in a psychological phenomenon may seem to have the properties of a bifurcation, but until one specifies what type of bifurcation it represents and develops appropriate means for documenting its occurrence, this observation does not qualify as a meaningful hypothesis. As usually happens with the introduction of a new paradigm, there is presently an imbalance between theory and data regarding the dynamical perspective in social psychology. For this approach to fulfill its promise, it is imperative that new data sets be generated in the context of research strategies designed to provide explicit tests of dynamical predictions.

In view of the generative power of the dynamical systems perspective, there is reason to believe that such research programs will in fact develop with increasing frequency in the years to come. Through repeated iterations of this ongoing process, some ideas are certain to be supported at the expense of others. Looking to the future, the field of social psychology may well undergo a transition not unlike that revealed in dynamical analyses of individual and social change. The dynamical systems perspective provides common ground for otherwise distinct areas of science, after all, and it has an especially natural fit with the subject matter of social psychology. In this light, it is not unreasonable to suggest that as we enter the 21st century, dynamical social psychology will emerge as an integrative framework for capturing the elusive and highly diverse aspects of personal and interpersonal experience. By revealing the dynamics underlying phenomena at different levels of social reality, this perspective holds promise for imposing theoretical order on the many degrees of freedom in the minds, actions, and interactions of human beings.

References

Abelson, R. P. (1979). Social clusters and opinion clusters. In P. W. Holland & S. Leinhardt (Eds.), *Perspectives in social network research* (pp. 239–256). New York: Academic Press.

Abelson, R. P., Aronson, E., McGuire, W. J., Newcomb, T. M., Rosenberg, M. J., & Tannenbaum, P. H. (Eds.). (1968). *Theories of cognitive consistency: A sourcebook.* Chicago: Rand McNally.

Abraham, F. D. (1990). *A visual introduction to dynamical systems for psychology.* Santa Cruz, CA: Aerial Press.

Abraham, F. D., & Gilgen, A. (1995). *Chaos theory in psychology.* Westport, CT: Greenwood Publishing Group.

Abramson, L. Y., Metalsky, G. I., & Alloy, L. B. (1989). Hopelessness depression: A theory-based subtype of depression. *Psychological Review, 96,* 358–372.

Adams, J. S. (1965). Inequity in social exchange. In L. Berkowitz (Ed.), *Advances in experimental social psychology* (Vol. 2, pp. 267–299). New York: Academic Press.

Ajzen, I. (1977). Intuitive theories of events and the effects of base-rate information on prediction. *Journal of Personality and Social Psychology, 35,* 303–314.

Allport, G. W. (1935). Attitudes. In C. Murchison (Ed.), *Handbook of social psychology* (pp. 798–884). Worcester, MA: Clark University Press.

Allport, G. W. (1954). *The nature of prejudice.* Cambridge, MA: Addison-Wesley.

Amit, D. J. (1989). *Modeling brain function: The world of attractor neural networks.* Cambridge,UK: Cambridge University Press.

Anderson, C. A., Lepper, M. R., & Ross, L. (1980). Perseverance of social theories: The role of explanation in the persistence of discredited information. *Journal of Personality and Social Psychology, 39*, 1037–1049.

Anderson, J. R. (1990). *Cognitive psychology and its implications* (3rd ed.). New York: Freeman.

Anderson, N. H. (1968). Likableness ratings of 555 personality-trait words. *Journal of Personality and Social Psychology, 9*, 272–279.

Anderson, N. H. (1981). *Foundations of information integration theory*. New York: Academic Press.

Aronson, E. (1992). The return of the oppressed: Dissonance theory makes a comeback. *Psychological Inquiry, 3*, 303–311.

Asch, S. E. (1946). Forming impressions of personalities. *Journal of Abnormal and Social Psychology, 41*, 258–290.

Asch, S. E. (1956). Studies of independence and conformity: A minority of one against a unanimous majority. *Psychological Monographs, 70*(9, Whole No. 416).

Atkinson, J. W. (1957). Motivational determinants of risk-taking behavior. *Psychological Review, 64*, 359–372.

Atkinson, J. W. (1964). *An introduction to motivation*. Princeton, NJ: Van Nostrand.

Axelrod, R. (1984). *The evolution of cooperation*. New York: Basic Books.

Baars, B. J. (1988). *A cognitive theory of consciousness*. New York: Cambridge University Press.

Baddeley, A. D. (1986). *Working memory*. Oxford, UK: Oxford University Press.

Bandura, A. (1986). *Social foundations of thought and action*. Englewood Cliffs, NJ: Prentice-Hall.

Bargh, J. A. (1989). Conditional automaticity: Varieties of automatic influence in social perception and cognition. In J. S. Uleman & J. A. Bargh (Eds.), *Unintended thought* (pp. 3–51). New York: Guilford Press.

Bargh, J. A. (1997). The automaticity of everyday life. In R. S. Wyer, Jr. (Ed.), *Advances in social cognition* (Vol. 10, pp. 1–61). Mahwah, NJ: Erlbaum.

Baron, R. M., Amazeen, P. G., & Beek, P. J. (1994). Local and global dynamics of social relations. In R. R. Vallacher & A. Nowak (Eds.), *Dynamical systems in social psychology* (pp. 111–138). San Diego: Academic Press.

Bartlett, R. A. (1932). *A study in experimental and social psychology*. New York: Cambridge University Press.

Barton, S. (1994). Chaos, self-organization, and psychology. *American Psychologist, 49*, 5–14.

Basar, E. (1990). *Chaos in brain function*. Berlin: Springer.

Bassingthwaighte, J. B., Liebovitch, L. J., & West, B. J. (1994). *Fractal physiology*. New York: Oxford University Press.

Baumeister, R. F. (1982). A self-presentational view of social phenomena. *Psychological Bulletin, 91*, 3–26.

Baumeister, R. F. (1984). Choking under pressure: Self-consciousness and paradoxical effects of incentives on skillful performance. *Journal of Personality and Social Psychology, 46*, 610–620.

Baumeister, R. F. (1991). *Escaping the self.* New York: Basic Books.

Baumeister, R. F. (Ed.) (1993). *Self-esteem: The puzzle of low self-regard.* New York: Plenum.

Baumeister, R. F., & Heatherton, T. F. (1996). Self-regulation failure: An overview. *Psychological Inquiry, 7*, 1–15.

Baumeister, R. F., Smart, L., & Bowden, J. M. (1996). Relation of threatened egotism to violence and aggression: The dark side of self-esteem. *Psychological Review, 103*, 5–33.

Baumgardner, A. (1990). To know oneself is to like oneself: Self-certainty and self-affect. *Journal of Personality and Social Psychology, 58*, 1062–1072.

Beckmann, J., & Gollwitzer, P. M. (1987). Deliberative versus implemental states of mind: The issue of impartiality in predecisional and postdecisional information processing. *Social Cognition, 5*, 259–279.

Beek, P. J., & Hopkins, B. (1992). Four requirements for a dynamical systems approach to the development of social coordination. *Human Movement Science, 11*, 425–442.

Beek, P. J., Verschoor, F., & Kelso, J. A. S. (1997). Requirements for the emergence of a dynamical social psychology. *Psychological Inquiry, 8*, 100–104.

Bem, D. J. (1967). Self-perception: An alternative interpretation of cognitive dissonance phenomena. *Psychological Review, 74*, 183–200.

Bem, D. J., & Allen, A. (1974). On predicting some of the people some of the time: The search for cross-situational consistencies in behavior. *Psychological Review, 81*, 506–520.

Berkowitz, L. (1988). Frustrations, appraisals, and aversively stimulated aggression. *Aggressive Behavior, 14*, 3–12.

Bernieri, F., Reznick, J. S., & Rosenthal, R. (1988). Synchrony, psuedosynchrony, and dissynchrony: Measuring the entrainment process in mother–infant dyads. *Journal of Personality and Social Psychology, 54*, 243–253.

Berscheid, E. (1983). Emotion. In H. H. Kelley, E. Berscheid, A. Christensen, J. Harvey, T. Huston, G. Levinger, E. McClintock, L. A. Peplau, & D. Peterson (Eds.), *Close relationships* (pp. 110–168). New York: Freeman.

Biddle, B. S., & Thomas, E. J. (Eds.). (1966). *Role theory: Concepts and research.* New York: Wiley.

Bieri, J., Atkins, A. L., Briar, S., Leaman, R. L., Miller, H., & Tripodi, T. (1966). *Clinical and social judgment.* New York: Wiley.

Bodenhausen, G. V. (1990). Stereotypes as judgmental heuristics: Evidence of circadian rhythms in discrimination. *Psychological Science, 1,* 319–322.

Boninger, D. S., Krosnick, J. A., & Berent, M. K. (1995). Origins of attitude importance: Self-interest, social identification, and value relevance. *Journal of Personality and Social Psychology, 68,* 61–80.

Bower, G. (1981). Mood and memory. *American Psychologist, 36,* 129–148.

Brehm, S. (1992). *Intimate relationships* (Vol. 2). New York: McGraw-Hill.

Brehm, S. S., & Brehm, J. W. (1981). *Psychological reactance: A theory of freedom and control.* New York: Academic Press.

Brewer, M. B. (1988). A dual process model of impression formation. In T. K. Srull & R. S. Wyer, Jr. (Eds.), *Advances in social cognition* (Vol. 1, pp. 1–36). Hillsdale, NJ: Erlbaum.

Brewer, M. B., Dull, V., & Lui, L. (1981). Perceptions of the elderly: Stereotypes and prototypes. *Journal of Personality and Social Psychology, 41,* 656–670.

Brewer, M. B., & Kramer, R. M. (1985). The psychology of intergroup attitudes and behavior. *Annual Review of Psychology, 36,* 219–243.

Brown, F. M., & Graeber, R. C. (Eds.). (1982). *Rhythmic aspects of behavior.* Hillsdale, NJ: Erlbaum.

Brown, K. W., & Moskowitz, D. S. (1998). Dynamic stability of behavior: The rhythms of our interpersonal lives. *Journal of Personality, 66,* 105–134.

Buder, E. H. (1991). A nonlinear dynamic model of social interaction. *Communication Research, 18,* 174–198.

Burgess, R. L., & Huston, T. L. (Eds.). (1979). *Social exchange in developing relationships.* New York: Academic Press.

Busemeyer, J. R., & Townsend, J. T. (1993). Decision field theory: A dynamic–cognitive approach to decision making in an uncertain environment. *Psychological Review, 100,* 432–459.

Byrne, D. (1971). *The attraction paradigm.* New York: Academic Press.

Byrne, D., Clore, G. L., & Smeaton, G. (1986). The attraction hypothesis: Do similar attitudes affect anything? *Journal of Personality and Social Psychology, 51,* 1167–1170.

Cacioppo, J. T., & Berntson, G. G. (1994). Relationship between attitudes and evaluative space: A critical review, with emphasis on the separability of positive and negative substrates. *Psychological Bulletin, 115,* 401–423.

Cacioppo, J. T., Gardner, W. L., & Berntson, G. G. (1997). Beyond bipolar conceptualizations and measures: The case of attitudes and evaluative space. *Personality and Social Psychology Review, 1,* 3–25.

Campbell, J. D. (1990). Self-esteem and clarity of the self-concept. *Journal of Personality and Social Psychology, 59,* 538–549.

Cantor, N., & Kihlstrom, J. F. (1987). *Personality and social intelligence*. Englewood Cliffs, NJ: Prentice-Hall.

Cantor, N., & Mischel, W. (1979). Prototypes in person perception. In L. Berkowitz (Ed.), *Advances in experimental social psychology* (Vol. 12, pp. 3–52). New York: Academic Press.

Caporael, L. R., & Brewer, M. B. (1995). Hierarchical evolutionary theory: There is an alternative, and it's not creationism. *Psychological Inquiry, 6,* 31–34.

Cartwright, D., & Zander, A. (Eds.). (1968). *Group dynamics: Research and theory* (3rd ed.). New York: Harper & Row.

Carver, C. S. (1997). Dynamical social psychology: Chaos and catastrophe for all. *Psychological Inquiry, 8,* 110–119.

Carver, C. S., & Scheier, M. F. (1981). *Attention and self-regulation: A control-theory approach to human behavior*. New York: Springer-Verlag.

Carver, C. S., & Scheier, M. F. (1990). Origins and functions of positive and negative affect: A control-process view. *Psychological Review, 97,* 19–35.

Carver, C. S., & Scheier, M. F. (1998). *On the self-regulation of behavior*. New York: Cambridge University Press.

Carver, C. S., & Scheier, M. F. (in press). Themes and issues in the self-regulation of behavior. In R. S. Wyer, Jr. (Ed.), *Advances in social cognition* (Vol. 12). Mahwah, NJ: Erlbaum.

Casti, J. L. (1994). *Complexification*. New York: HarperCollins.

Chaiken, S. (1980). Heuristic versus systematic information processing and the use of source versus message cues in persuasion. *Journal of Personality and Social Psychology, 39,* 752–766.

Cialdini, R. B. (1988). *Influence: Science and practice* (2nd ed.). New York: HarperCollins.

Cialdini, R. B., & Kenrick, D. T. (1976). Altruism as hedonism: A social development perspective on the relationship of negative mood state and helping. *Journal of Personality and Social Psychology, 34,* 907–914.

Clark, M. S., & Mills, J. (1979). Interpersonal attraction in exchange and communal relationships. *Journal of Personality and Social Psychology, 37,* 12–24.

Cohen, J., & Stewart, I. (1994). *The collapse of chaos: Discovering simplicity in a complex world*. New York: Viking.

Condon, W. S., & Ogston, W. D. (1967). A segmentation of behavior. *Journal of Psychiatric Research, 5,* 221–235.

Condry, J. (1977). Enemies of exploration: Self-initiated versus other-initiated learning. *Journal of Personality and Social Psychology, 35,* 459–477.

Converse, P. (1964). The nature of belief systems in mass public. In D. E. Apter (Ed.), *Ideology and discontent* (pp. 206–261). New York: Free Press.

Cooley, C. H. (1902). *Human nature and the social order*. New York: Scribner.

Coovert, M. D., & Reeder, G. D. (1990). Negativity effect in impression formation: The role of unit formation and schematic expectation. *Journal of Personality and Social Psychology, 26,* 49–62.

Cottrell, N. B. (1972). Social faciliation. In C. G. McClintock (Ed.), *Experimental social psychology* (pp. 185–236). New York: Holt, Rinehart & Winston.

Craik, F. I. M., & Lockhart, R. S. (1972). Levels of processing: A framework for memory research. *Journal of Verbal Learning and Verbal Behavior, 11,* 671–684.

Crowne, D. P., & Marlowe, D. (1964). *The approval motive: Studies in evaluative dependence.* New York: Wiley.

Csikszentmihalyi, M. (1982). Towards a psychology of optimal experience. In L. Wheeler (Ed.), *Review of personality and social psychology* (Vol. 2, pp. 13–36). Beverly Hills, CA: Sage.

Csikszentmihalyi, M. (1990). *Flow: The psychology of optimal experience.* New York: Harper & Row.

Csikszentmihalyi, M., & Figurski, T. J. (1982). Self-awareness and aversive experience in everyday life. *Journal of Personality, 50,* 15–28.

Davies, P. (1988). *The cosmic blueprint: New discoveries in nature's creative ability to order the universe.* New York: Simon & Schuster.

Deci, E. L. (1975). *Intrinsic motivation.* New York: Plenum.

Deci, E. L., & Ryan, R. M. (1985). *Intrinsic motivation and self-determination in human behavior.* New York: Plenum.

Dennett, D. C. (1991). *Consciousness explained.* Boston: Little, Brown.

Devine, P. (1989). Stereotypes and prejudice: Their automatic and controlled components. *Journal of Personality and Social Psychology, 56,* 5–18.

Diener, E. (1980). Deindividuation: The absence of self-awareness and self-regulation in group members. In P. Paulus (Ed.), *The psychology of group influence* (pp. 209–242). Hillsdale, NJ: Erlbaum.

Dittman, A. T., & Llewellyn, L. G. (1969). Body movement and speech rhythm in social conversation. *Journal of Personality and Social Psychology, 11,* 98–106.

Dornbusch, S. M., Hastorf, A. H., Richardson, S. A., Muzzy, R. E., & Vreeland, R. S. (1965). The perceiver and the perceived: Their relative influence on the categories of interpersonal perception. *Journal of Personality and Social Psychology, 1,* 434–440.

Dovidio, J. F., & Gaertner, S. L. (Eds.). (1986). *Prejudice, discrimination, and racism.* Orlando, FL: Academic Press.

Dreben, E. K., Fiske, S. T., & Hastie, R. (1979). The independence of evaluative and item information: Impression and recall order effects in behavior-based impression formation. *Journal of Personality and Social Psychology, 37,* 1758–1768.

Duck, S. (1988). *Relating to others.* Chicago: Dorsey Press.

Duncan, B. L. (1976). Differential social perception and attribution of inter-group violence: Testing the lower limits of stereotyping of blacks. *Journal of Personality and Social Psychology, 34*, 590–598.

Dunn, J., & Plomin, R. (1990). *Separate lives: Why siblings are so different.* New York: Basic Books.

Durkheim, E. (1938). *The rules of sociological method.* Chicago: University of Chicago Press.

Duval, S., & Wicklund, R. A. (1972). *A theory of objective self awareness.* New York: Academic Press.

Eckmann, J. P., & Ruelle, D. (1985). Ergodic theory of chaos and strange attractors. *Review of Modern Physics, 57*, 617–656.

Edelman, G. M. (1992). *Bright air, brilliant fire.* New York: Basic Books.

Edwards, A. L. (1957). *The social desirability variable in personality assessment and research.* New York: Dryden.

Eiser, J. R. (1990). *Social judgment.* Pacific Grove, CA: Brooks/Cole.

Eiser, J. R. (1994a). *Attitudes, chaos, and the connectionist mind.* Oxford, UK: Blackwell.

Eiser, J. R. (1994b). Toward a dynamic conception of attitude consistency and change. In R. R. Vallacher & A. Nowak (Eds.), *Dynamical systems in social psychology* (pp. 197–218). San Diego: Academic Press.

Elman, J. L. (1995). Language as a dynamical system. In R. F. Port & T. van Gelder (Eds.), *Mind as motion: Explorations in the dynamics of cognition* (pp. 195–225). Cambridge, MA: MIT Press.

Epstein, S. (1979). The stability of behavior: I. On predicting most of the people much of the time. *Journal of Personality and Social Psychology, 37*, 1097–1126.

Erber, R., Wegner, D. M., & Thierrault, N. (1996). On being cool and collected: Mood regulation in anticipation of social interaction. *Journal of Personality and Social Psychology, 70*, 757–766.

Feigenbaum, M. J. (1978). Quantitative universality for a class of nonlinear transformations. *Journal of Statistical Physics, 19*, 25–52.

Fenigstein, A., Scheier, M. F., & Buss, A. H. (1975). Public and private self-consciousness: Assessment and theory. *Journal of Consulting and Clinical Psychology, 43*, 522–527.

Festinger, L. (1957). *A theory of cognitive dissonance.* Evanston, IL: Row, Peterson.

Festinger, L., & Carlsmith, J. M. (1959). Cognitive consequences of forced compliance. *Journal of Abnormal and Social Psychology, 58*, 203–210.

Festinger, L., Schachter, S., & Back, K. (1950). *Social pressures in informal groups.* Stanford, CA: Stanford University Press.

Fischer, K. W., & Bidell, T. R. (1997). Dynamic development of psychological structures in action and thought. In R. Lerner (Ed.), *Handbook of child psychology: Vol. 1. Theoretical models of human development* (pp. 467–561). (Series Ed: W. Damon). New York: Wiley.

Fiske, S. T., & Neuberg, S. L. (1990). A continuum of impression formation, from category-based to individuating processes: Influences of information and motivation on attention and interpretation. *Advances in Experimental Social Psychology, 23*, 1–74.

Fiske, S. T., & Taylor, S. E. (1991). *Social cognition* (2nd ed.). McGraw-Hill.

Flache, A., & Macy, M. (1996). The weakness of strong ties: Collective action failure in a highly cohesive group. *Journal of Mathematical Sociology, 21*, 3–28.

Freedman, J. L., & Fraser, S. C. (1966). Compliance without pressure: The foot-in-the-door technique. *Journal of Personality and Social Psychology, 4*, 195–202.

Freud, S. (1937). *The ego and the mechanisms of defense*. London: Hogarth.

Friedkin, N. E., & Johnson, E. C. (1990). Social influence and opinions. *Journal of Mathematical Sociology, 15*, 193–205.

Gallistel, C. R. (1980). *The organization of action*. Hillsdale, NJ: Erlbaum.

Gardner, E. (1988). The space of interactions in neural network models. *Journal of Physics A, 21*, 257–270.

Gardner, M. (1983). *Wheels, life and other mathematical amusements*. San Francisco: Freeman.

Gell-Mann, M. (1994). *The quark and the jaguar*. New York: Freeman.

Gergen, K. J. (1971). *The concept of self*. New York: Holt.

Gergen, K. J. (1985). The social constructionist movement in modern psychology. *American Psychologist, 40*, 266–275.

Gergen, K. J. (1994). *Realities and relationships: Soundings in social construction*. Cambridge, MA: Harvard University Press.

Gilbert, D. T. (1993). The ascent of man: Mental representation and the control of belief. In D. M. Wegner & J. W. Pennebaker (Eds.), *Handbook of mental control* (pp. 57–87). Englewood Cliffs, NJ: Prentice-Hall.

Gilbert, D. T. (1995). Attribution and interpersonal perception. In A. Tesser (Ed.), *Advanced social psychology* (pp. 99–147). New York: McGraw-Hill.

Gilden, D. L. (1991). On the origins of dynamical awareness. *Psychological Review, 98*, 554–568.

Glass, L., & Mackey, M. C. (1988). *From clocks to chaos: The rhythms of life*. Princeton, NJ: Princeton University Press.

Gleick, J. (1987). *Chaos: The making of a new science*. New York: Viking–Penguin.

Goffman, E. (1959). *The presentation of self in everyday life*. Garden City, NY: Doubleday/Anchor Books.

Goldman, A. I. (1970). *A theory of human action*. Princeton, NJ: Princeton University Press.

Gollwitzer, P. M. (1990). Action phases and mind-sets. In E. T. Higgins & R. M. Sorrentino (Eds.), *Handbook of motivation and cognition: Foundations of social behavior* (Vol. 2, p. 53–92). New York: Guilford Press.

Gollwitzer, P. M. (1996). The volitional benefits of planning. In P. M. Gollwitzer & J. A. Bargh (Eds.), *The psychology of action:Linking cognition and motivation to behavior* (pp. 287–312). New York: Guilford Press.

Gottman, J. M. (1993). A theory of marital dissolution and stability. *Journal of Family Psychology, 7,* 57–75.

Gottman, J. M. (1979). Detecting cyclicity in social interaction. *Psychological Bulletin, 86,* 338–348.

Gottman, J. M. (1983). *Time series analysis: A comprehensive introduction for social scientists.* Cambridge, UK: Cambridge University Press.

Graeber, R. C. (1982). Alternations in performance following rapid transmeridian flight. In F. M. Brown & R. C. Graeber (Eds.), *Rhythmic aspects of behavior* (pp. 173–212). Hillsdale, NJ: Erlbaum

Grassberger, P., & Procaccia, I. (1983). On the characterization of strange attractors. *Physical Review Letters, 50,* 346–350.

Gur, R. C., & Sackheim, H. A. (1979). Self-deception: A concept in search of a phenomenon. *Journal of Personality and Social Psychology, 37,* 147–169.

Gutowitz, H. (1991). *Cellular automata: Theory and experiment.* Cambridge, MA: MIT Press.

Guzik, A. (1996). *Dynamic versus static integration of information and the consequences for the relationship between attitudes and behavior.* Unpublished master's thesis, Warsaw University.

Haken, H. (1978). *Synergetics.* Berlin: Springer.

Haken, H. (Ed.). (1982). *Order and chaos in physics, chemistry, and biology.* Berlin: Springer.

Haken, H., & Stadler, M. (1990). *Synergetics of cognition.* New York: Springer.

Hall, E. T. (1966). *The hidden dimension.* New York: Doubleday.

Hamilton, D. L., & Trolier, T. K. (1986). Stereotypes and stereotyping: An overview of the cognitive approach. In J. F. Dovidio & S. L. Gaertner (Eds.), *Prejudice, discrimination, and racism* (pp. 127–163). Orlando, FL: Academic Press.

Hamilton, D. L., & Zanna, M. P. (1972). Differential weighting of favorable and unfavorable attributes in impressions of personality. *Journal of Experimental Research in Personality, 6,* 204–212.

Hanges, P. J., Braverman, E. P., & Rentsch, J. R. (1991). Changes in raters' perceptions of subordinates: A catastrophe model. *Journal of Applied Psychology, 76,* 878–888.

Harackiewicz, J., Abrahams, S., & Wageman, R. (1987). Performance evaluation and intrinsic motivation: The effects of evaluative focus, rewards, and achievement orientation. *Journal of Personality and Social Psychology, 53*, 1015–1023.

Hardin, G. (1968). The tragedy of the commons. *Science, 162*, 1243–1248.

Harré, R., & Gillett, G. (1994). *The discursive mind.* Thousand Oaks, CA: Sage.

Harré, R., & Secord, P. F. (1973). *The explanation of social behaviour.* Oxford,UK: Blackwell.

Harvey, O. J., Hunt, D. E., & Schroder, H. H. (1961). *Conceptual systems and personality organization.* New York: Wiley.

Hastie, R. (1980). Memory for behavioral information that confirms or contradicts a personality impression. In R. Hastie, T. M. Ostrom, E. B. Ebbesen, R. S. Wyer, Jr., D. L. Hamilton, & D. E. Carlston (Eds.), *Person memory: The cognitive basis of social perception* (pp. 141–172). Hillsdale, NJ: Erlbaum.

Hastie, R., & Park, B. (1986). The relationship between memory and judgment depends on whether the judgment task is memory-based or online. *Psychological Review, 93*, 258–268.

Hastie, R., Penrod, S. D., & Pennington, N. (1983). *Inside the jury.* Cambridge, MA: Harvard University Press.

Hastorf, A. H., Schneider, D. J., & Zebrowitz, L. (1977). *Person perception* (2nd ed.). Reading, MA: Addison-Wesley.

Hatfield, E., Utne, M. K., & Traupmann, J. (1979). Equity theory and intimate relationships. In R. L. Burgess & T. L. Huston (Eds.), *Social exchange in developing relationships* (pp. 99–103). New York: Academic Press.

Hegselman, R. (1994). Zur selbstoganisation von solidarnetzwerken unter ungleichen—ein simulationsmodell. In K. Homann (Ed.), *Wirtschaftsethische Perspektiven I: Theorie, Ordnungsfragen, Internationale Institutuionen* (pp. 105–129). Berlin: Duncker & Humblot.

Hegselman, R. (1998). Modeling social dynamics with cellular automata. In W. B. Liebrand, A. Nowak, & R. Hegselman (Eds.), *Computer modeling of social processes.* London: Sage.

Hegselman, R., Troitzch, K., & Muller, U. (Eds.). (1996). *Modeling and simulation in the social sciences from the philosophy of science point of view.* The Netherlands: Kluwer Academic Publishers.

Heider, F. (1944). Social perception and phenomenal causality. *Psychological Review, 51*, 358–374.

Heider, F. (1958). *The psychology of interpersonal relations.* New York: Wiley.

Henchy, T., & Glass, D. (1968). Evaluation apprehension and the social facilitation of dominant and subordinate responses. *Journal of Personality and Social Psychology, 10*, 446–454.

Higgins, E. T. (1987). Self-discrepancy: A theory relating self and affect. *Psychological Review, 94*, 319–340.

Higgins, E. T. (1996). Ideals, oughts, and regulatory focus: Affect and motivation from distinct pains and pleasures. In P. M. Gollwitzer & J. A. Bargh (Eds.), *The psychology of action: Linking cognition and motivation to behavior* (pp. 91–114). New York: Guilford Press.

Higgins, E. T., & Bargh, J. A. (1987). Social cognition and social perception. In M. R. Rosenzweig & L. W. Porter (Eds.), *Annual review of psychology* (Vol. 38, pp. 369–425). Palo Alto, CA: Annual Reviews.

Hobson, J. A. (1988). *The dreaming brain.* New York: Basic Books.

Hock, H. S., Kelso, J. A. S., & Schöner, G. (1993). Bistability and hysteresis in the organization of apparent motion pattern. *Journal of Experimental Psychology: Human Perception and Performance, 19,* 63–80.

Hock, H. S., Schöner, G., & Voss, A. (1997). The influence of adaptation and stochastic fluctuations on spontaneous perceptual changes for bistable stimuli. *Perception and Psychophysics, 59,* 509–522.

Hodges, B. H. (1974). Effect of valence on relative weighting in impression formation. *Journal of Personality and Social Psychology, 30,* 378–381.

Hoffer, E. (1951). *The true believer.* New York: Harper & Row.

Hoffman, M. L. (1981). Is altruism part of human nature? *Journal of Personality and Social Psychology, 40,* 121–137.

Hofstadter, D. R. (1979). *Godel, Escher, Bach.* New York: Basic Books.

Holland, J. H. (1975). *Adaptation in natural and artificial systems.* Ann Arbor: University of Michigan Press.

Holland, J. H. (1989). Using classifier systems to study adaptive nonlinear networks. In D. Stein (Ed.), *Complex systems, SFI studies in the sciences of complexity.* Redwood City, CA: Addison-Wesley.

Homans, G. C. (1961). *Social behavior: Its elementary forms.* New York: Harcourt.

Hopfield, J. J. (1982). Neural networks and physical systems with emergent collective computational abilities. *Proceedings of the National Academy of Sciences, 79,* 2554–2558.

Hopfield, J. J. (1984). Neurons with graded response have collective computational properties like those of two-state neurons. *Proceedings of National Academy of Sciences USA, 81,* 3088–3092.

Hovland, C., Janis, I., & Kelley, H. H. (1953). *Communication and persuasion.* New Haven, CT: Yale University Press.

Hovland, C., & Weiss, R. (1951). The influence of source credibility on communication effectiveness. *Public Opinion Quarterly, 15,* 635–650.

Hsee, C. K., & Abelson, R. P. (1991). The velocity relation: Satisfaction as a function of the first derivative of outcome over time. *Journal of Personality and Social Psychology, 60,* 341–347.

Hsee, C. K., Abelson, R. P., & Salovey, P. (1991). The relative weighting of position and velocity in satisfaction. *Psychological Science, 2,* 263–266.

Hull, J. G., & Levy, A. S. (1979). The organizational functions of the self:

An alternative to the Duval and Wicklund model of self-awareness. *Journal of Personality and Social Psychology, 37*, 756–768.

Hull, J. G., & Young, R. D. (1983). The self-awareness-reducing effects of alcohol: Evidence and implications. In J. Suls & A. G. Greenwald (Eds.), *Psychological perspectives on the self* (Vol. 2, pp. 159–190). Hillsdale, NJ: Erlbaum.

Innes, J. M., & Young, R. R. (1975). The effect of presence of an audience, evaluation apprehension, and objective self-awareness on learning. *Journal of Experimental Social Psychology, 11*, 35–42.

Jaffe, J., & Feldstein, S. (1970). *Rhythms of dialogue*. New York: Academic Press.

James, W. (1890). *Principles of psychology*. New York: Holt.

Janis, I. L. (1982). *Groupthink*. Boston: Houghton Mifflin.

Jones, E. E. (1964). *Ingratiation*. New York: Appleton–Century–Crofts.

Jones, E. E., & Davis, K. E. (1965). From acts to dispositions: The attribution process in person perception. In L. Berkowitz (Ed.), *Advances in experimental social psychology* (Vol. 2, pp. 220–266). New York: Academic Press.

Jones, E. E., & Gerard, H. B. (1967). *Foundations of social psychology*. New York: Wiley.

Jones, E. E., Rock, L., Shaver, K. G., Goethals, G. R., & Ward, L. M. (1968). Patterns of performance and ability attribution: An unexpected primacy effect. *Journal of Personality and Social Psychology, 10*, 317–340.

Jones, M. R. (1976). Time, our lost dimension: Toward a new theory of perception, attention, and memory. *Psychological Review, 83*, 323–355.

Jones, M. R., & Boltz, M. (1989). Dynamic attending and responses to time. *Psychological Review, 96*, 459–491.

Jones, S. C. (1973). Self- and interpersonal evaluations: Esteem theories versus consistency theories. *Psychological Bulletin, 79*, 185–189.

Kaneko, K. (1984). Like structures and spatiotemporal intermittency of coupled logistic lattice: Toward a field theory of chaos. *Progress in Theoretical Physics, 72*, 480.

Kaneko, K. (1989). Chaotic but regular Posi-Nega Switch among coded attractors by clustersize variation. *Physical Review Letters, 63*, 219–223.

Kaneko, K. (Ed.). (1993). *Theory and applications of coupled map lattices*. Singapore: World Scientific.

Kanouse, D. E., & Hanson, L. R. (1971). *Negativity in evaluations*. Morristown, NJ: General Learning Press.

Kaplan, D. T., & Glass, L. (1992). Direct test for determinism in a time series. *Physics Review Letters, 68*, 427–430.

Kaplowitz, S. A., & Fink, E. L. (1992). Dynamics of attitude change. In R. L. Levine & H. E. Fitzgerald (Eds.), *Analysis of dynamic psychological systems* (Vol. 2, pp. 341–369). New York: Plenum.

Katz, I., & Hass, R. G. (1988). Racial ambivalence and American value conflict: Correlational and priming studies of dual cognitive structures. *Journal of Personality and Social Psychology, 55*, 893–905.

Kauffman, S. (1995). *At home in the universe*. New York: Oxford University Press.

Kaufman, J., Vallacher, R. R., & Nowak, A. (1993). *Procedural variations in the mouse paradigm*. Unpublished research data.

Kelley, H. H., & Thibaut, J. W. (1978). *Interpersonal relations: A theory of interdependence*. New York: Wiley–Interscience.

Kelly, G. A. (1955). *The psychology of personal constructs*. New York: Norton.

Kelman, H. C., & Hovland, C. I. (1953). "Reinstatement" of the communicator in delayed measurement of attitude change. *Journal of Abnormal and Social Psychology, 48*, 327–335.

Kelso, J. A. S. (1984). Phase transitions and critical behavior in human bimanual coordination. *American Journal of Physiology: Regulatory, Integrative and Comparative Physiology, 15*, R1000–R1004.

Kelso, J. A. S. (1995). *Dynamic patterns: The self-organization of brain and behavior*. Cambridge, MA: MIT Press.

Kelso, J. A. S., & DeGuzman, G. C. (1991). An intermittency mechanism for coherent and flexible brain and behavioral function. In J. Requin & G. E. Stalmach (Eds.), *Tutorials in motor neuroscience* (pp. 305–310). Dordrecht, The Netherlands: Kluwer.

Kelso, J. A. S., Ding, M., & Schöner, G. (1991). Dynamic pattern formation: A primer. In A. B. Baskin & J. E. Mettenthal (Eds.), *Principles of behavior in organisms* (pp. 397–439). New York: Addison-Wesley.

Kelso, J. A. S., Scholz, J. P., & Schöner, G. (1986). Nonequilibrium phase transitions in coordinated biological motion: Critical fluctuations. *Physics Letters, 118*, 279–284.

Kernis, M. H. (1993). The roles of stability and level of self-esteem in psychological functioning. In R. Baumeister (Ed.), *Self-esteem: The puzzle of low self-regard* (pp. 167–182). New York: Plenum.

Kernis, M. H. (1995). *Efficacy, agency, and self-esteem*. New York: Plenum.

Kerr, N. L. (1983). Motivation losses in small groups: A social dilemma analysis. *Journal of Personality and Social Psychology, 45*, 819–828.

Kiesler, C. A. (1971). *The psychology of commitment*. New York: Academic Press.

Kilpatrick, S., Gelatt, C. D., & Vecchi, M. P. (1983). Optimization by simulated annealing. *Science, 220*, 671–680.

Kim, M. P., & Rosenberg, S. (1980). Comparison of two structural models of implicit personality theory. *Journal of Personality and Social Psychology, 38*, 375–389.

Kimble, G. A., & Perlmuter, L. C. (1970). The problem of volition. *Psychological Review, 77*, 361–384.

Klinger, E., Barta, S. G., & Maxeiner, M. E. (1980). Motivational correlates of thought content frequency and commitment. *Journal of Personality and Social Psychology, 39,* 1222–1237.

Köhler, W. (1947). *Gestalt psychology: An introduction to new concepts in modern psychology* (rev. ed.). New York: Liveright.

Kozlowska, M., Nowak, A., & Kus, M. (1997). *Nonlinear dynamics of close relationships.* Manuscript in preparation.

Krech, D., & Crutchfield, R. S. (1948). *Theory and problems of social psychology.* New York: McGraw-Hill.

Kruglanski, A. W., Clement, R. W., & Jost, J. T. (1997). The new wave of dynamism: Will it engulf the field? *Psychological Inquiry, 8,* 132–135.

Kuhn, T. S. (1970). *The structure of scientific revolutions* (2nd ed.). Chicago: University of Chicago Press.

Kunda, Z., & Oleson, K. C. (1995). Maintaining stereotypes in the face of disconfirmation: Constructing grounds for subtyping deviants. *Journal of Personality and Social Psychology, 68,* 565–579.

Kunda, Z., & Thagard, P. (1996). Forming impressions from stereotypes, traits, and behaviors: A parallel-constraint-satisfaction theory. *Psychological Review, 103,* 284–308.

Lam, L., & Noris, H. C. (Eds.). (1990). *Nonlinear structures in dynamical systems.* New York: Springer-Verlag.

Landau, L. D., & Lifshitz, E. M. (1964). *Statistical physics.* Oxford, UK: Pergamon Press.

Langer, E. J. (1978). Rethinking the role of thought in social interaction. In J. H. Harvey, W. Ickes, & R. F. Kidd (Eds.), *New directions in attribution research* (Vol. 2, pp. 35–58). Hillsdale, NJ: Erlbaum.

Langer, E. J., & Imber, L. G. (1979). When practice makes imperfect: Debilitating effects of overlearning. *Journal of Personality and Social Psychology, 37,* 2014–2024.

Larsen, R. J. (1987). The stability of mood variability: A spectral analytic approach to daily mood assessments. *Journal of Personality and Social Psychology, 52,* 1195–1204.

Larsen, R. J., & Kasimatis, M. (1990). Individual differences in entrainment of mood to the weekly calendar. *Journal of Personality and Social Psychology, 58,* 164–171.

Latané, B. (1981). The psychology of social impact. *American Psychologist, 36,* 343–356.

Latané, B., & Darley, J. M. (1968). Group inhibition of bystander intervention in emergencies. *Journal of Personality and Social Psychology, 10,* 215–221.

Latané, B., Liu, J., Nowak, A., Bonavento, M., & Zheng, L. (1995). Distance matters: Physical space and social influence. *Personality and Social Psychology Bulletin, 21,* 795–805.

Latané, B., & Nowak, A. (1994). Attitudes as catastrophes: From dimensions to categories with increasing involvement. In R. R. Vallacher & A. Nowak (Eds.), *Dynamical systems in social psychology* (pp. 219–249). San Diego: Academic Press.

Latané, B., & Nowak, A. (1997). The causes of polarization and clustering in social groups. *Progress in Communication Sciences, 13*, 43–75.

Latané, B., Nowak, A., & Liu, J. (1994). Measuring emergent social phenomena: Dynamism, polarization and clustering as order parameters of social systems. *Behavioral Science, 39*, 1–24.

Latané, B., Williams, K., & Harkins, S. (1979). Many hands make light the work: The causes and consequences of social loafing. *Journal of Personality and Social Psychology, 37*, 823–832.

LeDoux, J. E. (1989). Cognitive-emotional interactions in the brain. *Cognition and Emotion, 3*, 267–289.

Lepore, L., & Brown, R. (1997). Category and stereotype activation: Is prejudice inevitable? *Journal of Personality and Social Psychology, 72*, 275–287.

Lepper, M. R., & Greene, D. (Eds.). (1978). *The hidden costs of reward.* Hillsdale, NJ: Erlbaum.

Lepper, M. R., Greene, D., & Nisbett, R. E. (1973). Undermining children's intrinsic interest with extrinsic reward: A test of the overjustification hypothesis. *Journal of Personality and Social Psychology, 28*, 129–137.

Lerner, M. J., Miller, D. T., & Holmes, J. G. (1976). Deserving and the emergence of forms of social justice. In L. Berkowitz (Ed.), *Advances in experimental social psychology* (Vol. 9, pp. 133–162). New York: Academic Press.

Levine, J. M. (1996, October). *Solomon Asch's legacy for group research.* Paper presented in Plenary Session (S. Fiske, Chair) Honoring the Memory of Solomon Asch, Society of Experimental Social Psychology, Toronto, Canada.

Levinger, G. (1980). Toward the analysis of close relationships. *Journal of Experimental Social Psychology, 16*, 510–544.

Lewenstein, M., & Nowak, A. (1989a). Fully connected neural networks with self-control of noise levels. *Physics Review Letter, 62*, 225–229.

Lewenstein, M., & Nowak, A. (1989b). Recognition with self-control in neural networks. *Physical Review* A, *40*, 4652–4664.

Lewenstein, M., Nowak, A., & Latané, B. (1993). Statistical mechanics of social impact. *Physics Review A, 45*, 703–716.

Lewin, K. (1936a). *A dynamic theory of personality.* New York: McGraw-Hill.

Lewin, K. (1936b). *Principles of topological psychology.* New York: McGraw-Hill.

Lewin, K. (1951). *Field theory in social psychology.* New York: Harper.

Liberman, A., & Chaiken, S. (1991). Value conflict and thought-induced attitude change. *Journal of Experimental Social Psychology, 27*, 203–216.

Lingle, J. H., & Ostrom, T. M. (1979). Retrieval selectivity in memory-based impression judgments. *Journal of Personality and Social Psychology, 37,* 180–194.

Linville, P. W. (1985). Self-complexity and affective extremity: Don't put all your eggs in one cognitive basket. *Social Cognition, 3,* 94–120.

Linville, P. W., Fischer, G. W., & Salovey, P. (1989). Perceived distributions of the characteristics of in-group and out-group members: Empirical evidence and a computer simulation. *Journal of Personality and Social Psychology, 57,* 165–188.

Lomborg, B. (1992). *Evolution of strategies in PDG with noise.* Paper presented at 5th International Conference on Social Dilemmas, Bielefeld, Germany.

Lorenz, E. (1963). Deterministic nonperiodic flow. *Journal of Atmospheric Science, 20,* 282–293.

Losada, M., & Markovitch, S. (1990). Group Analyzer: A system for dynamic analysis of group interaction. *Proceedings of the 23rd Annual Hawaii International Conference on System Sciences* (pp. 101–110). Washington, DC: IEEE Computer Society Press.

Luce, R. D., & Raiffa, H. (1957). *Games and decisions: Introduction and critical survey.* New York: Wiley.

Luchins, A. S. (1957). Primacy–recency in impression formation. In C. Hovland (Ed.), *The order of presentation in persuasion* (pp. 62–75). New Haven, CT: Yale University Press.

MacLachlan, J., & Siegel, M. H. (1980). Reducing the costs of TV commercials by use of time compressions. *Journal of Marketing Research, 17,* 52–57.

Macrae, C. N., Bodenhausen, G. V., & Milne, A. B. (1995). The dissection of selection in person perception: Inhibitory processes in social stereotyping. *Journal of Personality and Social Psychology, 69,* 397–407.

Macy, M., Skvoretz, J., & Bainbridge, W. (1995). *Telltale signs: Learning to cooperate with strangers.* Paper presented at annual meeting of American Sociological Association, Washington, DC.

Mandelbrot, B. B. (1982). *The fractal geometry of nature.* New York: Freeman.

Mandell, A. J., & Selz, K. A. (1994). The new statistical dynamics: An informal look at invariant measures of psychological time series. In R. R. Vallacher & A. Nowak (Eds.), *Dynamical systems in social psychology* (pp. 55–69). San Diego: Academic Press.

Mandler, G. (1975). *Mind and emotion.* New York: Wiley.

Markus, H. (1980). The self in thought and memory. In D. M. Wegner & R. R. Vallacher (Eds.), *The self in social psychology* (pp. 102–130). New York: Oxford University Press.

Markus, H. (1983). Self-knowledge: An expanded view. *Journal of Personality, 51,* 543–565.

Markus, H., & Nurius, P. S. (1986). Possible selves. *American Psychologist, 41*, 954–969.

Markus, H. R., & Kitayama, S. (1991). Culture and the self: Implications for cognition, emotion, and motivation. *Psychological Review, 98,* 224–253.

Markus, H. R., Kitayama, S., & Heiman, R. J. (1996). Culture and basic psychological principles. In E. T. Higgins & A.W. Kruglanski (Eds.), *Social psychology: Handbook of basic principles* (pp. 857–913). New York: Guilford Press.

Markus, H., & Zajonc, R. B. (1985). The cognitive perspective in social psychology. In G. Lindzey & E. Aronson (Eds.), *The handbook of social psychology* (3rd ed. Vol. 1, pp. 137–230). New York: Random House.

Marten, R., & Landers, D. M. (1972). Evaluation potential as a determinant of coaction effects. *Journal of Experimental Social Psychology, 8,* 347–359.

Martin, L., & Tesser, A. (1989). Toward a motivational and structural model of ruminative thought. In J. S. Uleman & J. A. Bargh (Eds.), *Unintended thought* (pp. 306–326). New York: Guilford Press.

Martin, L. L., & Tesser, A. (1996). Some ruminative thoughts. In R. S. Wyer, Jr. (Ed.), *Advances in social cognition* (Vol. 9, pp. 1–47). Mahwah, NJ: Erlbaum.

McClelland, J. L., & Rumelhart, D. E. (Eds.). (1986). *Parallel distributed processing: Explorations in the microstructure of cognition* (Vol. 2). Cambridge, MA: MIT Press.

McConahay, J. B. (1986). Modern racism, ambivalence, and the Modern Racism Scale. In J. F. Dovido & S. L. Gaertner (Eds.), *Prejudice, discrimination, and racism* (pp. 91–125). Orlando, FL: Academic Press.

McConahay, J. B. (1983). Modern racism and modern discrimination: The effects of race, racial attitudes, and context on simulated hiring decisions. *Personality and Social Psychology Bulletin, 9,* 551–558.

McGrath, J. E., & Kelly, J. R. (1986). *Time and human interaction: Toward a social psychology of time.* New York: Guilford Press.

McGraw, K. O. (1978). The detrimental effects of reward on performance: A literature review and a prediction model. In M. R. Lepper & D. Greene (Eds.), *The hidden costs of reward* (pp. 33–60). Hillsdale, NJ: Erlbaum.

Mead, G. H. (1934). *Mind, self, and society.* Chicago: University of Chicago Press.

Messick, D. M., & Liebrand, V. B. G. (1995). Individual heuristics and the dynamics of cooperation in large groups. *Psychological Review, 102,* 131–145.

Messick, D. M., & Liebrand, V. B. G. (1997). The new dynamical social psychology. *Psychological Inquiry, 8,* 135–137.

Milgram, S. (1974). *Obedience to authority: An experimental view.* New York: Harper & Row.

Miller, G. A. (1956). The magical number seven, plus or minus two: Some limits on our capacity for processing information. *Psychological Review, 63,* 81–97.

Miller, G. A., Galanter, E., & Pribram, K. (1960). *Plans and the structure of behavior.* New York: Holt.

Miller, N., & Campbell, D. T. (1959). Recency and primacy in persuasion as a function of the timing of speeches and measurements. *Journal of Abnormal and Social Psychology, 59,* 1–9.

Miller, N., Maruyama, G., Beaber, R. J., & Valone, K. (1976). Speed of speech and persuasion. *Journal of Personality and Social Psychology, 48,* 615–624.

Miller, N. E. (1944). Experimental studies of conflict. In J. M. Hunt (Ed.), *Personality and the behavior disorders* (pp. 431–465). New York: Ronald.

Minsky, M. (1985). *The society of mind.* New York: Simon & Schuster.

Mischel, W., & Peake, P. K. (1982). Beyond deja-vu in the search for cross-situational consistency. *Psychological Review, 89,* 730–755.

Mischel, W., & Shoda, Y. (1995). A cognitive–affective system theory of personality: Reconceptualizing situations, dispositions, dynamics, and invariance in personality structure. *Psychological Review, 102,* 246–268.

Moscovici, S., & Zavalloni, M. (1969). The group as a polarizer of attitudes. *Journal of Personality and Social Psychology, 12,* 124–135.

Myers, D. G., & Diener, E. (1995). Who is happy? *Psychological Science, 6,* 10–19.

Myers, D. G., & Lamm, H. (1976). The group polarization phenomenon. *Psychological Bulletin, 83,* 602–627.

Naitoh, P. (1982). Chronobiologic approach for optimizing human performance. In F. M. Brown & R. C. Graeber (Eds.), *Rhythmic aspects of behavior* (pp. 173–212). Hillsdale, NJ: Erlbaum.

Newcomb, T. M. (1961). *The acquaintance process.* New York: Holt, Rinehart & Winston.

Newston, D. (1973). Attribution and the unit of perception of ongoing behavior. *Journal of Personality and Social Psychology, 28,* 28–38.

Newtson, D. (1994). The perception and coupling of behavior waves. In R. R. Vallacher & A. Nowak (Eds.), *Dynamical systems in social psychology* (pp. 139–167). San Diego: Academic Press.

Newtson, D., Hairfield, J., Bloomingdale, J., & Cutino, S. (1987). The structure of action and interaction. *Social Cognition, 5,* 48–82.

Nezlek, J. B. (1993). The stability of social interaction. *Journal of Personality and Social Psychology, 65,* 930–941.

Nezlek, J. B., & Wheeler, L. (1984). RIRAP: Rochester Interaction Record Analysis Package. *Psychological Documents, 14*(6), 2610.

Nisbett, R. E., & Ross, L. (1980). *Human inference: Strategies and shortcomings of social judgment.* Englewood Cliffs, NJ: Prentice-Hall.

Nisbett, R. E., & Wilson, T. D. (1977). Telling more than we can know: Verbal reports on mental processes. *Psychological Review, 84*, 231–259.

Noelle-Neumann, E. (1984). *The spiral of silence: Public opinion—our social skin*. Chicago: University of Chicago Press.

Nowak, A., & Borkowski, W. (1995). *Competition among socially defined strategies in the Prisoner's Dilemma Game*. Unpublished research data.

Nowak, A., Latané, B., & Lewenstein, M. (1994). Social dilemmas exist in space. In U. Schulz, W. Albers, & U. Mueller (Eds.), *Social dilemmas and cooperation* (pp. 114–131). Heidelberg: Springer-Verlag.

Nowak, A., & Lewenstein, M. (1994). Dynamical systems: A tool for social psychology? In R. R. Vallacher & A. Nowak (Eds.), *Dynamical systems in social psychology* (pp. 17–53). San Diego: Academic Press.

Nowak, A., & Lewenstein, M. (1996). Modeling social change with cellular automata. In R. Hegselmann, K. Troitzch, & U. Muller (Eds.), *Modeling and simulation in the social sciences from the philosophy of science point of view* (pp. 249–285). Dordrecht, The Netherlands: Kluwer Academic.

Nowak, A., Lewenstein, M., & Frejlak, P. (1996). Dynamics of public opinion and social change. In R. Hegselman & H. O. Pietgen (Eds.), *Modeling social dynamics: Order, chaos, and complexity* (pp. 54–78). Vienna: Helbin.

Nowak, A., Lewenstein, M., & Szamrej, J. (1993). Social transitions occur through bubbles. *Scientific American* (Polish version), *12*, 16–25.

Nowak, A., Lewenstein, M., & Tarkowski, W. (1994). Repellor neural networks. *Physical Review E, 48*, 4091–4094.

Nowak, A., Lewenstein, M., & Vallacher, R. R. (1994). Toward a dynamical social psychology. In R. R. Vallacher & A. Nowak (Eds.), *Dynamical systems in social psychology* (pp. 279–293). San Diego: Academic Press.

Nowak, A., Szamrej, J., & Latané, B. (1990). From private attitude to public opinion: A dynamic theory of social impact. *Psychological Review, 97*, 362–376.

Nowak, A., & Vallacher, R. R. (1998). Toward computational social psychology: Cellular automata and neural network models of interpersonal dynamics. In S. J. Read & L. C. Miller (Eds.), *Connectionist models of social reasoning and social behavior* (pp. 277–311). Mahwah, NJ: Erlbaum.

Nowak, A., Vallacher, R. R., & Burnstein, E. (1998). Computational social psychology: A neural network approach to interpersonal dynamics. In W. Liebrand, A. Nowak, & R. Hegselman (Eds.), *Computer modeling of social processes* (pp. 97–125). London: Sage.

Nowak, A., Vallacher, R. R., Tesser, A., & Borkowski, W. (1997). *Society of self: The collective properties of self-structure*. Unpublished research data.

Nowak, A., Zochowski, M., Borkowski, W., & Vallacher, R. R. (1997). *Coupled maps: The synchronization of personal dynamics in close relationships*. Unpublished research data.

Oatley, K., & Johnson-Laird, P. N. (1987). Toward a cognitive theory of emotions. *Cognition and Emotion, 1,* 29–50.

Osgood, C. E., Suci, G. J., & Tannenbaum, P. H. (1957). *The measurement of meaning.* Urbana: University of Illinois Press.

Ostrom, T. M., Skowronsky, J. J., & Nowak, A. (1994). The cognitive foundations of attitudes: It's a wonderful construct. In P. G. Levine, D. L. Hamilton, & T. M. Ostrom (Eds.), *Social cognition: Impact on social psychology* (pp. 195–258). San Diego: Academic Press.

Othmer, H. G. (Ed.). (1986). *Lecture notes in mathematics: Vol. 66. Nonlinear oscillations in biology and chemistry.* Berlin: Springer.

Ott, E., Grebogi, C., & York, J. A. (1990). Controlling chaos. *Physics Review Letter, 64,* 1196–1199.

Pagels, H. (1988). The dreams of reason: *The computer and the rise of the sciences of complexity.* New York: Simon & Schuster.

Parker, I., & Shotter, J. (Eds.). (1990). *Deconstructing social psychology.* London: Routledge & Kegan Paul.

Peeters, G., & Czapinski, J. (1990). Positive–negative asymmetry in evaluations: The distinction between affective and informational negativity effects. In W. Stroebe & M. Hewstone (Eds.), *European review of social psychology* (Vol. 1, pp. 33–60). London: Wiley.

Pelham, B. W. (1991). On confidence and consequences: The certainty and importance of self-knowledge. *Journal of Personality and Social Psychology, 60,* 518–530.

Pennebaker, J. W. (1988). *Opening up.* New York: Morrow.

Pennebaker, J. W., Hughes, C. F., & O'Heeron, R. C. (1987). The psychophysiology of confession: Linking inhibitory and psychosomatic processes. *Journal of Personality and Social Psychology, 52,* 781–793.

Penner, L. A., Shiffman, S., Paty, A., & Fritzche, B. A. (1994). Individual differences in intraperson variability in mood. *Journal of Personality and Social Psychology, 66,* 712–721.

Petitot, J. (1995). Morphodynamics and attractor syntax: Constituency in visual perception and cognitive grammar. In R. F. Port & T. van Gelder (Eds.), *Mind as motion: Explorations in the dynamics of cognition* (pp. 227–281). Cambridge, MA: MIT Press.

Petty, R. E., & Cacioppo, J. T. (1984). The effects of involvement on responses to argument quantity and quality: Central and peripheral routes to persuasion. *Journal of Personality and Social Psychology, 46,* 69–81.

Petty, R. E., & Cacioppo, J. T. (1986). The elaboration likelihood model of persuasion. In L. Berkowitz (Ed.), *Advances in experimental social psychology* (Vol. 19, pp. 123–205). New York: Academic Press.

Pettigrew, T. F. (1958). The measurement and correlates of category width as a cognitive variable. *Journal of Personality, 6,* 532–544.

Petty, R. E., Ostrom, T. M., & Brock, T. C. (Eds.). (1981). *Cognitive responses in persuasion*. Hillsdale, NJ: Erlbaum.

Piaget, J. (1971). *Biology and knowledge*. Chicago: University of Chicago Press.

Pietgen, H. O., & Richter, P. H. (1986). *The beauty of fractals*. Berlin: Springer.

Pittman, T. S., & Heller, J. F. (1987). Social motivation. *Annual Review of Psychology, 38,* 461–489.

Plutchik, R. (1980). *Emotion: A psychoevolutionary synthesis*. New York: Harper & Row.

Polanyi, M. (1969). *Knowing and being*. Chicago: University of Chicago Press.

Pope, K. S., & Singer, J. L. (Eds.). (1978). *The stream of consciousness: Scientific investigations into the flow of human experience*. New York: Plenum.

Port, R. F., & van Gelder, T. (Eds.). (1995). *Mind as motion: Explorations in the dynamics of cognition*. Cambridge, MA: MIT Press.

Poston, T., & Stewart, I. (1978). *Catastrophe theory and its applications*. Boston: Pitman.

Powers, W. T. (1973). *Behavior: The control of perception*. Chicago: Aldine.

Pratkanis, A. R., Greenwald, A. G., Leippe, M. R., & Baumgardner, M. H. (1988). In search of reliable persuasion effects: III. The sleeper effect is dead. Long live the sleeper effect. *Journal of Personality and Social Psychology, 54,* 203–218.

Pratto, F., & John, O. P. (1991). Automatic vigilance: The attention grabbing power of negative information. *Journal of Personality and Social Psychology, 61,* 380–391.

Prigogine, I., & Stengers, I. (1984). *Order out of chaos*. Toronto: Bantam Books.

Quattrone, G. A. (1986). On the perception of a group's variability. In S. Worchel & W. Austin (Eds.), *The psychology of intergroup relations* (Vol. 2, pp. 25–48). Chicago: Nelson-Hall.

Read, S. J., & Miller, L. C. (Eds.). (1998). *Connectionist models of social reasoning and social behavior*. Mahwah, NJ: Erlbaum.

Read, S. J., Vanman, E. J., & Miller, L. C. (1997). Connectionism, parallel constraint satisfaction processes, and Gestalt principles: (Re)Introducing cognitive dynamics to social psychology. *Personality and Social Psychology Review, 1,* 26–53.

Richards, D. (1990). Is strategic decision making chaotic? *Behavioral Science, 35,* 219–232.

Rogers, C. R. (1961). *On becoming a person*. Boston: Houghton Mifflin.

Rogers, T. B., Kuiper, N. A., & Kirker, W. S. (1977). Self-reference and the encoding of personal information. *Journal of Personality and Social Psychology, 35,* 677–688.

Rokeach, M. (1964). *The three Christs of Ypsilanti: A psychological study.* New York: Columbia University Press.

Rosenberg, M. (1965). *Society and the adolescent self-image.* Princeton, NJ: Princeton University Press.

Rosenberg, S., Nelson, C., & Vivekananthan, P. S. (1968). A multidimensional approach to the structure of personality impressions. *Journal of Personality and Social Psychology, 22,* 283–294.

Rosenberg, S., & Sedlak, A. (1972). Structural representations of implicit personality theory. In L. Berkowitz (Ed.), *Advances in experimental social psychology* (Vol. 6, pp. 235–297). New York: Academic Press.

Rosenblum, L. D., & Turvey, M. T. (1988). Maintenance tendency in coordinated rhythmic movements: Relative fluctuations and phase. *Neuroscience, 27,* 289–300.

Rosnow, R. L. (1981). *Paradigms in transition: The methodology of social inquiry.* New York: Oxford University Press.

Ross, L. D., Lepper, M. R., Strack, F., & Steinmetz, J. (1977). Social explanation and social expectation: Effects of real and hypothetical explanations on subjective likelihood. *Journal of Personality and Social Psychology, 35,* 817–829.

Rothbart, M., & Lewis, S. (1988). Inferring category attributes from exemplar attributes: Geometric shapes and social categories. *Journal of Personality and Social Psychology, 55,* 861–872.

Rotter, J. B. (1966). Generalized expectancies for internal versus external control of reinforcement. *Psychological Monographs, 80*(1, Whole No. 609).

Ruelle, D. (1989). *Elements of differentiable dynamics and bifurcation theory.* New York: Academic Press.

Ruelle, D., & Takens, F. (1971). On the nature of turbulence. *Communications in Mathematical Physics, 20,* 167–192.

Rumelhart, D. E., & Ortony, A. (1977). The representation of knowledge in memory. In R. C. Anderson, R. J. Spiro, & W. E. Montague (Eds.), *Schooling and the acquisition of knowledge* (pp. 99–136). Hillsdale, NJ: Erlbaum.

Rusbult, C. E. (1980). Commitment and satisfaction in romantic associations: A test of the investment model. *Journal of Experimental Social Psychology, 16,* 172–186.

Rusbult, C. E. (1983). A longitudinal test of the investment model: The development (and deterioration) of satisfaction and commitment in heterosexual involvement. *Journal of Personality and Social Psychology, 45,* 101–117.

Rusbult, C. E., & Martz, J. M. (1995). Remaining in an abusive relationship: An investment model analysis of nonvoluntary dependence. *Personality and Social Psychology Bulletin, 21,* 558–571.

Russell, J. A. (1991). Culture and the categorization of emotions. *Psychological Bulletin, 110*, 426–450.

Ryle, G. (1949). *The concept of mind*. London: Hutchinson.

Salovey, P., & Mayer, J. D. (1990). Emotional intelligence. *Imagination, Cognition, and Personality, 9*, 185–211.

Saltzman, E. L. (1995). Dynamics and coordinate systems in skilled sensorimotor activity. In R. F. Port & T. van Gelder (Eds.), *Mind as motion: Explorations in the dynamics of cognition* (pp. 149–173). Cambridge, MA: MIT Press.

Saltzman, E. L., & Kelso, J. A. S. (1987). Skilled actions: A task dynamic approach. *Psychological Review, 94*, 84–106.

Sanders, G. S., Baron, R. S., & Moore, D. L. (1978). Distraction and social comparison as mediators of social facilitation. *Journal of Experimental Social Psychology, 14*, 291–303.

Sarason, I. G. (1972). Experimental approaches to test anxiety: Attention and the uses of information. In C. D. Spielberger (Ed.), *Anxiety: Current trends in theory and research* (Vol. 2, pp. 383–403). New York: Academic Press.

Sarbin, T. R., & Allen, V. L. (1968). Role theory. In G. Lindzey & E. Aronson (Eds.), *The handbook of social psychology* (2nd ed., Vol. 1, pp. 488–567). Reading, MA: Addison-Wesley.

Schank, R. C., & Abelson, R. P. (1977). *Scripts, plans, goals, and understanding*. Hillsdale, NJ: Erlbaum.

Scheier, M. F., & Carver, C. S. (1983). Two sides of the self: One for you and one for me. In J. Suls & A. G. Greenwald (Eds.), *Psychological perspectives on the self* (Vol. 2, pp. 123–157). Hillsdale, NJ: Erlbaum.

Schein, E. (1956). The Chinese indoctrination program for prisoners of war: A study of attempted "brainwashing." *Psychiatry, 19*, 149–172.

Schmidt, R. C., Beek, P. J., Treffner, P. J., & Turvey, M. T. (1991). Dynamical substructure of coordinated rhythmic movements. *Journal of Experimental Psychology: Human Perception and Performance, 17*, 635–651.

Schöner, G., & Kelso, J. A. S. (1988). Dynamic pattern generation in behavioral and neural systems. *Science, 239*, 1513–1520.

Schroeck, F. E., Jr. (1994). New mathematical techniques for pattern recognition. In R. R. Vallacher & A. Nowak (Eds.), *Dynamical systems in social psychology* (pp. 71–93). San Diego: Academic Press.

Schuster, H. G. (1984). *Deterministic chaos*. Vienna: Physik Verlag.

Schwartz, B. (1982). Reinforcement-induced behavioral stereotypy: How not to teach people to discover rules. *Journal of Experimental Psychology: General, 111*, 23–59.

Scott, W. A., Osgood, D. W., & Peterson, C. (1979). *Cognitive structure: Theory and measurement of individual differences*. Washington, DC: Winston.

Sedikides, C., & Skowronski, J. J. (1997). The symbolic self in evolutionary context. *Personality and Social Psychology Review, 1*, 80–102.

Seligman, M. E. P. (1975). *Helplessness: On depression, development and death.* San Francisco: Freeman.

Selz, K. A., & Mandell, A. J. (1994). A family of autocorrelation graph equivalence classes on symbolic dynamics as models of individual differences in behavioral style. In R. R. Vallacher & A. Nowak (Eds.), *Dynamical systems in social psychology* (pp. 169–196). San Diego: Academic Press.

Shelling, T. (1969). Models of segregation. *American Economic Review, 59*, 488–493.

Shelling, T. (1971). Dynamic models of segregation. *Journal of Mathematical Sociology, 1*, 143–186.

Sherif, M., & Hovland, C. (1961). *Social judgment: Assimilation and contrast effects in communication and attitude change.* New Haven, CT: Yale University Press.

Sherman, J. W. (1996). Development and mental representation of stereotypes. *Journal of Personality and Social Psychology, 70*, 1126–1141.

Shinbrot, T. (1994). Synchronization of coupled maps and stable windows. *Physics Review E, 50*, 3230–3233.

Shoda, Y., Mischel, W., & Wright, J. C. (1994). Intraindividual stability in the organization and patterning of behavior: Incorporating psychological situations into the idiographic analysis of personality. *Journal of Personality and Social Psychology, 67*, 674–687.

Shrauger, J. S. (1975). Responses to evaluation as a function of initial self-perceptions. *Psychological Bulletin, 82*, 581–596.

Shultz, T. R., & Lepper, M. R. (1996). Cognitive dissonance reduction as constraint satisfaction. *Psychological Review, 103*, 219–240.

Siegman, A. W., & Feldstein, S. (Eds.). (1987). *Nonverbal behavior and communication.* Hillsdale, NJ: Erlbaum.

Sigmund, K. (1993). *Games of life.* New York: Penguin.

Simon, H. A. (1967). Motivational and emotional controls of cognition. *Psychological Review, 74*, 29–39.

Singer, J. L. (1988). Sampling ongoing consciousness and emotional experience: Implications for health. In M. J. Horowitz (Ed.), *Psychodynamics and cognition* (pp. 297–346). Chicago: University of Chicago Press.

Singer, J. L., & Bonnano, G. A. (1990). Personality and private experience: Individual variations in consciousness and in attention to subjective phenomena. In L. A. Pervin (Ed.), *Handbook of personality: Theory and research* (pp. 419–444). New York: Guilford Press.

Skarda, C. A., & Freeman, W. J. (1987). How brains make chaos in order to make sense of the world. *Behavioral and Brain Sciences, 10*, 161–195.

Skowronski, J. J., & Carlston, D. E. (1989). Negativity and extremity biases in impression formation: *A review of explanations*. *Psychological Bulletin*, *105*, 131–142.

Smith, E. R. (1996). What do connectionism and social psychology offer each other? *Journal of Personality and Social Psychology*, *70*, 893–912.

Smith, E. R., Fazio, R. H., & Cejka, M. A. (1996). Accessible attitudes influence categorization of multiply categorizable objects. *Journal of Personality and Social Psychology*, *71*, 888–898.

Smith, L. B., & Thelen, E. (1993). *A dynamic systems approach to development: Applications*. Cambridge, MA: MIT Press.

Smolensky, P. (1988). On the proper treatment of connectionism. *Behavioral and Brain Sciences*, *11*, 1–23.

Snyder, M. (1974). The self-monitoring of expressive behavior. *Journal of Personality and Social Psychology*, *30*, 526–537.

Staats, A. W. (1975). *Social behaviorism*. Homewood, IL: Dorsey Press.

Staats, A. W. (1991). Unified positivism and unification psychology: Fad or new field? *American Psychologist*, *46*, 899–912.

Steele, C. M. (1988). The psychology of self-affirmation: Sustaining the integrity of the self. In L. Berkowitz (Ed.), *Advances in experimental social psychology* (Vol. 21, pp. 261–302). New York: Academic Press.

Stevens, S. S. (1961). To honor Fechner and repeal his law. *Science*, *133*, 80–86.

Strack, F., Martin, L. L., & Stepper, S. (1988). Inhibiting and facilitating conditions of the human smile: A nonobtrusive test of the facial feedback hypothesis. *Journal of Personality and Social Psychology*, *54*, 768–777.

Sullivan, H. S. (1953). *The interpersonal theory of psychiatry*. New York: Horton.

Suls, J., & Greenwald, A. G. (Eds.). (1983). *Psychological perspectives on the self* (Vol. 2). Hillsdale, NJ: Erlbaum.

Sussman, K., Vallacher, R. R., Nowak, A., & Wade, J. (1997). *Static versus dynamic integration in stereotyping*. Unpublished research data.

Swann, W. B., Jr. (1990). To be adored or to be known? The interplay of self-enhancement and self-verification. In E. T. Higgins & R. M. Sorrentino (Eds.), *Handbook of motivation and cognition: Foundations of social behavior* (Vol. 2, pp. 408–448). New York: Guilford Press.

Swann, W. B., Jr., Ely, R. J. (1984). A battle of wills: Self-verification versus behavioral confirmation. *Journal of Personality and Social Psychology*, *46*, 1287–1302.

Swann, W. B., Giuliano, T., & Wegner, D. M. (1982). Where leading questions can lead: The power of conjecture in social interaction. *Journal of Personality and Social Psychology*, *42*, 1025–1035.

Swann, W. B., Griffin, J. J., Predmore, S. C., & Gaines, B. (1987). The cognitive-affective crossfire: When self-consistency confronts self-enhancement. *Journal of Personality and Social Psychology, 52*, 881–889.

Szamrej, J. (1989). *Dynamics of social influence and relocation in social space: A simulation model.* Unpublished research data.

Szamrej, J., Nowak, A., & Latané, B. (1992). Self-organizing structures in society: Visual display of dynamic social processes. Paper presented at the 25th International Congress of Psychology, Brussels, Belgium.

Tajfel, H., & Turner, J. C. (1986). The social identity theory of intergroup behavior. In S. Worchel & W. G. Austin (Eds.), *Psychology of intergroup relations* (2nd ed., pp. 33–47). Monterey, CA: Nelson-Hall.

Takens, F. (1981). Detecting strange attractors in turbulescence. In D. A. Rand & L. S. Young (Eds.), *Lecture notes in mathematics* (Vol. 898, pp. 366–381). New York: Springer.

Tangney, J. P., & Fischer, K. W. (Eds.). (1995). *Self-conscious emotions: The psychology of shame, guilt, embarrassment, and pride.* New York: Guilford Press.

Taylor, S. E. (1991). Asymmetrical effects of positive and negative events: The mobilization-minimization hypothesis. *Psychological Bulletin, 103*, 193–210.

Taylor, S. E., & Brown, J. D. (1988). Illusion and well-being: A social psychological perspective on mental health. *Psychological Bulletin, 103*, 193–210.

Taylor, S. E., & Crocker, J. (1981). Schematic bases of social information processing. In E. T. Higgins, C. P. Herman, & M. P. Zanna (Eds.), *Social cognition: The Ontario symposium* (Vol. 1, pp. 89–134). Hillsdale, NJ: Erlbaum.

Tesser, A. (1978). Self-generated attitude change. In L. Berkowitz (Ed.), *Advances in experimental social psychology* (Vol. 11, pp. 85–117). New York: Academic Press.

Tesser, A. (1980). When individual dispositions and social pressure conflict: A catastrophe. *Human Relations, 33*, 393–407.

Tesser, A. (1988). Toward a self-evaluation maintenance model of social behavior. In L. Berkowitz (Ed.), *Advances in experimental social psychology* (Vol. 21, 181–227). New York: Academic Press.

Tesser, A., & Achee, J. (1994). Aggression, love, conformity, and other social psychological catastrophes. In R. R. Vallacher & A. Nowak (Eds.), *Dynamical systems in social psychology* (pp. 96–109). San Diego: Academic Press.

Tesser, A., & Campbell, J. (1983). Self-definition and self-evaluation maintenance. In J. Suls & A. G. Greenwald (Eds.), *Psychological perspectives on the self* (Vol. 2, pp. 1–31). Hillsdale, NJ: Erlbaum.

Tesser, A., & Leone, C. (1977). Cognitive schemas and thought as determinants of attitude change. *Journal of Experimental Social Psychology, 13,* 340–356.

Tesser, A., Martin, L., & Cornell, D. (1996). On the substitutability of self-protective mechanisms. In P. M. Gollwitzer & J. A. Bargh (Eds.), *The psychology of action: Linking motivation and cognition to behavior* (pp. 488–67). New York: Guilford Press.

Tesser, A., McMillen, R., & Collins, J. (1997). Chaos: On making a convincing case for social psychology. *Psychological Inquiry, 8,* 137–143.

Thelen, E. (1992). Development as a dynamic system. *Current Directions in Psychological Science, 1,* 189–193.

Thelen, E. (1995). Motor development: A new synthesis. *American Psychologist, 50,* 79–95.

Thelen, E., & Smith, L. B. (Eds.). (1994). *A dynamic systems approach to the development of cognition and action.* Cambridge, MA: MIT Press/Bradford Books.

Thibaut, J. W., & Kelley, H. H. (1959). *The social psychology of groups.* New York: Wiley.

Thom, R. (1975). *Structural stability and morphogenesis.* New York: Addison-Wesley.

Thorndike, E. L. (1920). A constant error in psychological ratings. *Journal of Applied Psychology, 4,* 25–29.

Thurstone, L. L. (1928). Attitudes can be measured. *American Journal of Sociology, 33,* 529–554.

Tickle-Degnen, L., & Rosenthal, R. (1987). Group rapport and nonverbal behavior. *Review of Personality and Social Psychology, 9,* 113–136.

Townsend, J. T., & Busemeyer, J. (1995). Dynamic representation of decision-making. In R. F. Port & T. van Gelder (Eds.), *Mind as motion: Explorations in the dynamics of cognition* (pp. 101–120). Cambridge, MA: MIT Press.

Treisman, A. M., & Schmidt, H. (1982). Illusory conjunction in the perception of objects. *Cognitive Psychology, 14,* 107–141.

Trope, Y. (1986). Identification and inferential processes in dispositional attribution. *Psychological Review, 93,* 239–257.

Tuller, B., Kelso, J. A. S., & Harris, K. S. (1983). Converging evidence for the relative role of timing in speech. *Journal of Experimental Psychology: Human Perception and Performance, 9,* 829–833.

Turner, R. H., & Killian, L. M. (1957). *Collective behavior.* Englewood Cliffs, NJ: Prentice-Hall.

Turvey, M. T. (1990). Coordination. *American Psychologist, 4,* 938–953.

Turvey, M. T., & Carello, J. (1995). Some dynamical themes in perception and action. In R. F. Port & T. van Gelder (Eds.), *Mind as motion: Explorations in the dynamics of cognition* (pp. 373–402). Cambridge, MA: MIT Press.

Ulam, S. (1952). Random processes and transformations. *Proceedings of International Congress of Mathematics*, 2, 264–275.

Uleman, J. S., & Bargh, J. A. (Eds.). (1989). *Unintended thought*. New York: Guilford Press.

Vallacher, R. R. (1978). Objective self awareness and the perception of others. *Personality and Social Psychology Bulletin*, 4, 63–67.

Vallacher, R. R. (1980). An introduction to self theory. In D. M. Wegner & R. R. Vallacher (Eds.), *The self in social psychology* (pp. 3–30). New York: Oxford University Press.

Vallacher, R. R. (1993). Mental calibration: Forging a working relationship between mind and action. In D. M. Wegner & J. W. Pennebaker (Eds.), *The handbook of mental control* (pp. 443–472). New York: Prentice-Hall.

Vallacher, R. R. (1995, June). *Mental dynamics in close relationships*. Paper presented at a symposium, "Dynamical and Temporal Systems in Personal Relationships," International Network on Personal Relationships, Williamsburg, VA.

Vallacher, R. R. (1998). Give science the chance. *Psychological Inquiry*, 9, 109–113.

Vallacher, R. R., & Kaufman, J. (1996). Dynamics of action identification: Volatility and structure in the mental representation of behavior. In P. M. Gollwitzer & J. A. Bargh (Eds.), *The psychology of action: Linking cognition and motivation to behavior* (pp. 260–282). New York: Guilford Press.

Vallacher, R. R., Markus, J., Nowak, A., & Strauss, J. (1996). *Intrinsic dynamics of emergent action identification*. Unpublished research data.

Vallacher, R. R., & Nowak, A. (Eds.). (1994a). *Dynamical systems in social psychology*. San Diego: Academic Press.

Vallacher, R. R., & Nowak, A. (1994b). The chaos in social psychology. In R. R. Vallacher & A. Nowak (Eds.), *Dynamical systems in social psychology* (pp. 1–16). San Diego: Academic Press.

Vallacher, R. R., & Nowak, A. (1994c). The stream of social judgment. In R. R. Vallacher & A. Nowak (Eds.), *Dynamical systems in social psychology* (pp. 251–277). San Diego: Academic Press.

Vallacher, R. R., & Nowak, A. (1997). The emergence of dynamical social psychology. *Psychological Inquiry*, 8, 73–99.

Vallacher, R. R., & Nowak, A. (in press). The dynamics of self-regulation. In R. S. Wyer, Jr. (Ed.), *Advances in social cognition* (Vol. 12). Mahwah, NJ: Erlbaum.

Vallacher, R. R., Nowak, A., Froehlich, M., & Borkowski, W. (1997). *The stream of self-evaluation*. Unpublished research data.

Vallacher, R. R., Nowak, A., & Kaufman, J. (1994). Intrinsic dynamics of social judgment. *Journal of Personality and Social Psychology*, 67, 20–34.

Vallacher, R. R., Nowak, A., Markus, J., & Strauss, J. (1998). Dynamics in the coordination of mind and action. In M. Kofta, G. Weary, & G. Sedlek (Eds.), *Personal control in action: Cognitive and motivational mechanisms* (pp. 27–59). New York: Plenum.

Vallacher, R. R., & Selz, K. (1991). Who's to blame? Action identification in allocating responsibility for alleged rape. *Social Cognition, 9,* 194–219.

Vallacher, R. R., & Solodky, M. (1979). Objective self awareness, standards of evaluation, and moral behavior. *Journal of Experimental Social Psychology, 15,* 254–262.

Vallacher, R. R., & Wegner, D. M. (1985). *A theory of action identification.* Hillsdale, NJ: Erlbaum.

Vallacher, R. R., & Wegner, D. M. (1987). What do people think they're doing? Action identification and human behavior. *Psychological Review, 94,* 1–15.

Vallacher, R. R., & Wegner, D. M. (1989). Levels of personal agency: Individual variation in action identification. *Journal of Personality and Social Psychology, 57,* 660–671.

Vallacher, R. R., Wegner, D. M., & Somoza, M. P. (1989). That's easy for you to say: Action identification and speech fluency. *Journal of Personality and Social Psychology, 56,* 199–208.

van Geert, P. (1991). A dynamic systems model of cognitive and language growth. *Psychological Review, 98,* 3–53.

van Geert, P. (1995). Growth dynamics in development. In R. F. Port & T. van Gelder (Eds.), *Mind as motion: Explorations in the dynamics of cognition* (pp. 313–337). Cambridge, MA: MIT Press.

van Geert, P. (1997). Time and theory in social psychology. *Psychological Inquiry, 8,* 143–151.

von Cranach, M., & Harré, R. (1982). *The analysis of action.* Cambridge: Cambridge University Press.

von Neumann, J. (1966). *Theory of self-reproducing automata.* Champaign: University of Illinois Press.

Wasserman, S., & Faust, K. (1994). *Social network analysis: Methods and applications.* New York: Cambridge University Press.

Weber, R., & Crocker, J. (1983). Cognitive processes in the revision of stereotypic beliefs. *Journal of Personality and Social Psychology, 45,* 961–977.

Webster, D. M., & Kruglanski, A. W. (1994). Individual differences in need for cognitive closure. *Journal of Personality and Social Psychology, 67,* 1049–1062.

Wegner, D. M. (1986). Transactive memory: A contemporary analysis of the group mind. In B. Mullen & G. R. Goethals (Eds.), *Theories of group behavior* (pp. 185–208). New York: Springer-Verlag.

Wegner, D. M. (1989). *White bears and other unwanted thoughts.* New York: Viking.

Wegner, D. M. (1994). Ironic processes of mental control. *Psychological Review, 101*, 34–52.

Wegner, D. M. (1996). Why the mind wanders. In J. D. Cohen & J. W. Schooler (Eds.), *Scientific approaches to consciousness* (pp. 295–315). Hillsdale, NJ: Erlbaum.

Wegner, D. M., & Bargh, J. A. (1998). Control and automaticity in social life. In D. T. Gilbert, S. T. Fiske, & G. Lindzey (Eds.), *The handbook of social psychology* (vol. 1, pp. 446–496). Boston, MA: McGraw-Hill.

Wegner, D. M., Coulton, G., & Wenzlaff, R. (1985). The transparency of denial: Briefing in the debriefing paradigm. *Journal of Personality and Social Psychology, 49*, 338–346.

Wegner, D. M., & Giuliano, T. (1980). Arousal-induced attention to self. *Journal of Personality and Social Psychology, 38*, 719–726.

Wegner, D. M., & Pennebaker, J. W. (Eds.). (1993). *Handbook of mental control*. Englewood Cliffs, NJ: Prentice-Hall.

Wegner, D. M., Schneider, D. J., Carter, S., III, & White, L. (1987). Paradoxical effects of thought suppression. *Journal of Personality and Social Psychology, 58*, 409–418.

Wegner, D. M, Shortt, J. W., Blake, A. W., & Page, M. S. (1990). The suppression of exciting thoughts. *Journal of Personality and Social Psychology, 58*, 409–418.

Wegner, D. M., & Vallacher, R. R. (1977). *Implicit psychology*. New York: Oxford University Press.

Wegner, D. M., & Vallacher, R. R. (Eds.). (1980). *The self in social psychology*. New York: Oxford University Press.

Wegner, D. M., & Vallacher, R. R. (1981). Common-sense psychology. In J. P. Forgas (Ed.), *Social cognition: Perspectives on everyday understanding* (pp. 225–246). London: Academic Press.

Wegner, D. M., & Vallacher, R. R. (1986). Action identification. In R. M. Sorrentino & E. T. Higgins (Eds.), *Handbook of motivation and cognition: Foundations of social behavior* (Vol. 1, pp. 550–582). New York: Guilford Press.

Wegner, D. M., & Vallacher, R. R. (1987). The trouble with action. *Social Cognition, 5*, 179–190.

Wegner, D. M., Vallacher, R. R., Kiersted, G., & Dizadji, D. (1986). Action identification in the emergence of social behavior. *Social Cognition, 4*, 18–38.

Wegner, D. M., Vallacher, R. R., Macomber, G., Wood, R., & Arps, K. (1984). The emergence of action. *Journal of Personality and Social Psychology, 46*, 269–279.

Weidlich, W. (1991). Physics and social science: The approach of synergetics. *Physics Reports, 204*, 1–163.

Weidlich, W., & Haag, G. (1983). *Concepts and models of quantitative sociology*. Berlin: Springer.

Weisbuch, G. (1992). *Complex systems dynamics*. Redwood City, CA: Addison-Wesley.

Werner, H. (1957). *Comparative psychology of mental development* (3rd ed.). New York: International Universities Press.

Wever, R. A. (1982). Behavioral aspects of circadian rhythmicity. In F. M. Brown & R. C. Graeber (Eds.), *Rhythmic aspects of behavior* (pp. 173–212). Hillsdale, NJ: Erlbaum.

White, R. W. (1959). Motivation reconsidered: The concept of competence. *Psychological Review, 66*, 297–333.

Wicklund, R. A. (1986). Orientation to the environment versus preoccupation with human potential. In R. M. Sorrentino & E. T. Higgins (Eds.), *Handbook of motivation and cognition: Foundations of social behavior* (Vol. 1, pp. 64–95). New York: Guilford Press.

Wicklund, R. A., & Brehm, J. W. (1976). *Perspectives on cognitive dissonance*. Hillsdale, NJ: Erlbaum.

Wicklund, R. A., & Frey, D. (1980). Self-awareness theory: When the self makes a difference. In D. M. Wegner & R. R. Vallacher (Eds.), *The self in social psychology* (pp. 31–54). New York: Oxford University Press.

Wiggins, J. A. (1979). Dynamic theories of social relationships and resulting research strategies. In R. L. Burgess & T. L. Huston (Eds.), *Social exchange in developing relationships* (pp. 381–407). New York: Academic Press.

Wilson, M., & Daly, M. (1992). The man who mistook his wife for chattel. In J. H. Barkow, L. Cosmides, & J. Tooby (Eds.), *The adapted mind* (pp. 289–322). New York: Oxford University Press.

Wine, J. D. (1971). Test anxiety and the direction of attention. *Psychological Bulletin, 76*, 92–104.

Witkin, H. A., Dyk, R. B., Faterson, H. F., Goodenough, D. R., & Karp, S. A. (1962). *Psychological differentiation*. New York: Wiley.

Wittenbrink, B., Judd, C. M., & Park, B. (1997). Evidence for racial prejudice at the implicit level and its relationship with questionnaire measures. *Journal of Personality and Social Psychology, 72*, 262–274.

Wolfram, S. (Ed.). (1986). *Theory and applications of cellular automata*. Singapore: World Scientific.

Yerkes, R. M., & Dodson, J. D. (1908). The relation of strength of stimulus to rapidity of habit formation. *Journal of Comparative Neurology and Psychology, 18*, 459–482.

Zajonc, R. B. (1960). The process of cognitive tuning in communication. *Journal of Abnormal and Social Psychology, 61*, 159–167.

Zajonc, R. B. (1980). Cognition and social cognition: A historical perspective. In L. Festinger (Eds.), *Retrospections on social psychology* (pp. 180–204). New York: Oxford University Press.

Zebrowitz, L. A. (1990). *Social perception*. Pacific Grove, CA: Brooks/Cole.

Zeeman, E. C. (1976). Catastrophe theory. *Scientific American, 234*, 65–83.

Zimbardo, P. G. (1970). The human choice: Individuation, reason, and order versus deindividuation, impulse, and chaos. In W. J. Arnold & D. Levine (Eds.), *Nebraska Symposium on Motivation, 1969* (pp. 237–307). Lincoln: University of Nebraska Press.

Zimbardo, P. G. (1977). Shyness: *What it is and what you can do about it.* Reading, MA: Addison-Wesley.

Zochowski, M., Lewenstein, M., & Nowak, A. (1993). Memory that tentatively forgets. *Journal of Physics A, 26,* 2453–2460.

Zochowski, M., Lewenstein, M., & Nowak, A. (1995). SMARTNET: A neural network with self-controlled learning. *Network, 6,* 93–101.

Zochowski, M., & Liebovitch, L. (1997). Synchronization of trajectory as a way to control the dynamics of the coupled system. *Physics Review E, 56,* 3701.

Zubek, J. P. (Ed.). (1969). *Sensory deprivation: Fifteen years of research.* New York: Appleton–Century–Crofts.

Zukier, H. (1990). Aspects of narrative thinking. In I. Rock (Ed.), *The legacy of Solomon Asch: Essays in cognition and social psychology* (pp. 195–209). Hillsdale, NJ: Erlbaum.

Zukier, H. (1986). The paradigmatic and narrative modes in goal-guided inference. In R. M. Sorrentino & E. T. Higgins (Eds.), *Handbook of motivation and cognition: Foundations of social behavior* (Vol. 1, pp. 465–502). New York: Guilford Press.

Index